Clinical Management of Ovarian Cancer

To our patients, who have taught us so much

Clinical Management of Ovarian Cancer

Edited by

Jonathan A Ledermann MD, FRCP
Department of Oncology
Royal Free and University College Medical School
University College London
London, UK

William J Hoskins MD
Gynecology Service, Department of Surgery
& Disease Management Teams
Memorial Sloan-Kettering Cancer Center
New York, USA

Stanley B Kaye MD, FRCP
CRC Department of Medical Oncology
The Royal Marsden Hospital
Sutton, Surrey, UK

Ignace B Vergote MD, PhD
Gynecologic Oncology
University Hospital Leuven
Leuven, Belgium

MARTIN DUNITZ

© Martin Dunitz Ltd 2001

First published in the United Kingdom in 2001 by
Martin Dunitz Ltd
The Livery House
7–9 Pratt Street
London NW1 0AE

Tel: +44-(0)20-7482-2202
Fax: +44-(0)20-7267-0159
E-mail: info.dunitz@tandf.co.uk
Website: http://www.dunitz.co.uk

Although every effort has been made to ensure that all owners of
copyright material have been acknowledged in this publication, we
would be glad to acknowledge in subsequent reprints or editions
any omissions brought to our attention.

A CIP catalogue record for this book is available from
the British Library

ISBN 1-85317-704-0

Distributed in the United States by:
Blackwell Science Inc.
Commerce Place, 350 Main Street
Malden, MA 02148, USA
Tel: 1-800-215-1000

Distributed in Canada by:
Login Brothers Book Company
324 Salteaux Cresent
Winnipeg, Manitoba R3J 3T2
Canada
Tel: 1-204-224-4068

Distributed in Brazil by:
Ernesto Reichmann Distribuidora de Livros, Ltda
Rua Coronel Marques 335, Tatuape 03440-000
Sao Paulo,
Brazil

*Cover illustration courtesy of Dr D Timmerman, Department of
Obstetrics and Gynaecology, University Hospitals, Leuven, Belgium.*

Composition by Wearset, Boldon, Tyne and Wear.
Printed and bound in Great Britain by
Biddles Ltd, Guildford and King's Lynn

Contents

Section 3: Relapsed Ovarian Cancer

Section 4: Diagnostic Aspects in Ovarian Cancer

Section 5: Psychosocial Issues and Palliative Care

Section 6: Management of the Internet Surfer

Preface

Ovarian cancer accounts for 5% of all cancer deaths, and is the fourth most common cause of cancer–related death in women. Oncologists and gynaecologists will almost certainly encounter patients with the disease, and there are few women who do not know about the importance of the condition. Like many other malignancies, ovarian cancer is not a single disease entity and its manifestations are diverse.

Over the last 30 years, diagnosis and therapeutic advances have altered the way ovarian cancer is treated. Such changes generate controversies in management and demand evidence to support new therapeutic approaches. Increasing awareness of ovarian cancer amongst healthcare workers and the public raises issues about early diagnosis, screening and the genetic predisposition to cancer. However, the investigation and treatment of such individuals remains controversial. Management of advanced disease has become more complex: surgery for primary and relapsed disease, and its relationship to combination chemotherapy, are areas of continuing research. The last decade has seen the introduction of several new chemotherapeutic agents that require careful evaluation. Open discussion about the treatment of advanced ovarian cancer requires a better understanding of palliation and the effect of the disease on the patient and her family. Patients are living longer, and need help to adjust to what is often a chronic disease.

Management of ovarian cancer requires input from a multidisciplinary team comprising gynaecologists, oncologists, pathologists, radiologists, palliative care physicians and nurse specialists. For some of these healthcare professionals, ovarian cancer is only one of many conditions they manage, and they are often faced with complicated management decisions. Therefore, when we set out to write this book, we decided to use clinical cases taken from our own practice to discuss these complex clinical problems. Each chapter is devoted to one aspect of the management of ovarian cancer, and the clinical cases are used as a basis for discussion, integrating published data to provide a complete review.

This book has been specifically written to assist oncologists, gynaecologists and other healthcare professionals in dealing with the clinical management of ovarian cancer from three continents. We would also like to thank Martin Dunitz and Alison Campbell for their enthusiastic support and guidance throughout this project.

JAL
WJH
SBK
IBV

Contributors

Anca C Ansink MD
Department of Oncology
Academic Medical Center of the
University of Amsterdam
Meibergdreef 9
1100 DD Amsterdam
The Netherlands

Joke JM Bais MD
Department of Gynecology
Academic Medical Center of the
University of Amsterdam
Meibergdreef 9
1100 DD Amsterdam
The Netherlands

Richard R Barakat MD
Gynecology Service
Department of Surgery
Memorial Sloan-Kettering Cancer Center
1275 York Avenue
New York, NY 10021
USA

Maria EL van der Burg MD, PhD
Department of Medical Oncology
University Hospital Rotterdam
Dr Molewaterplein 40
3015 GD Rotterdam
The Netherlands

Nicoletta Colombo MD
Isituto Europeo di Oncologia
via Ripamonti 435
20141 Milan
Italy

Ilora Finlay FRCGP, FRCP
Department of Palliative Medicine
University of Wales College of Medicine
and Marie Curie Centre
Holme Tower
Bridgeman Road
Penarth
Valley of Glamorgan CF64 3YR
UK

Michael L Friedlander PhD
Department of Medical Oncology
Prince of Wales Hospital
High Street
Randwick, NSW 2031
Australia

Martin Gore PhD, FRCP
Institute of Cancer Research
237 Fulham Road
London SW3 6JB
UK

Neville F Hacker MD
Gynaecologic Cancer Centre
Royal Hospital for Women
Barker Street
Randwick, NSW 2031
Australia

Andrea B Hamilton PhD
Attending Psychologist
Gynecology Service
Department of Surgery
Memorial Sloan-Kettering Cancer Center
1275 York Avenue
New York, NY 10021
USA

Jonathan JO Herod MRCOG
Department of Gynaecology and Oncology
Liverpool Women's Hospital
Crown Street
Liverpool L8 7S3
UK

William Hoskins MD
Gynecology Service
Department of Surgery
Memorial Sloan-Kettering Cancer Center
1275 York Avenue
New York, NY 10021
USA

Dwight D Im MD
The Gynecologic Oncology Center
Mercy Medical Center
301 St. Paul Place
Baltimore, MD 21202
USA

Frank-Willem Jansen MD
University Medical Center
Department of Gynaecology
2300 RC Leiden
The Netherlands

Janne Kaern MD, PhD
Chemotherapy Section
The Gynecologic Department
The Norwegian Radium Hospital
Montebello
0310 Oslo
Norway

Stanley B Kaye MD, FRCP
CRC Department of Medical Oncology
The Royal Marsden Hospital
Downs Road
Sutton
Surrey SM2 5PT
UK

Jonathan A Ledermann MD, FRCP
Department of Oncology
Royal Free and University College
Medical School
University College London
91 Riding House Street
London W1P 8BT
UK

William P McGuire III MD
The Gynecologic Oncology Center
Mercy Medical Center
301 St. Paul Place
Baltimore, MD 21202
USA

Hans-Gerd Meerpohl MD
Obstetrics and Gynecology
St Vincentius-Krankenhäuser Karlsruhe
Frauenklinik mit Hebammenlehranstalt
Südendstrasse 32
76137 Karlsruhe
Germany

Mark A Morgan MD
Division of Gynecologic Oncology
University of Pennsylvania
Medical Center
3400 Spruce Street, 1000
Courtyard Bldg
Philadelphia, PA 19104
USA

Beth A Morrison MLS
Librarian
BC Cancer Agency
Vancouver, BC V52 4E6
Canada

Edward S Newlands PhD, FRCP
Department of Cancer Medicine
Division of Medicine
Hammersmith Hospital
Charing Cross Campus
Fulham Palace Road
London W6 8RF
UK

Kenneth Offit MD, MPH
Clinical Genetics Service
Memorial Sloan-Kettering Cancer Center
1275 York Avenue
New York, NY 10021
USA

Timothy John Perren MD, FRCP
ICRF Cancer Medicine Research Unit
St James's University Hospital
Leeds Teaching Hospitals NHS Trust
Beckett Street
Leeds LS9 7TF
UK

Elizabeth A Poynor MD
Gynecology Service
Department of Surgery
Memorial Sloan-Kettering Cancer Center
1275 York Avenue
New York, NY 10021
USA

Jubilee B Robinson MD
The Gynecologic Oncology Center
Mercy Medical Center
301 St. Paul Place
Baltimore, MD 21202
USA

Neil B Rosenshein MD
The Gynecologic Oncology Center
Mercy Medical Center
301 St. Paul Place
Baltimore, MD 21202
USA

Stephen C Rubin MD
Division of Gynecologic Oncology
University of Pennsylvania
Medical Center
3400 Spruce Street, 1000
Courtyard Bldg
Philadelphia, PA 19104
USA

Marten S Schilthuis MD
Department of Oncology
Academic Medical Center of the
University of Amsterdam
Meiberdreef 9
1100 DD Amsterdam
The Netherlands

Michelle R Scurr BMed
Department of Medical Oncology
Prince of Wales Hospital
High Street
Randwick, NSW 2031
Australia

Kenneth D Swenerton MD, FRCPC
Clinical Professor of Medicine
University of British Columbia
Medical Oncologist
BC Cancer Agency
Vancouver, BC V5Z 4E6
Canada

Willem ten Bokkel Huinink MD
Antoni van Leeuwenhoekhuis
Plesmanlaan 121
1066 CX Amsterdam
The Netherlands

J Baptist Trimbos MD, PhD
Department of Gynaecology
University Medical Center
2300 RC Leiden
The Netherlands

Claes Tropé MD, PhD
Gynecology Department
The Norwegian Radium Hospital
Montebello
0310 Oslo
Norway

Paul A Vasey MRCP
University of Glasgow
Garscube Estate
Bearsden
Glasgow G61 1BD
UK

Ignace B Vergote MD, PhD
Gynecologic Oncology
University Hospital Leuven
Gasthuisberg
3000 Leuven
Belgium

Nafisa Wilkinson MA, MRCPath
Pathology
St James's University Hospital
Leeds Teaching Hospitals NHS Trust
Beckett Street
Leeds LS9 7TF
UK

SECTION 1: Epithelial Ovarian Cancer

1

Pelvic mass in a woman over 40 years

Martin Gore, Jonathan Herod

INTRODUCTION

Epithelial ovarian cancer is the commonest tumour of the female genital tract and the fourth most common cause of cancer-related mortality among women. It accounts for approximately 5% of all new cancers and 6% of cancer deaths in women. Its incidence rises with age, being rare under 30 years and most common in women aged 60–69 years. More than 80% of ovarian cancers occur in women over the age of 50 years.

Most women present with advanced disease. Symptoms are due to an enlarging pelvic mass and/or widespread dissemination throughout the peritoneal cavity or beyond. In about 70% of cases, the tumour has spread beyond the ovary and pelvis. Prompt and appropriate investigations are required to make a preoperative diagnosis of ovarian cancer. The type of pelvic mass seen on ultrasonography, the age of the patient and the presence of an elevated serum CA125 level all help to make a preoperative diagnosis.

In this chapter, the surgical and chemotherapeutic management of a typical case of operable advanced ovarian cancer in a postmenopausal women is discussed.

CASE HISTORY

A 56-year-old woman was referred by her general practitioner, having presented with a four-month history of intermittent pain in her left iliac fossa radiating into her back. The pain had been increasing in frequency and was now present on most days; it particularly occurred when the patient was lying in bed at night. The pain was associated with constipation and she had also noted lower abdominal distension, with her clothes becoming 'tight'.

Her past health was good. She had had one pregnancy and no history of gynaecological problems. She had had a single uncomplicated pregnancy with a normal vaginal delivery resulting in the birth of a healthy daughter. She had undergone the menopause four years earlier at the age of 52. At that time, she commenced combined oestrogen–progesterone hormone replacement therapy, which she was still taking. She had no significant family history of cancer, except that an aunt had died of breast cancer in old age. The patient was divorced, worked as a receptionist for a local dentist and lived with her 23-year-old daughter. She smoked 10 cigarettes a day and had no history of excessive alcohol intake.

The patient appeared to be in good health, with a ECOG (Esterna Cooperative Oncology Group) performance status of 0 (see Appendix 3). Her breasts were normal and there was no cervical or axillary lymphadenopathy. Examination of her abdomen revealed a minor degree of distension, a scar in the right iliac fossa from a previous appendicectomy in childhood and mild tenderness in the lower abdomen, particularly on the left. A 16-week gestational-size mass in the area of the tenderness was palpated and appeared to be arising from the pelvis. No other masses were palpable and there was no inguinal lymphadenopathy. Bimanual examination confirmed the presence of a large, firm, cystic mass filling the pelvis. The mass was mobile and appeared to be separate from the uterus, which was of normal size. Rectal examination was normal.

What investigations should be performed?

The first investigation that this patient underwent was transabdominal ultrasonography, which had been ordered by her general practitioner and revealed the presence of a complex 10 cm pelvic mass, possibly arising from the ovary. Further investigation was aimed at confirming that the origin of the mass was the ovary and establishing whether the tumour was malignant. Other investigations included a full blood count, serum urea, creatinine, electrolytes and liver function tests. Blood was also taken for serum tumour markers – in particular CA125, but also carcinoembryonic antigen (CEA). The latter may help differentiate between a gastrointestinal malignancy and primary ovarian cancer, although CEA may be elevated in ovarian cancer, particularly the mucinous subtype. A chest radiograph was performed to exclude the presence of intrathoracic disease such as a pleural effusion.

The most important initial investigation in this case is transvaginal ultrasonography, but this is a very operator-dependent investigation and must be performed by someone with adequate experience. Colour flow Doppler is a useful adjunct to standard transvaginal ultrasonography, and should be performed if available. Women who have a pelvic mass where the index of suspicion of malignancy is high should also have a computed tomography (CT) scan of abdomen and pelvis in order to define any obvious intraabdominal metastases and to help assess operability. Mammography is not routinely performed unless there are clinical signs of breast disease. Similarly, barium enema, sigmoidoscopy, colonoscopy or intravenous urography are only ordered if indicated from the history or clinical examination or as a result of one of the previous examinations; for example, the gastrointestinal tract should be investigated if the serum CEA is much higher than the CA125. The results of the investigations showed a thickening of the peritoneum over the liver surface, right-upper quadrant, anteriorly, and in the pelvis. The omentum was replaced by tumour, and a bilateral ovarian mass was seen. Ascites was present throughout the abdominal cavity, but the liver, spleen and kidney were normal. There was a mass arising out of the pelvis (Figure 1.1). The CA125 was raised at 51 U/ml (normal <35 U/ml) and the CEA level was 1.9 µg/ml (normal <5 µg/l). The chest radiograph was normal. These results strongly suggest a diagnosis of ovarian cancer. This is because the CA125 is raised, the CEA is normal, and the transvaginal ultrasonography suggests that the mass is arising from the ovary and has features associated with malignancy.

How sure can one be that a pelvic mass is malignant?

A simple method of estimating the likelihood that a pelvic mass is malignant has been described by Jacobs and his colleagues.[1] The risk of malignancy index (RMI) is the product of the serum concentration of CA125, the menopausal status of the patient and a numerical score given to the transvaginal ultrasound assessment. A

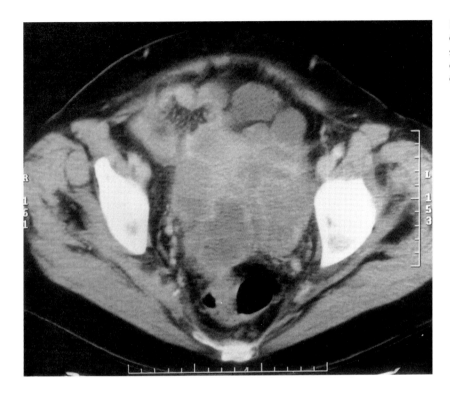

Figure 1.1
Computed tomography (CT) scan showing the mass arising out of the pelvis; see text for other findings.

score of 0 is given for a normal investigation, and then one point is added for each of the following features: multilocular cyst, evidence of solid areas, evidence of metastases, presence of ascites, bilateral lesions. A value of 1 is allocated to the score in premenopausal women and 3 if the patient is postmenopausal (Table 1.1). A value greater than 200 has an 85% specificity and 97% sensitivity for discriminating between ovarian cancer and benign ovarian disease. In this case, the RMI of 612 was highly suggestive of ovarian cancer:

51 (serum CA125 concentration) × 3 (post-menopausal) + 4 (ultrasound score) = 612

The presumptive diagnosis in this woman was therefore ovarian cancer, and she was informed and counselled accordingly. She consented to a standard management plan of laparotomy for diagnosis, staging of the disease and cytoreduction of the tumour; this was to be followed by chemotherapy. A CT scan was performed preoperatively to help assess operability.

OPERATION REPORT

A midline incision was made from above the symphysis pubis to above the umbilicus. The findings were as follows: a large volume of ascites, multiple nodules (diameter <0.5 cm) on the under-surface of both hemidiaphragms and on the peritoneal and mesenteric surfaces, tumour replacing the infracolic omentum, and a mass arising from the left ovary adherent to the posterior aspect of the uterus and sigmoid colon. The liver, spleen, gall bladder and both kidneys were normal, there was no evidence of para-aortic or pelvic lymphadenopathy, and

Table 1.1   The sensitivity, specificity and likelihood ratio for malignancy given a positive or negative result for different levels of the risk of malignancy index (RMI)[1]

RMI score	Sensitivity		Specificity		Likelihood ratio for malignancy if result is	
	%	95% CI	%	95% CI	Positive	Negative
25	100.0	91.4–100.0	62.2	51.9–71.8	2.7	0.00
50	95.1	83.5–99.4	76.5	66.9–84.5	4.1	0.06
75	92.7	80.1–98.5	84.7	76.0–91.2	6.1	0.09
100	85.4	70.8–94.4	87.8	79.6–93.5	7.0	0.17
150	85.4	70.8–94.4	93.9	87.2–97.7	14.0	0.16
200	85.4	70.8–94.4	96.9	91.3–99.4	42.1	0.15
250	78.0	62.4–89.4	99.0	94.5–100.0	79.9	0.22

95% CI, 95% confidence interval.

although the right ovary was bulky, it had no obvious macroscopic features of malignancy. Ascitic fluid was sent for cytology, and a total abdominal hysterectomy, bilateral salpingo-oophorectomy and infracolic omentectomy was performed. The estimated blood loss from the procedure was 750 ml. There was residual tumour of 0.5 cm (maximum diameter) remaining after the surgery. The patient made an excellent postoperative recovery and was discharged eight days following her surgery.

A diagnosis of FIGO stage IIIc ovarian cancer was made (see Appendix 1). The histology of the tumour was reported as a moderately differentiated serous papillary adenocarcinoma of the ovary with metastatic disease in the omentum. The ascitic fluid contained malignant cells.

How should this patient be managed?

Ovarian cancer is sensitive to chemotherapy, and although many patients eventually die from their disease, some are long-term survivors – especially if they have small-volume residual disease after laparotomy. In those who are not, chemotherapy can provide good palliation. Thus, there is a clear indication for chemotherapy following cytoreductive surgery. Response to chemotherapy is an important prognostic indicator of survival, and the question arises as to the optimal agent/agents that should be given, and their dose, schedule and method of administration.

The first effective chemotherapy to be used in ovarian cancer involved alkylating agents, which were first introduced during the 1970s. Early reports[2] suggested that there was an improved survival when these drugs were given compared with untreated patients, but there were wide variations in the response rates reported, 35–65%. The median survival for patients with advanced ovarian cancer treated with alkylating agents was 10–14 months, with a five-year survival rate of 6–9%.[3] In the mid-1970s, cisplatin was introduced, and demonstrated activity against a wide range of tumours. It was shown to be the most active agent in the treatment of ovarian cancer, with response rates of 25–40% in patients who had relapsed after alkylating agent therapy.[3] In previously untreated patients, there was a clear advantage of cisplatin over alkylating agent therapy; response rates were higher and randomized trials showed prolongation of progression-free survival, and in one early trial an overall survival benefit.[4] This study showed that patients treated with a combination of cisplatin and cyclophosphamide had a two-year survival rate of 52%, compared with 19% for patients treated with cyclophosphamide alone. Subsequently, two population-based studies demonstrated a clear survival benefit for platinum-based therapies,[5,6] and a recent updated meta-analysis has confirmed the survival benefit of platinum-based chemotherapy.[7]

Should cisplatin or carboplatin be used?

Survival rates are now double that obtained in the pre-platinum era, with a median survival of 20–30 months, five-year survival rate of 20–30% and 10-year survival rate of 10–20% consistently being reported.[8,9] In the early 1980s, the platinum analogue carboplatin was developed and was clearly shown to be less toxic than cisplatin, with less neurotoxicity, ototoxicity and renal toxicity, as well as producing considerably less emesis. However, carboplatin was shown to cause more myelosuppression, particularly thrombocytopenia, but its overall toxicity profile was so favourable that it was substituted for cisplatin when single-agent therapy was utilized.[10] A number of randomized trials have shown that cisplatin and carboplatin are equivalent in efficacy, and this has been confirmed by meta-analyses.[7,11]

Should patients receive a single drug or combination therapy?

A major controversy during the 1980s and early 1990s was whether single-agent platinum was as effective as platinum-based combinations. The overall response rate with combination therapy is 60–90%, which is higher than those of single-agent therapy, and complete response rates are between 20% and 40%.[10] However, there was controversy as to whether overall survival was improved. The Advanced Ovarian Cancer Trialists Group reviewed all the available data in a meta-analysis in 1991, and showed that there was a small but statistically significant survival advantage to the use of combination platinum-based therapies as compared with single-agent platinum.[11] Meta-analyses of randomized trials involving doxorubicin supported this view,[12] although a more recent randomized trial comparing single-agent carboplatin with a cisplatin–doxorubicin–cyclophosphamide combination has failed to confirm this.[13]

In the early 1990s, prior to the introduction of the taxanes, a combination of cyclophosphamide and cisplatin or carboplatin, with or without doxorubicin, was considered by many oncologists in mainland Europe and the USA to be standard first-line therapy for fit patients. Single-agent carboplatin was reserved for poor-risk patients, although it remained standard for all patients in the UK.

Are higher doses of platinum more effective?

A recurring research question in the 1980s and 1990s has been the optimal dose intensity of platinum. Levin and Hryniuk[14] published an analysis of 65 trials, and determined the outcome relative to the dose of platinum used. They concluded that dose intensity was an important determinant of survival. Ten randomized trials investigating the dose intensity of platinum have now reported, and the results are disappointing.[15–24] Seven trials failed to show an effect, two very small trials did show a survival benefit, and a large trial from the Scottish Cooperative Group showed a survival benefit for doubling the dose of cisplatin when the trial was initially reported – but on further follow-up this difference virtually disappeared.[25,26] There was a significant increase in toxicity when the dose of cisplatin was doubled from 50 mg/m^2 to 100 mg/m^2, with only a marginal survival benefit. The authors therefore recommended that the standard dose of cisplatin should be 75 mg/m^2. The conclusion from all these trials is that doubling the dose of platinum does not significantly increase survival.

What is the current standard chemotherapy for advanced ovarian cancer?

In the mid-1990s, standard therapy for advanced ovarian cancer changed with the introduction of paclitaxel (Taxol). Paclitaxel is a compound derived from the bark of the Pacific yew tree (*Taxus brevifolia*). It was isolated and screened for activity during a US National Cancer Institute programme that involved over 35 000 plant species from 1958 to 1980. Paclitaxel is a spindle poison that exerts its effect by promoting the aggregation of microtubules during mitosis. It also has a number of other biological effects, including antiangiogenic properties.[27] Early phase II data suggested that paclitaxel had considerable activity in relapsed ovarian cancer, and in 1993 an overview of the available data from five separate phase II studies suggested that in 184 patients the overall response rate was 31%, with a median duration of 7.2 months.[28] These early results led to a large randomized European–Canadian multicentre trial in relapsed ovarian cancer, in which patients were randomized to two different schedules and doses of paclitaxel, namely, 3- versus 24-hour infusion and 135 mg/m^2 versus 175 mg/m^2. There was a modest dose–response effect, which was not sta-

tistically significant, and the shorter infusion was associated with a slightly lower incidence of neutropenia.[29]

In 1996, the Gynaecologic Oncology Group (GOG) in the USA reported a randomized trial of cisplatin–cyclophosphamide versus cisplatin–paclitaxel in previously untreated suboptimally debulked patients with stage III (>1 cm residual disease) or stage IV ovarian cancer. There was a statistically significant advantage to women treated with cisplatin–paclitaxel; the response rates were 73% and 60%, the progression-free survivals were 18 months and 13 months, and the median survivals were 38 months and 24 months (Figures 1.2 and 1.3).[30] This statistically significant survival advantage was confirmed by a large Scottish, Canadian and European Intergroup trial, which demonstrated an almost identical advantage in progression-free and overall survival for cisplatin–paclitaxel.[31] In this study, paclitaxel was given at the higher dose of 175 mg/m^2 as a 3-hour infusion. As a result, the combination of a platinum compound and paclitaxel has become standard first-line therapy for advanced ovarian cancer. There remains some controversy over whether or not carboplatin can be substituted for cisplatin in the context of paclitaxel combination therapy, and there are currently three large randomized trials addressing this issue. Recently reported results from these trials suggest that it is safe to substitute carboplatin for cisplatin in the context of paclitaxel.[32–34]

Is there a role for intraperitoneal chemotherapy?

There is a substantial body of literature on the use of cytotoxic agents intraperitoneally. The rationale for treating patients with ovarian cancer by this route is that the disease is confined to the peritoneal cavity for the greater part of its natural history, and that, for some drugs, a clear pharma-

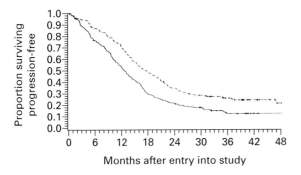

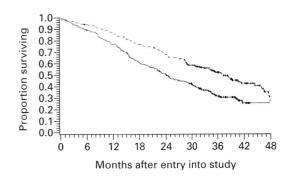

Treatment	No. progression-free	No. with treatment failure	Total	Median progression-free survival (months)
—— Cisplatin + cyclophosphamide	28	174	202	13
- - - Cisplatin + paclitaxel	45	139	184	18

Figure 1.2
Progression-free survival according to treatment group. (Reproduced with permission from McGuire et al, *N Engl J Med* 1996; **334**: 1–6. © 1996 Massachusetts Medical Society. All rights reserved.)

Treatment	No. alive	No. dead	Total	Median survival (months)
—— Cisplatin + cyclophosphamide	65	137	202	24
- - - Cisplatin + paclitaxel	86	98	184	38

Figure 1.3
Survival according to treatment group. (Reproduced with permission from McGuire et al, *N Engl J Med* 1996; **334**: 1–6. © 1996 Massachusetts Medical Society. All rights reserved.)

cokinetic advantage can be demonstrated for this method of administration. This advantage differs from agent to agent, but, for instance, there is a 20-fold advantage with platinum compounds and a 1000-fold advantage with paclitaxel.[35]

However, it is clear that chemotherapy delivered intraperitoneally can only penetrate 1–2 mm from the peritoneal surface into tumours and that this route of administration is inappropriate for tumour nodules greater than 1–2 cm.[36] In addition, there are specific problems associated with intraperitoneal therapy, such as the technique of catheter insertion, its aftercare, abdominal pain consequent on the instillation of fluid, poor distribution of the cytotoxic agent within the peritoneum, infection associated with an indwelling catheter, and adhesion formation with subsequent intestinal obstruction.

In 1995, the Southwest Oncology Group (SWOG) published the results of a study in optimally debulked patients receiving cisplatin and cyclophosphamide.[37] There was a randomization to the mode of administration of the cisplatin: intravenous versus intraperitoneal. There was a significant survival advantage to patients treated with intraperitoneal cisplatin, and this led to a further study by the GOG, which has recently been reported. This second trial has shown a trend towards a survival advantage for intraperitoneally delivered therapy, although this just fails to reach statistical significance.[38] There is now considerable controversy as to whether this study confirms or negates the use of intraperitoneal therapy as first-line treatment in ovarian cancer, and further studies are required before this mode of administration becomes part of standard care. In particular, the role of intraperitoneal paclitaxel with or without intraperitoneal cisplatin needs to be assessed. A trial, GOG 172, is currently underway comparing intravenous cisplatin–paclitaxel with intravenous paclitaxel and intraperitoneal paclitaxel and cisplatin.

CONCLUSIONS

The amount of residual disease following initial surgery remains the most powerful prognostic factor in advanced ovarian cancer after stage of disease. The Goldie–Coldman hypothesis suggests that the number of tumour cells and the length of time they are present is directly related to the emergence of chemotherapy-resistant clones. The hypothesis gives support to the observation that the less disease is present following surgery, the more likely is the patient to gain a survival benefit from chemotherapy. This has led to the concept that for patients who cannot be optimally debulked, surgery should be performed after two or three cycles of chemotherapy in order to reduce the likelihood of the development of chemotherapy-resistant disease during cytotoxic treatment (see Chapter 3). Randomized trials have now defined the standard chemotherapy regimen that should be used in ovarian cancer, and this has been set out in several consensus statements that advise a combination of platinum and paclitaxel.[39–44] The recently reported data from randomized trials described above confirm that carboplatin can be safely substituted for cisplatin in the context of paclitaxel therapy.

LEARNING POINTS

❊ Ovarian cancer is an important cause of non-specific abdominal symptoms such as discomfort and bloating in a postmenopausal woman.
❊ The risk of malignancy index (RMI) can be calculated from the results of transvaginal ultrasonography, CA125 measurement and menopausal status.
❊ A higher response rate to chemotherapy and an increase in survival are seen in patients who have small-volume residual disease following debulking surgery.

❊ The highest response rate to chemotherapy is seen with platinum-based drugs. Platinum–paclitaxel combinations are associated with the best outcome, and have become the standard of care for advanced ovarian cancer.

REFERENCES

1. Jacobs I, Oram D, Fairbanks J et al, A risk of malignancy index incorporating CA 125, ultrasound and menopausal status for the accurate preoperative diagnosis of ovarian cancer. *Br J Obstet Gynaecol* 1990; **97**: 922–9.
2. Masterton J, Management of ovarian cancer: surgery, irradiation and chemotherapy. *Am J Obstet Gynecol* 1967; **98**: 374–6.
3. Young RC, Chemotherapy of ovarian cancer: past and present. *Semin Oncol* 1975; **2**: 267–76.
4. Decker DG, Fleming TR, Malkasian GD Jr et al, Cyclophosphamide plus cis-platinum in combination: treatment program for stage III or IV ovarian carcinoma. *Obstet Gynecol* 1982; **60**: 481–7.
5. Hunter RW, Alexander ND, Soutter WP, Meta-analysis of surgery in advanced ovarian carcinoma: is maximum cytoreductive surgery an independent determinant of prognosis? *Am J Obstet Gynecol* 1992; **166**: 504–11.
6. Junor EJ, Hole DJ, Gillis CR, Management of ovarian cancer: referral to a multidisciplinary team matters. *Br J Cancer* 1994; **70**: 363–70.
7. Advanced Ovarian Cancer Trialists Group, Chemotherapy in advanced ovarian cancer: for systematic meta-analyses of individual patient data from 37 randomised trials. *Br J Cancer* 1998; **78**: 1479–87.
8. Neijt JP, ten Bokkel Huinink WW, van der Burg ME et al, Long-term survival in ovarian cancer. Mature data from The Netherlands Joint Study Group for Ovarian Cancer. *Eur J Cancer* 1991; **27**: 1367–72.
9. Sutton GP, Stehman FGB, Einhorn LH et al, Ten-year follow-up of patients receiving cis-platin, doxorubicin, and cyclophosphamide

chemotherapy for advanced epithelial ovarian carcinoma. *J Clin Oncol* 1989; **7**: 223–9.

10. Taylor AE, Wiltshaw E, Gore ME et al, Long-term follow-up of the first randomized study of cisplatin versus carboplatin for advanced epithelial ovarian cancer. *J Clin Oncol* 1994; **12**: 2066–70.

11. Advance Ovarian Cancer Trialists Group, Chemotherapy in advanced ovarian cancer: an overview of randomised clinical trials. *BMJ* 1991; **303**: 884–93.

12. AHern RP, Gore ME, Impact of doxorubicin on survival in advanced ovarian cancer. *J Clin Oncol* 1995; **13**: 726–32.

13. ICON Collaborators, ICON2: randomised trial of single-agent carboplatin against three-drug combination of CAP (cyclophosphamide, doxorubicin, and cisplatin) in women with ovarian cancer. ICON Collaborators. International Collaborative Ovarian Neoplasm Study. *Lancet* 1998; **352**: 1571–6.

14. Levin L, Hryniuk WM, Dose intensity analysis of chemotherapy regimens in ovarian carcinoma. *J Clin Oncol* 1987; **5**: 756–67.

15. Ngan HYS, Choo YC, Cheung M et al, A randomised study of high-dose versus low-dose cisplatin combined with cyclophosphamide in the treatment of advanced ovarian cancer. *Chemotherapy* 1989; **35**: 221–7.

16. Conte PF, Bruzzone M, Carnino F, High dose versus low dose cisplatin in combination with cyclophosphamide and epidoxorubicin in suboptimal ovarian cancer: a randomised study of the Gruppo Oncologico Nord-Ovest. *J Clin Oncol* 1996; **14**: 351–6.

17. Kaye SB, Paul J, Cassidy J et al, Mature results of a randomised trial of two doses of cisplatin for the treatment of ovarian cancer. *J Clin Oncol* 1996; **14**: 2113–19.

18. Jakobsen A, Bertelsen K, Andersen JE, Dose effect study of carboplatin in ovarian cancer: a Danish Ovarian Cancer Group study. *J Clin Oncol* 1997; **15**: 193–8.

19. Columbo N, Pittelli MR, Parma G et al, Cisplatin dose intensity in advanced ovarian cancer: a randomised study of conventional dose vs dose intense cisplatin mono-chemotherapy. *Proc Am Soc Clin Oncol* 1993; **12**: 255.

20. Murphy D, Crowther D, Renninson J et al, A randomised dose intensity study in ovarian carcinoma comparing chemotherapy given at four week intervals for six cycles with half dose of chemotherapy given for twelve cycles. *Ann Oncol* 1993; **4**: 377–83.

21. Bella M, Cocconi G, Lotticci R, Mature results of a prospective randomised trial comparing two dose-intensity regimens of cisplatin in advanced ovarian carcinoma. *Ann Oncol* 1994; **5**(Suppl 8): 2.

22. McGuire WP, Hoskins WJ, Brady MF et al, Assessment of dose intensive therapy in suboptimally debulked ovarian cancer: a GOG study. *J Clin Oncol* 1995; **13**: 1589–99.

23. Gore ME, Mainwaring PN, Macfarlane V et al, A randomised study of high versus standard dose carboplatin in patients with advanced epithelial ovarian cancer. *Proc Am Soc Clin Oncol* 1996; **15**: 769.

24. Dittrich C, Obermair A, Kurz C et al, Prospective randomised trial of cisplatin/carboplatin versus conventional cisplatin/cyclophosphamide in epithelial ovarian cancer: first results of the impact of platinum dose intensity on patient outcome. *Proc Am Soc Clin Oncol* 1996; **15**: 749.

25. Kaye SB, Lewis C, Paul J et al, Randomised study of two doses of cisplatin and cyclophosphamide in epithelial ovarian cancer. *Lancet* 1992; **340**: 329–33.

26. Kaye SB, Paul J, Cassidy J et al, Mature results of a randomised trial of two doses of cisplatin for the treatment of ovarian cancer. Scottish Gynaecology Cancer Trials Group. *J Clin Oncol* 1996; **14**: 2113–19.

27. Klauber N, Parangi S, Flynn E et al, Inhibition of angiogenesis and breast cancer in mice by the microtubule inhibitors 2-methoxyestradiol and Taxol. *Cancer Res* 1997; **57**: 81–6.

28. Hansen HH, Eisenhauer EA, Hansen M et al,

New cytostatic drugs in ovarian cancer. *Ann Oncol* 1993; 4(Suppl 4): 63–70.

29. Eisenhauer EA, ten Bokkel Huinink WW, Swenerton KD et al, European–Canadian randomized trial of paclitaxel in relapsed ovarian cancer: high-dose versus low-dose and long versus short infusion. *J Clin Oncol* 1994; **12**: 2654–66.

30. McGuire WP, Hoskins WJ, Brady MF et al, Cyclophosphamide and cisplatin compared with paclitaxel and cisplatin in patients with stage III and stage IV ovarian cancer. *N Engl J Med* 1996; **334**: 1–6.

31. Piccart MJ, Bertelsen K, James K et al, Randomised intergroup trial of cisplatin–paclitaxel versus cisplatin–cyclophosphamide in women with advanced epithelial ovarian cancer: three-year results. *J Natl Cancer Inst* 2000: **92**: 699–708.

32. du Bois A, Lueck HJ, Meier W et al, Cisplatin/paclitaxel vs carboplatin/paclitaxel in ovarian cancer: update of an Arbeitsgemeinschaft Gynaekologische Onkologie (AGO) Study Group Trial. *Proc Am Soc Clin Oncol* 1999; **18**: 1374.

33. Neijt JP, Hansen M, Hansen SW et al, Randomized phase III study in previously untreated epithelial ovarian cancer FIGO stage IIB, IIC, III, IV, comparing paclitaxel–cisplatin and paclitaxel–carboplatin. *Proc Am Soc Clin Oncol* 1997; **16**: 1259.

34. Ozols RF, Bundy BN, Fowler J et al, Randomized phase III study of cisplatin (CIS)/paclitaxel (PAC) versus carboplatin (CARBO)/PAC in optimal stage III epithelial ovarian cancer (OC): a Gynecologic Oncology Group trial (GOG 158). *Proc Am Soc Clin Oncol* 1999; **18**: 1373.

35. Markman M, Intraperitoneal chemotherapy. In: *Cancer of the Ovary* (Markman M, Hoskins WJ, eds). New York: Raven Press, 1993: 317–26.

36. Los G, Mutsaers PH, van der Vijgh WJ et al, Direct diffusion of *cis*-diamminedichloroplatinum(II) in intraperitoneal rat tumors after intraperitoneal chemotherapy: a comparison with systemic chemotherapy. *Cancer Res* 1989; **49**: 3380–4.

37. Alberts DS, Liu PY, Hannigan EV et al, Intraperitoneal cisplatin plus intravenous cyclophosphamide versus intravenous cisplatin plus intravenous cyclophosphamide for stage III ovarian cancer. *N Engl J Med* 1996; **335**: 1950–5.

38. Markman M, Bundy B, Benda J et al, Randomized phase 3 study of intravenous (iv) cisplatin (cis)/paclitaxel (pac) versus moderately high dose iv carboplatin (carb) followed by iv pac and intraperitoneal (ip) cis in optimal residual ovarian cancer (OC): an intergroup trial (COG, SWOG, ECOG). *Proc Am Soc Clin Oncol* 1998; **17**: 1392.

39. Morgan RJ Jr, Copeland L, Gershenson D et al, NCCN Ovarian Cancer Practice Guidelines. The National Comprehensive Cancer Network. *Oncology (Huntingt)* 1996; **10**(11 Suppl): 293–310.

40. Berek JS, Bertelsen K, du Bois A et al, Advanced epithelial ovarian cancer: 1998 consensus statements. *Ann Oncol* 1999; **10**(Suppl 1): 87–92.

41. Joint Council for Clinical Oncology, The current role of paclitaxel in the first-line chemotherapy for ovarian cancer. In: The Royal Colleges of Physicians and Radiologists, London, 1998.

42. Adams M, Calvert AH, Carmichael J et al, Chemotherapy for ovarian cancer – a consensus statement on standard practice. *Br J Cancer* 1998; **78**: 1404–6.

43. National Institute for Clinical Excellence, NHS. *Guidance on the use of taxanes for ovarian cancer*. www.nice.org.uk.

44. NHS Executive. *Guidance on commissioning cancer services. Improving outcomes in gynaecological cancers: the manual*. NHS Executive, London, 1999: 30–4.

2
Pelvic mass in a woman under 40 years

Mark A Morgan, Stephen C Rubin

INTRODUCTION

Although infrequent, epithelial ovarian cancer can occur in young patients. Below the age of 30 years, the incidence is approximately 1.5 per 100 000 and it rises to about 15 per 100 000 by age 40 years (the peak incidence is 57 per 100 000). Because of the possibility of ovarian cancer, an adnexal mass in a young woman must be thoroughly evaluated, and many of these patients will require surgery, either by laparoscopy or laparotomy. Screening programs, particularly for women with a family history of ovarian cancer, are now available, although their value is uncertain. These assessments are likely to lead to more surgical explorations in young women. Some of these women will have ovarian cancer. For patients with early disease, conservative fertility-sparing surgery may be possible. This raises issues about follow-up, since the remaining ovary is at risk. The role of 'second-look' surgery needs to be considered. In patients with early disease, the value of adjuvant therapy is still unclear. In some cases, these young patients will be found to have advanced disease, and both surgical therapy and chemotherapy must be aggressive.

CASE HISTORY 1

A 32-year-old gravida 2, para 2 was referred to the gynecologic oncology service after evaluation of a pelvic mass and rectal bleeding revealed papillary serous carcinoma on transrectal biopsy. Computerized tomography (CT) of the abdomen and pelvis demonstrated a large soft tissue mass in the cul-de-sac as well as a 3.8 cm cyst on the right ovary and multiple, <2 cm cysts, on the left ovary. There was no ascites.

The patient had a six-month history of constipation and abdominal bloating. She was on oral contraceptives at the time of diagnosis. Her family history was significant for a maternal grandmother who died of 'intraabdominal cancer'.

Preoperatively, the patient had a barium enema, which revealed a mass impinging on the rectum as well as a mass effect on the transverse colon, but no evidence of mucosal involvement. The rest of the colon appeared normal. A chest X-ray was normal and the CA125 level was 211 U/ml.

The abdomen was explored through a midline incision, and she was found to have multiple nodules in the omentum and a large tumor in the cul-de-sac. A total omentectomy was performed. In the pelvis, the peritoneum was opened lateral to the ovarian vessels bilaterally to facilitate the dissection because the tumor infiltrated into the retroperitoneum. A total abdominal hysterectomy, bilateral salpingoopherectomy, and a sigmoid colectomy with end colostomy were performed because of infiltration of the tumor into the bowel wall muscularis. At the completion of surgery, there were no residual tumor nodules greater than 1 cm. Final pathology confirmed papillary serous carcinoma arising in the left ovary with metastases to the omentum, uterus, other ovary, and sigmoid colon, with involvement of the muscularis and submucosa. The distal margin of the colonic resection was microscopically positive. Postoperatively, various chemotherapeutic options were discussed with the patient, and she agreed to participate in a Gynecologic Oncology Group (GOG) trial for patients with advanced ovarian cancer with minimal residual disease randomizing patients to intraperitoneal cisplatin and paclitaxel (Taxol) plus intravenous paclitaxel versus cisplatin and paclitaxel intravenously. She was randomized to the intraperitoneal arm, and had an intraperitoneal catheter placed prior to beginning therapy two weeks after surgery.

What are the epidemiologic risk factors for ovarian cancer?

This is an unusual case of advanced epithelial ovarian cancer presenting as a pelvic mass in a woman under 40 years of age. It illustrates many important points in the evaluation and treatment of advanced ovarian cancer.

The median age of diagnosis of epithelial ovarian cancer is 61 years. Approximately 12% of all ovarian cancers occur below the age 40, and, of those, malignant epithelial tumors make up about one-third.[1] Borderline epithelial and germ cell tumors make up most of the rest, with malignant germ cell tumors being much more common in woman under age 20. Epidemiologic studies have demonstrated that prior pregnancy and oral contraceptives reduce the risk of ovarian cancer. These epidemiologic findings support the

'incessant ovulation' hypothesis for the development of ovarian cancer. This theory suggests that ovarian cancer develops as an aberrant repair process from repeated ovulation, so that decreasing the number of ovulating cycles should decrease the risk of ovarian cancer.[2] Interestingly, this patient had two children and was using oral contraceptives at the time of diagnosis. In addition, she had breast-fed both her children, which is also associated with a decreased risk.[3]

Is there a benefit for screening for ovarian cancer?

The early onset of ovarian cancer in this woman raises the possibility of an inherited genetic predisposition. The fact that her maternal grandmother died of 'intraabdominal cancer' points out the difficulty in determining the accuracy of family history. Frequently, family histories are incomplete or accurate diagnoses may not be available.[4] Women with mutations in the BRCA1 gene may have an estimated lifetime risk of ovarian cancer as high as 45%, while BRCA2 mutations may convey a 15–20% lifetime risk. Without knowledge of specific mutations, a woman with a single family member with ovarian cancer has a 4–5% risk of developing the disease. Two involved relatives increase the risk to 7%, and women with at least two first-degree relatives may have as high as a 50% chance of developing ovarian cancer.[5] It has been postulated that oral contraceptives may not be as protective in women with an inherited predisposition to cancer; however, a case–control study of women with either BRCA1 or BRCA2 mutations did demonstrate an approximately 50% reduced risk of ovarian cancer with oral contraceptive use,[6] which is similar to the degree of reduction seen in the general population.

Could this disease have been detected earlier? Currently, there is no accepted method of screening the general population for ovarian cancer, and the patient's family history would not have made a strong case for an inherited syndrome. Although there is no conclusive survival benefit, studies of transvaginal ultrasound in the general population and in patients with a family history have detected cases of early ovarian cancer.[7,8] Although sensitivity and specificity have been greater than 90%, the positive predictive value has been low (<10%) owing to the low prevalence of the disease in both populations. The combination of ultrasound and CA125 increased the positive predictive value to 26.8% in one study.[9] The addition of color flow Doppler, statistically derived morphologic indices, and serial studies may further reduce the false-positive rate and make screening strategies acceptable in high-risk groups, such as those women known to be from families with *BRCA1* or *BRCA2* mutations. It should be noted, however, that most studies in ovarian cancer screening have dealt with postmenopausal populations, and false-positive tests are likely to be higher in women under 40. Although this patient did not appear to fit into a clear-cut high-risk group to target for screening, it is interesting that she was followed for six months with vague abdominal complaints and bowel symptoms, and was not referred to a gynecologist until a transrectal biopsy revealed a papillary serous malignancy. Although symptoms often do not develop until the disease has metastasized, the length of time that symptoms were present in this woman suggests that earlier evaluation of the pelvis may have detected disease at a point where such extensive surgery may not have been required.

This patient's preoperative evaluation included CT of the abdomen and pelvis, a barium enema, a chest X-ray, and a CA125 blood test. All of these tests could be justified based on the unusual presentation and the need to search for other sources of cancer. A barium enema is particularly useful when colonic involvement is suspected and bowel resection may be necessary. A preoperative mechanical bowel preparation is indicated, and has been shown to decrease the incidence of infectious complications.[10,11] Either a standard three-day regimen or one-day whole-gut lavage with a polyethylene glycol–electrolyte solution could be used. Oral neomycin sulfate and erythromycin on the day prior to surgery further decrease the bowel bacterial count. In the absence of a biopsy showing papillary carcinoma, it would have also been prudent to measure serum α-fetoprotein (AFP) β human chorionic gonadotropin (βhCG), and lactate dehydrogenase (LDH) levels, since germ cell tumor of the ovary would have been a possibility in this 32-year-old woman.

What is appropriate surgical therapy and chemotherapy for patients with advanced ovarian cancer?

Exploration of the abdomen should be performed through a vertical incision starting at the pubis with extension above the umbilicus. When advanced, bulky intraabdominal cancer is found, an attempt at maximal surgical cytoreduction should be made. Since 1975,[12] it has been known that the size of residual disease after debulking is directly related to prognosis in epithelial ovarian cancer. This has been shown in many studies since then,[13] and has made aggressive surgical cytoreduction the standard of care in the primary management of advanced ovarian cancer in the USA.[14] Despite this, the issue of surgical debulking and its impact on prognosis is still debated. Hoskins et al[15] showed that, in the GOG experience, the superior survival of 'optimally debulked' stage III patients is due largely to the inclusion of patients who either started with optimal (<1 cm) disease or required minimal effort to achieve optimal status. In suboptimally debulked patients, the extensive debulking was beneficial only if it approached 'optimal residual disease'.[16] Although a randomized controlled trial has not been performed comparing aggressive primary cytoreductive surgery with less aggressive surgery, a randomized trial of interval cytoreduction by the European Organization for Research and Treatment of Cancer (EORTC) after a planned three courses of chemotherapy in suboptimally debulked patients did demonstrate a significant survival benefit to debulking surgery.[17]

This patient had extensive pelvic disease, infiltrating the retroperitoneum and involving the bowel wall. Optimal (<1 cm residual) debulking was obtained by taking a retroperitoneal approach and performing a sigmoid resection with an end colostomy. In general, colon resection and colostomy should be done rarely in the primary surgical management of ovarian cancer, and usually only when the other sites of disease can be resected, as was the case here. Although sigmoid colectomy can be performed safely in most cases, its effect on survival is not clear.[18] Frequently, when sigmoid colectomy is performed, low reanastomosis is possible, especially using surgical staplers.

In addition to possibly providing a survival benefit, cytoreductive surgery can influence decisions regarding subsequent treatment. In the USA, the standard chemotherapeutic regimen used to treat advanced ovarian cancer consists of cisplatin and paclitaxel, based primarily on the results of a randomized trial reported by the GOG. This trial demonstrated improved progression-free and overall survival in patients with suboptimally debulked stage III and IV ovarian cancer treated with cisplatin and paclitaxel versus cisplatin and cyclophosphamide.[19] A recently completed trial reported by the GOG and the Southwest Oncology Group (SWOG) demonstrated superior survival in patients treated with intraperitoneal cisplatin and intravenous cyclophosphamide versus the same two drugs given intravenously.[20] This patient was entered on a current GOG trial testing not only whether intraperitoneal cisplatin but also intraperitoneal paclitaxel will add to the efficacy of intravenous paclitaxel. The addition of intraperitoneal paclitaxel to this regimen was based on phase II data from the GOG that demonstrated a 61% complete surgical response rate in patients with microscopic disease at second-look surgery.[21]

Is there a benefit for second-look surgical reassessment in patients who have complete primary chemotherapy?

If this patient achieves a complete clinical response, she would be a good candidate for second-look surgery and reversal of her colostomy. Although a clear-cut survival benefit has not been demonstrated, second-look surgery remains the most accurate technique in assessing completeness of disease response. One study from Memorial Sloan-Kettering Cancer Center found persistent disease in 62% of patients with a normal CA125 at the time of second-look surgery.[22] All of these patients had an elevated CA125 at initial presentation. Since a survival benefit has not been demonstrated with currently available second-line therapies, second-look surgery should be reserved for instances where an innovative trial of second-line treatment is available. Second-look surgery for this patient is reasonable not only to assess disease status and institute aggressive second-line therapy, but also to reverse her colostomy.

LEARNING POINTS

❊ There are no proven methods for effective screening for ovarian cancer.
❊ When advanced epithelial ovarian cancer is found in a young patient, conservative therapy is not an option.

✳ The management of advanced epithelial ovarian cancer in a young patient involves aggressive cytoreductive surgery and chemotherapy.

✳ Although controversial, many authorities recommend second-look laparoscopy or laparotomy following primary chemotherapy.

CASE HISTORY 2

A 34-year-old gravida 1, para 1, with a history of chronic pelvic pain and endometriosis, was found to have an enlarged right ovary on routine pelvic examination. An ultrasound was performed that showed a 5 cm × 6 cm complex cystic mass on the right ovary. There were thick septations but no solid areas. Diffuse internal echoes suggested hemorrhage. The patient was placed on oral contraceptives. After two months, the mass was found to be the same size and the thick septations persisted. A CA125 was obtained, which was found to be elevated at 95 U/ml. The patient had no family history of cancer, but her mother and maternal aunt had had hysterectomies for 'female problems'.

Laparoscopy was performed, and a mobile right ovarian mass was identified with several small external excrescences. The other ovary, uterus, and the rest of the abdomen appeared normal. There was no ascites or signs of endometriosis. The right tube and ovary were removed laparoscopically and were placed in a retrieval bag prior to rupturing the cyst to prevent spillage. Frozen section revealed poorly differentiated carcinoma with clear cell features. The laparoscopic instruments were removed and a laparotomy was performed. A total abdominal hysterectomy with left salpingo-oopherectomy was performed, in addition to an omentectomy, pelvic and paraaortic lymph node sampling, and peritoneal and diaphragmatic biopsies. The gastrointestinal tract was carefully examined, and there was no gross evidence of metastatic disease. Final pathology revealed a clear cell carcinoma of the ovary with disease on the surface of the ovarian capsule, but all other biopsies and peritoneal cytology were negative, making her tumor a stage IC. The patient was then started on chemotherapy with carboplatin and paclitaxel for a planned six courses.

What is the appropriate evaluation of an adnexal mass in a woman under the age of 40 years?

An adnexal mass presenting in a woman under 40 years of age is likely to be benign. Predicting which masses are neoplastic or malignant is difficult by examination unless there is obvious evidence of metastatic disease. Functional cysts are most common, especially when they are less than 10 cm, and although hormonal suppression is often used in these cases, its value is controversial.[23] Certainly, an endometrioma could have an identical presentation, including a slightly elevated CA125 level. Morphologic scoring systems have been devised using ultrasound to discriminate benign from inadequate lesions more clearly,[24] and the serum CA125 has also been used to help predict malignancy. Unfortunately, about half of early ovarian cancers will have a normal CA125 level, and a falsely elevated CA125 level is more common in premenopausal women owing to conditions such as benign cysts, endometriosis, pelvic inflammatory disease, and fibroids. In a young woman, serum AFP and βhCG should be measured preoperatively, especially when the mass is solid, which suggests a possible germ cell tumor.

Can some adnexal masses in young patients be managed by laparoscopy and conservative surgery?

The initial surgical management of an adnexal mass suspicious for malignancy has traditionally been via laparotomy. Recently, however, there has been a trend towards the laparoscopic approach. This approach has been criticized because of the potential for spill and subsequent spread of tumor, as well as delay in instituting appropriate staging and therapy. The vast majority of adnexal masses approached laparoscopically will be benign, especially in non-oncologic practices.[25–27] Even in an oncologic referral practice, however, adnexal masses without gross obvious evidence of metastatic disease are likely to be benign.[28] In this case, the use of a bag to prevent spill of tumor, and immediate conversion to laparotomy, obviates some of the early criticism aimed at the laparoscopic approach.[29] Although several studies have not shown intraoperative rupture to be an independent adverse factor for prognosis,[30–32] rupture and morcellation have been shown to be capable of causing tumor dissemination.[33] Scientific evidence aside, it can be reasonably assumed that intentional rupture of an intact malignancy is not a good thing, and should be avoided where possible. If the decision is made to perform a cystectomy rather than oophorectomy, every attempt should be made to remove the cyst intact. If malignancy is found at the time of laparoscopy, the current standard dictates laparotomy with complete surgical staging as described. The GOG is currently evaluating the role of laparoscopic staging in incompletely staged ovarian cancers. Previous studies with laparotomy have found occult metastases in 20–30% of cases felt to have local disease at initial surgery.[34] Unilateral adnexectomy with complete surgical staging in women who wish to preserve reproductive potential has been retrospectively evaluated, and does not appear to worsen prognosis.[35,36] This is most appropriate in stage IA and low-grade lesions. Occult bilaterality may occasionally be present, however, so wedge biopsy of the contralateral ovary may be reasonable prior to conservative therapy.[37]

Should a patient with early ovarian cancer receive adjuvant therapy?

The choice of postoperative therapy in stage I ovarian cancer is controversial. Since only 10–15% of comprehensively staged cases of epithelial ovarian cancer are early-stage, and recurrence and death are infrequent, it is difficult to do randomized trials. Many older studies did not involve careful surgical staging, and are probably not relevant. In 1990, Young et al[38] reported two randomized trials in surgically staged patients with early disease. They found no benefit to adjuvant melphalan in stage I well- and moderately well-differentiated tumors, with a greater than 90% five-year survival rate in either arm. In patients with stage I poorly differentiated tumors or stage II disease, they found no difference in survival between intraperitoneal ^{32}P or melphalan (about an 80% five-year survival rate). They did find that clear cell tumors were associated with a greater risk of recurrence, even in early disease – a finding that has been supported in subsequent studies.[39,40] Previous trials may have failed to show any benefit for adjunctive therapy because the sample size was too small. The ICON (International Collaborative Group for Ovarian Neoplasia) has just completed a large trial of almost 2000 patients (ICON I) comparing immediate carboplatin treatment versus observation in patients where there is uncertainty about the need for adjunctive treatment. The first analysis of results will take place in 2000.

The current trend in the USA is to treat patients with high-risk (high-grade, external excrescences, or positive cytology) early disease with multiagent platinum-based chemotherapy because of a 20–30% chance of recurrence. Although an Italian trial demonstrated a benefit in recurrence-free survival with immediate therapy with cisplatin versus observation in stage I patients with grade 2 and 3 tumors, overall survival was not different, because of salvage therapy with cisplatin when patients in the no-treatment group recurred.[41] With longer follow-up, it is likely that many patients in the recurrent group will not be cured, and we may see a survival difference. The GOG compared radioactive phosphorus (^{32}P) versus three courses of cisplatin and cyclophosphamide in patients with high-risk stage I and any stage II disease, and have not shown a statistically significant difference in survival, but there was a 31% decrease in recurrence with chemotherapy.[42] Since platinum and paclitaxel combination regimens have produced superior results in advanced disease, it is certainly possible that these combinations will also be superior in early disease, where there is less of a tumor burden and, theoretically, there are fewer resistant clones. A recently completed GOG trial compared three versus six courses of carboplatin and paclitaxel in high-risk early disease, but it is too early to report results.

SUMMARY

Although most cases of epithelial ovarian cancer will occur in patients beyond childbearing age, some young patients will develop ovarian cancer, and currently there are no proven methods of screening for the disease. When the disease is found to be advanced, therapy must be aggressive, but for patients with early disease it may be possible to preserve childbearing capacity. Postoperative chemotherapy is indicated for patients with high-risk early disease, even in those cases where surgical therapy has been conservative.

LEARNING POINTS

❋ A persistent or suspicious adnexal mass in a young woman requires surgical evaluation.
❋ When performed appropriately, initial surgical evaluation may be performed by laparoscopy.
❋ If an ovarian mass is found to be malignant on frozen section, the surgical procedure should be converted to an open laparotomy to allow appropriate surgical staging.
❋ Conservative surgery (unilateral salpingo-oophorectomy and surgical staging) is appropriate for early ovarian cancer if the patient desires further childbearing.
❋ Postoperative chemotherapy for high-risk early epithelial ovarian cancer with a platinum compound and paclitaxel is being studied in ongoing trials.

REFERENCES

1. Partridge EE, Phillips JL, Menck HE, The National Cancer Data Base report on ovarian cancer treatment in United States hospitals. *Cancer* 1996; **78**: 2236–46.
2. Casagrande JT, Louie EW, Pike MC et al, 'Incessant ovulation' and ovarian cancer. *Lancet* 1979; **ii**: 170–3.
3. Whitemore AS, Characteristics relating to ovarian cancer risk: implications for prevention and detection. *Gynecol Oncol* 1994; **55**: S15–19.
4. Koch M, Hill GB, Problems in establishing accurate family history in patients with ovarian cancer of epithelial origin. *Cancer Detect Prev* 1987; **10**: 279–83.
5. Whittemore AS, Harris R, Itnyre J, Characteristics relating to ovarian cancer risk: collaborative analysis of 12 US case–control studies. II. Invasive epithelial ovarian cancers in white women. Collaborative Ovarian Cancer Group. *Am J Epidemiol* 1992; **136**: 1184–203.
6. Narod SA, Risch H, Moslehi R et al, Oral contraceptives and the risk of hereditary ovarian cancer. Hereditary Ovarian Cancer Clinical Study Group. *N Engl J Med* 1998; **339**: 424–8.
7. DePriest PD, van Nagell JR Jr, Gallion HH et al, Ovarian cancer screening in asymptomatic postmenopausal women. *Gynecol Oncol* 1993; **51**: 205–9.
8. Jacobs I, Davies AP, Bridges J et al, Prevalence

screening for ovarian cancer in post-menopausal women by CA125 measurement and ultrasonography. *BMJ* 1993; **306**: 1030–4.

9. Burke W, Daly M, Garber J et al, Recommendations for follow-up care of individuals with an inherited predisposition to cancer. II. BRCA1 and BRCA2. Cancer Genetics Studies Consortium. *JAMA* 1997; **277**: 997–1003.

10. Coppa GF, Eng K, Gouge TH et al, Parenteral and oral antibiotics in elective colon and rectal surgery. A prospective, randomized trial. *Am J Surg* 1983; **145**: 62–5.

11. Condon RE, Bowel preparation for colorectal operations. *Arch Surg* 1982; **117**: 265.

12. Griffiths CT, Surgical resection of tumor bulk in the primary treatment of ovarian carcinoma. *Natl Cancer Inst Monogr* 1975; **42**: 101–4.

13. Hoskins WJ, Perez CA, Young RC, *Principles and Practice of Gynecologic Oncology*, 2nd edn. Philadelphia: Lippincott-Raven, 1997: 941–2.

14. Morgan RJ Jr, Copeland L, Gershenson D et al, NCCN Ovarian Cancer Practice Guidelines. The National Comprehensive Cancer Network. *Oncology* 1996; **10**: 293–310.

15. Hoskins WJ, Bundy BN, Thigpen JT et al, The influence of cytoreductive surgery on recurrence-free interval and survival in small-volume stage III epithelial ovarian cancer: a Gynecologic Oncology Group study. *Gynecol Oncol* 1992; **47**: 159–66.

16. Hoskins WJ, McGuire WP, Brady MF et al, The effect of diameter of largest residual disease on survival after primary cytoreductive surgery in patients with suboptimal residual epithelial ovarian carcinoma. *Am J Obstet Gynecol* 1994; **170**: 974–9 (discussion 979–80).

17. van der Burg ME, van Lent M, Buyse M et al, The effect of debulking surgery after induction chemotherapy on the prognosis in advanced epithelial ovarian cancer. Gynecological Cancer Cooperative Group of the European Organization for Research and Treatment of Cancer. *N Engl J Med* 1995; **332**: 629–34.

18. Soper JT, Couchman G, Berchuck A et al, The role of partial sigmoid colectomy for debulking epithelial ovarian carcinoma. *Gynecol Oncol* 1991; **41**: 239–44.

19. McGuire WP, Hoskins WJ, Brady MF et al, Cyclophosphamide and cisplatin compared with paclitaxel and cisplatin in patients with stage III and stage IV ovarian cancer. *N Engl J Med* 1996; **334**: 1–6.

20. Alberts DS, Liu PY, Hannigan EV et al, Intraperitoneal cisplatin plus intravenous cyclophosphamide versus intravenous cisplatin plus intravenous cyclophosphamide for stage III ovarian cancer. *N Engl J Med* 1996; **335**: 1950–5.

21. Markman M, Brady MF, Spirtos NM et al, Phase II trial of intraperitoneal paclitaxel in carcinoma of the ovary, tube, and peritoneum: a Gynecologic Oncology Group Study. *J Clin Oncol* 1998; **16**: 2620–4.

22. Rubin SC, Hoskins WJ, Hakes TB et al, Serum CA 125 levels and surgical findings in patients undergoing secondary operations for epithelial ovarian cancer. *Am J Obstet Gynecol* 1989; **160**: 667–71.

23. Curtin JP, Management of the adnexal mass. *Gynecol Oncol* 1994; **55**: S42–6.

24. Lerner JP, Timor-Tritsch IE, Federman A et al, Transvaginal ultrasonographic characterization of ovarian masses with an improved, weighted scoring system. *Am J Obstet Gynecol* 1994; **170**: 81–5.

25 Parker WH, Levine RL, Howard FM et al, A multicenter study of laparoscopic management of selected cystic adnexal masses in post-menopausal women. *J Am Coll Surg* 1994; **179**: 733–7.

26. Shalev E, Eliyahu S, Peleg D et al, Laparoscopic management of adnexal cystic masses in postmenopausal women. *Obstet Gynecol* 1994; **83**: 594–6.

27. Hulka JF, Hulka CA, Preoperative sonographic evaluation and laparoscopic management of persistent adnexal masses: a 1994 review. *J Am Assoc Gynecol Laparosc* 1994; **1**: 197–205.

28. Dottino PR, Levine DA, Ripley DL et al, Laparoscopic management of adnexal masses in premenopausal and postmenopausal women. *Obstet Gynecol* 1999; **93**: 223–8.

29. Maiman M, Seltzer V, Boyce J, Laparoscopic excision of ovarian neoplasms subsequently found to be malignant. *Obstet Gynecol* 1991; 77: 563–5.

30. Dembo AJ, Davy M, Stenwig AE et al, Prognostic factors in patients with stage I epithelial ovarian cancer. *Obstet Gynecol* 1990; **75**: 263–73.

31. Sevelda P, Dittrich C, Salzer H, Prognostic value of the rupture of the capsule in stage I epithelial ovarian carcinoma. *Gynecol Oncol* 1989; **35**(3): 321–2.

32. Sjovall K, Nilsson B, Einhorn N, Different types of rupture of the tumor capsule and the impact on survival in early ovarian carcinoma. *Int J Gynecol Cancer* 1994; **4**: 333–6.

33. Kindermann G, Maassen V, Kuhn W, Laparoscopic management of ovarian tumors subsequently diagnosed as malignant: a survey from 127 German departments of obstetrics and gynecology. *J Pelvic Surg* 1996; **2**: 245–51.

34. Benjamin I, Rubin SC, Management of early-stage epithelial ovarian cancer. *Obstet Gynecol Clin North Am* 1994; **21**: 107–19.

35. Munnell EW, Is conservative therapy ever justified in stage I (A) cancer of the ovary? *Am J Obstet Gynecol* 1969; **103**: 641–53.

36. Parker RT, Parker CH, Wilbanks GD, Cancer of the ovary. Survival studies based upon operative therapy, chemotherapy, and radiotherapy. *Am J Obstet Gynecol* 1970; **108**: 878–88.

37. Benjamin I, Morgan MA, Rubin SC, Occult bilateral involvement in stage I epithelial ovarian cancer. *Gynecol Oncol* 1999; **72**: 288–91.

38. Young RC, Walton LA, Ellenberg SS et al, Adjuvant therapy in stage I and stage II epithelial ovarian cancer. Results of two prospective randomized trials. *N Engl J Med* 1990; **322**: 1021–7.

39. Behbakht K, Randall TC, Benjamin I et al, Clinical characteristics of clear cell carcinoma of the ovary. *Gynecol Oncol* 1998; **70**: 255–8.

40. Jenison EL, Montag AG, Griffiths CT et al, Clear cell adenocarcinoma of the ovary: a clinical analysis and comparison with serous carcinoma. *Gynecol Oncol* 1989; **32**: 65–71.

41. Bolis G, Colombo N, Pecorelli S et al, Adjuvant treatment for early epithelial ovarian cancer: results of two randomised clinical trials comparing cisplatin to no further treatment or chromic phosphate (^{32}P). G.I.C.O.G.: Gruppo Interregionale Collaborativo in Ginecologia Oncologica. *Ann Oncol* 1995; **6**: 887–93.

42. Young RC, Brady MF, Nieberg RM et al, Randomized clinical trial of adjuvant treatment of women with early (FIGO I–IIA high risk) ovarian cancer – GOG 95. In: *Proceedings of the Sixth Biennial Meeting of the International Gynecologic Cancer Society*. Fukuoka, Japan: Blackwell Science, 1997: 17 (Abst 047).

3

Aggressive or conservative surgery for ovarian cancer?

Jubilee B Robinson, Dwight D Im, Neil B Rosenshein, William P McGuire III

INTRODUCTION

The principle of surgical treatment for many solid tumors of the abdominopelvic cavity involves an en bloc excision of the tumor, but the pattern of spread of epithelial ovarian cancer does not usually permit such an approach. It is common for the surgeon to find the pelvis extensively involved by tumor, associated with diffuse peritoneal carcinomatosis, omental and diaphragmatic involvement, and multiple large tumor masses involving the bowel and mesentery (Figure 3.1).[1] The surgical treatment of epithelial ovarian cancer often involves cytoreductive surgery, an attempt to achieve the greatest possible degree of tumor removal. This approach is based on data indicating significantly higher rates of survival, clinical response, and pathological response in patients with minimal residual disease following surgery.[2] Cytoreductive surgery may employ surgical procedures such as small or large bowel resection or techniques such as ultrasonic surgical aspiration.

This chapter will examine the available scientific evidence underlying the theory and practice of reducing tumor burden. This should enable the surgeon to determine the operative approach and treatment regimen most beneficial for the patient with ovarian cancer.

CASE HISTORY

A 59-year-old woman presented to her physician with a six-week history of abdominal bloating, vague abdominal pain, and a decrease in appetite. In the previous week, she had noted a significant increase in abdominal girth and had had nausea and vomiting. Examination revealed a moderately ill woman with a distended abdomen. On pelvic examination, a large irregular mass was palpable, which was compressing the rectum. A computed tomography (CT) scan revealed a large volume of ascites, bilateral pelvic masses, and an apparent omental cake. A chest X-ray revealed a left pleural effusion and a moderate right pleural effusion. The CA125 level was 3575 U/ml. A medical evaluation judged the patient to be at increased but acceptable risk for surgery.

How does the initial surgical procedure affect survival, quality of life, mortality, and morbidity?

Primary cytoreductive surgery is defined as the removal of as much tumor as possible at the time of the initial operative procedure.[2] The development of effective chemotherapeutic modalities over the past several decades has allowed primary but incomplete cytoreductive surgery to

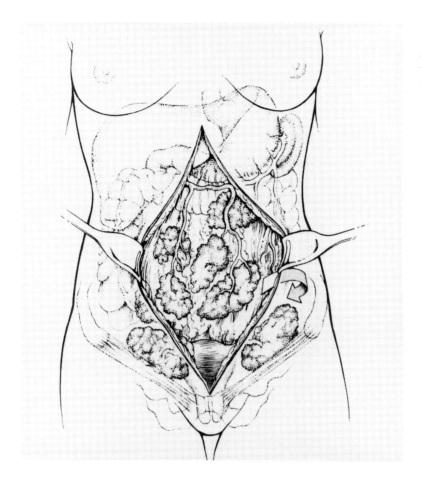

Figure 3.1
Extensive involvement of pelvis by ovarian carcinoma, obliterating the normal pelvic anatomy. (Reproduced from Wharton JT, Edwards C, *Clin Obstet Gynecol* 1983; **10**: 235–44.[1])

become an integral part of the treatment of ovarian cancer, since tumor remaining after surgery is subject to eradication by subsequent chemotherapy.

The utility of reducing tumor burden in ovarian cancer was documented as early as 1967, when Long et al[3] reported improved survival in patients who underwent radical surgery with radiotherapy compared with those undergoing oophorectomy or radiotherapy alone. In 1968, Munnell[4] first described cytoreductive surgery as a 'maximal surgical effort'. He reported that patients who underwent partial tumor removal survived longer than patients who underwent laparotomy and biopsy alone, despite the admin-

istration of postoperative whole-abdomen radiation in both groups. In 1969, Delclos and Quinlan[5] noted a correlation between initial tumor mass and survival. Surgically staged patients with stage II and III nonpalpable disease had a significant survival advantage over patients with palpable disease. The four-year survival rate was 72% versus 33% for stage II disease, and 25% versus 9% for stage III disease.

Evidence for the effectiveness of cytoreductive surgery continued with Griffiths' landmark paper[6] of 1975. The survival of 102 patients with stage II or III epithelial ovarian cancer was correlated with amount of residual tumor prior to the administration of single-agent alkylating

Table 3.1   Survival by diameter of largest residual disease

Size (cm)	No. of patients	Mean survival (months)
0	29	39
0–0.5	28	29
0.6–1.5	16	18
>1.5	29	11

Table 3.2   Theoretical mechanisms of cytoreductive surgery

Growth kinetics (recruitment of tumor cells into actively dividing pool)
Increased sensitivity to cytotoxic drugs
Decreased drug resistance (direct and indirect mechanisms)
Decreased tumor burden by a 'mass effect'
Relief of bowel obstruction
Enhanced host immunocompetence

chemotherapy. Survival improved as residual tumor volume decreased (Table 3.1). Griffiths and Fuller[7] published additional survival data in 1978. The survival of patients cytoreduced to 1.5 cm was similar to that of patients who presented with disease less than 1.5 cm. The 40-month survival rate for patients with less than 1.5 cm of residual tumor following cytoreductive surgery was 30%. No patient with residual tumor greater than 1.5 cm survived 40 months.

These findings spawned a worldwide accumulation of response and survival data supporting the benefit of primary cytoreductive surgery. This evidence has persisted through the era of platinum-based therapy. Primary cytoreductive surgery followed by platinum- and taxane-based combination chemotherapy has become the current cornerstone of therapy for patients with epithelial ovarian cancer.

Theoretical benefits of cytoreductive surgery

The rationale underlying primary cytoreductive surgery is based upon tumor growth kinetics and the susceptibility of ovarian cancer to cytotoxic agents. Surgical debulking affects tumor growth kinetics, drug resistance, cell number, nutrition, and immunocompetence, maximizing the effectiveness of cytotoxic chemotherapy (Table 3.2).[2,8,9]

The relationship between tumor size and growth rate follows Gompertzian kinetics.[2] As a tumor enlarges, its doubling time increases, presumably owing to a decrease in blood supply, oxygen, and nutrients. Larger tumors have a greater proportion of cells in the resting (G_0) phase, or nonproliferative phase. They are therefore relatively insensitive to cytotoxic chemotherapy, which typically inhibits the growth of cells actively undergoing DNA synthesis and cell division. The removal of large tumor masses during cytoreductive surgery results in the recruitment of resting tumor cells into the actively dividing pool of tumor cells. In small tumor implants of 0.1–0.5 cm^3, nearly every cell is in the actively dividing pool.[2] Thus, the residual tumor is potentially more susceptible to the cytotoxic effects of chemotherapy.[2]

The surgical removal of tumor may also influence drug sensitivity. As neoplasms enlarge, central necrosis often occurs, reflecting poor central blood supply. Cytoreductive surgery removes large tumor masses, which have a poor blood supply and would receive insufficient chemotherapy,[2] allowing for increased perfusion and cell kill of residual tumor.[10]

Drug resistance can be minimized through direct and indirect mechanisms. Through direct action, cytoreductive surgery can physically remove intrinsically resistant cell lines. However, resistant cell lines can also develop through spontaneous mutation (acquired resistance), decreasing the efficacy of the chemotherapy and the potential for cure. As suggested by the Goldie–Coldman hypothesis,[11] a tumor starts with intrinsic chemosensitivity, but develops spontaneous mutations to drug resistance at variable rates that are directly proportional to the cell number. With decreases in the tumor size and cell number, the probability of new mutations to drug resistance decreases. This decrease in the spontaneous development of new resistant phenotypes is an indirect but substantial potential benefit of cytoreductive surgery. This appears to be related to the amount of residual tumor at the completion of surgery, supporting an aggressive approach to cytoreductive surgery.[8]

The degree of cytoreduction is of theoretical importance in leaving fewer cells to be eradicated by chemotherapy. As described by Boente et al,[2] this 'mass effect' would only be significant in patients with no visible remaining tumor. Patients with bulky disease of 1 kg or more who undergo cytoreduction to leave a tumor burden of 1 cm^3 experience an exponential decrease in the number of tumor cells with surgery (10^9 to 10^6). By first-order kinetics, this would require seven 3-log cell kills to eradicate the last tumor cell. This model would predict possible cure only in those patients with one 1 cm^3 or less of residual disease for whom an extensive cytoreduction could achieve that goal and benefit the patient, again supporting aggressive cytoreduction.

Cytoreduction may also relieve or prevent symptoms of bowel obstruction or pain, have nutritional benefits,[9] and enhance host immunocompetence.[10] All of these theoretical advantages provide the scientific rationale for the observed improvement in outcome of patients who undergo successful cytoreductive surgery.

Clinical benefits of cytoreductive surgery
Outcome data
Cytoreductive surgery is based on strong indirect evidence of clinical benefit in patients who are left with minimal residual disease following cytoreductive surgery. Patients with an optimal cytoreduction, the presence of no tumor nodule that exceeds 1 cm in diameter after surgery, have a higher incidence of complete clinical response to chemotherapy, a higher incidence of negative findings at second-look laparotomy, an improved progression-free survival, and a prolonged median survival.[9] Although no prospective, randomized, controlled clinical trial has been performed to demonstrate the benefit of cytoreduction, this indirect evidence is convincing enough to dictate this as the standard of care in ovarian cancer. The relative contributions of surgical aggressiveness and expertise versus tumor biology in this outcome are discussed below.

The definition of optimal cytoreduction has

varied over the past three decades. In the 1970s, 'large residual disease' was defined as disease greater than 2 cm remaining after surgery.[12] In 1986, the Gynecologic Oncology Group (GOG) reported Protocol 47, in which suboptimal cytoreduction was defined as residual tumor greater than or equal to 3 cm in diameter.[13] Protocol 97, which was initiated in 1986, defined suboptimal disease as greater than 1 cm of tumor remaining after surgery, a definition used by all subsequent GOG protocols, and now generally accepted as the nodule size separating optimal and suboptimal disease.[12,14]

Many investigators have sought to determine the importance of the amount of residual tumor on the outcome of patients with an advanced ovarian malignancy. A summary of all published data evaluating outcome as a function of residual disease in groups of 50 or more patients is given in the Appendix to this chapter.[4,6,7,12,15–72] A meta-analysis by Allen et al[72] that examined the outcomes of 11 reports concluded that the amount of residual tumor significantly affected survival in patients with stage III disease. Patients with no macroscopic residual disease had a survival advantage over patients with macroscopic residual disease, and patients with 2 cm or less of residual disease had a survival advantage over patients with more than 2 cm of residual disease.[72] Boente et al[2] summarized 13 reports comparing optimal and suboptimal cytoreduction, and found that patients with optimal cytoreduction had higher rates of complete response (43% versus 24%), improved progression-free interval (31 months versus 13 months), and prolonged median survival (36 months versus 16 months). Likewise, Bertelsen et al[15] described a 46% five-year survival rate in patients with stage III or IV epithelial ovarian cancer and less than 1 cm of residual disease, compared with a 14% five-year survival rate in those patients with suboptimal residual disease.

Baker et al[16] agreed that a significant survival advantage and improved progression-free interval were documented in patients with less than 1 cm of residual disease.

Since the realization of the importance of cytoreductive surgery coincided with the development of modern platinum- and taxane-based chemotherapy, Hunter et al[73] performed a meta-analysis to determine the relative effects on outcome of debulking surgery and platinum-based chemotherapy. The outcomes of 6962 patients were tabulated, and cytoreduction was found to have a significant benefit on survival when a multivariate analysis was performed controlling for platinum-based chemotherapy. The effect of cytoreduction was small, however, when compared with the effect of platinum-based chemotherapy. A 4.1% increase in survival time was seen in patients who underwent 'maximum cytoreductive surgery', compared with a 53% increase in patients receiving platinum-containing chemotherapy.[73] Venesmaa and Ylikorkala[74] have confirmed these findings. Ozols[75] has since commented that the effect of cytoreduction seen in the meta-analysis by Hunter et al[73] is greater when patients with stage IV disease and patients who did not receive platinum-based chemotherapy are excluded. Regardless of the magnitude of the effect or of other variables, the literature consistently supports the significant survival advantage conferred by cytoreduction.

The degree of cytoreduction required in order to achieve clinical benefit has been investigated. Bertelsen et al[15] and Baker et al[16] agree that a survival advantage is detected only when the greatest diameter of residual tumor is less than 1 cm. GOG Protocols 52 and 97 have also addressed this question. In Protocol 52, which included only optimally debulked patients, Omura et al[17] found that patients with microscopic disease experienced a more favorable outcome than patients with macroscopic residual disease. In

Protocol 97, which included only suboptimally debulked patients, Hoskins et al[12] found that patients with 1–2 cm of residual disease had a survival advantage over patients with 2 cm or greater residual disease. On combining these two studies, no difference was seen between patients with less than 1 cm of residual disease and patients with 1–2 cm of residual disease. Thus, three groups were identified as having significantly different outcomes: microscopic residual disease, macroscopic residual disease measuring less than 2 cm, and macroscopic disease of 2 cm or more.[2]

Thus, the goal for the surgeon becomes clear. Every attempt should be made to remove all visible disease, since these patients have a significant survival advantage. If this is not possible, the benefit of aggressive surgery is evident when cytoreduction results in a small amount of residual tumor. Although the exact amount of residual tumor conferring benefit is not clear, less than 1–2 cm of residual tumor is an appropriate goal if removal of all visible disease is not possible. If neither of these goals can be met and suboptimal cytoreduction is inevitable, aggressive surgical procedures may not be warranted.

Tumor biology

Four studies have examined the relative effects of tumor biology and cytoreduction on patient outcome. In 1975, Griffiths[6] found that among patients with advanced ovarian cancer, those with residual disease less than 1.5 cm after cytoreduction had the same prognosis as patients with less than 1.5 cm of disease prior to cytoreduction. Wharton and Herson[18] found that the survival of patients who required extensive surgery to achieve optimal cytoreduction was the same as that of patients who did not require extensive surgery to reach an optimal disease state. These two studies suggest that the survival benefit may be related to the cytoreductive procedure itself rather than to the biology of a more indolent tumor that is intrinsically amenable to cytoreduction. These findings support aggressive cytoreductive surgery.

Two studies suggest that tumor biology may influence patient outcome. Potter et al[19] evaluated 163 patients with stage III or IV ovarian cancer, and found improved survival in patients who required a less extensive cytoreductive procedure to be considered 'optimal'. Hoskins et al[76] evaluated patients with optimally cytoreduced stage III ovarian cancer, and found the outcome among patients with less than 1 cm of tumor before surgery to be superior to that of patients who required extensive debulking procedures to achieve less than 1 cm of residual tumor. In the same study, Hoskins et al[76] noted that survival was correlated with patient age, tumor grade, and the number (not just the size) of tumor implants remaining after surgery. These findings suggest that a biologically less aggressive tumor may be more amenable to optimal cytoreduction, conferring an inherent survival advantage to patients achieving optimal disease status. This does not diminish the importance of cytoreduction, but suggests that tumor biology and other mechanisms may also influence patient outcome.

Stage IV disease

The role of cytoreductive surgery is less clear in patients with stage IV disease, since this indicates distant metastatic disease or intrahepatic metastases. The majority of studies do show a continued survival benefit among patients with stage IV disease who achieve optimal cytoreduction (Table 3.3).[77,78] Bristow et al[26] have recently confirmed this survival advantage in a retrospective analysis of 84 patients. Additionally, this study suggests that stage IV patients with less than 1 cm of residual intraperitoneal but greater than 1 cm of residual intraparenchymal liver disease have a survival advantage over patients with greater than 1 cm of residual disease in both the

Table 3.3   Outcome of stage IV patients based on residual tumor

Ref.	Endpoints[a]	Division of residual disease	n	p-value[b]	Benefit?
21	24-m survival	Microscopic; 0–1 cm; 1–2 cm; >2 cm	178	NP	Yes
	5-y survival		178	NP	Yes
22	24-m survival	2 cm	195	NP	Yes[c]
	Median survival		195	NP	Yes
23	24-m NED	Microscopic/macroscopic	27	NP	Trend
24	Median survival	2 cm	92	0.0136	Yes
25	Median survival	2 cm	92	<0.02	Yes
	DFI		92	0.1	No
26	Median survival	1 cm	84	0.0004	Yes
27	24-m survival	2 cm	14	NS	No
	5-y survival		14	NS	No
11	24-m survival	2 cm	35	NS	No
	5-y survival		35	NS	No
	Median survival		35	NS	No
18	Median survival	2 cm	47	0.0295	Yes

[a] m, month; y, year; NED, no evidence of disease; DFI, disease-free interval.
[b] NP, not provided; NS, not significant.
[c] Significant only for grades 1 and 4.

peritoneal cavity and the liver parenchyma (see also Chapter 7). This suggests a benefit from cytoreduction despite unresectable intra-parenchymal liver disease, but these findings have not yet been confirmed.[26]

Quality of life

The benefit of any therapy should not be measured by survival alone, but must also take quality of life into consideration. Optimal cytoreduction is associated with increased patient comfort. In one series, approximately 80% of patients who achieved optimal disease status after cytoreductive surgery subsequently reported 'enjoying life' and were able to conduct their normal activities, compared with only 46% of patients who were suboptimally cytoreduced.[79] The same series

found that optimally cytoreduced patients were more often able to return to work and less frequently admitted to the hospital. Optimal cytoreduction frequently relieved bowel obstruction, and decreased the number of subsequent episodes of bowel obstruction and paracentesis.[79] Cytoreductive surgery may also decrease adverse metabolic effects and allow the patient to maintain or improve her nutritional status.[9]

These benefits of an improved quality of life provide additional evidence that aggressive surgery may have positive effects if optimal disease status can be achieved. Quality-of-life issues may also influence the surgeon's decisions regarding aggressive procedures for reasons other than achieving optimal disease status. For example, if resection of the bowel will not result in an optimal disease status but will relieve bowel obstruction, such a procedure may be indicated not for survival benefit but for its projected impact on quality of life.

Consensus opinion

Review of the literature regarding the benefit of cytoreduction reveals overwhelming indirect evidence that it is of benefit to the patient. In order to address the body of evidence that has accrued, the US National Institutes of Health (NIH) held a Consensus Development Conference on Ovarian Cancer in 1994, and stated that 'aggressive efforts at maximal cytoreduction are important since minimal residual tumor is associated with improved survival'.[80]

How should the clinician determine the most appropriate surgery for a patient using evidence-based medicine?

Techniques of cytoreductive surgery

Advanced-stage epithelial ovarian carcinoma can significantly distort the pelvic anatomy, with obliteration of the normal anatomic planes and significant involvement of the pelvic and upper abdominal organs. The operating surgeon should be skilled in the surgical techniques of the pelvis, upper abdomen, and retroperitoneum, and should understand the clinical impact, tumor biology, and procedures involved in cytoreductive surgery.[9] This allows a patient-specific approach to operative intervention in advanced ovarian cancer.

Intraoperative assessment

The patient is positioned on the operating table in a semi-lithotomy position to permit access to the perineum and rectum. A generous vertical midline incision is made. Ascites is evacuated and the abdominopelvic cavity is systematically evaluated to determine the extent of disease. This involves palpation and inspection of all peri-toneal and mesenteric surfaces, including the pelvic contents and pelvic peritoneum, paracolic gutters, kidneys, liver, hemidiaphragms, omentum, lesser sac, stomach, spleen, small and large bowel, and pelvic and para-aortic lymph nodes. The surgeon should at this time determine the appropriate surgical approach and the extent of dissection and cytoreduction that he or she will pursue (Figure 3.2). This is perhaps the most difficult and important portion of the intraoperative process. The surgeon must assess the amount and location of disease, and determine the surgical procedures required to remove as much tumor as possible.

If the surgeon anticipates complete removal of all visible tumor, aggressive cytoreduction must be pursued regardless of the procedures required. The significant improvements in disease-free interval and survival mandate such an approach, assuming the patient can acutely withstand the surgery. Removal of all visible tumor is the ideal situation, with a significant improvement in outcome over patients with macroscopic residual disease.

In some situations, the surgeon may be able to remove all bulky disease but may be forced to leave macroscopic residual disease in which the largest implant is less than 1 cm. This may occur for many reasons, such as diffuse peritoneal studding, mesenteric implants, diaphragmatic disease, multiple capsular liver metastases, or intraparenchymal liver or distant metastases, as in the setting of stage IV disease. If the surgeon believes that optimal cytoreduction with macroscopic residual disease is possible, then aggressive surgical procedures are warranted. The improvement in the endpoints of disease-free interval, survival, and quality of life justify such aggressive surgery to achieve an optimal disease status.

If, however, the surgeon suspects that, despite the most aggressive surgical efforts, optimal

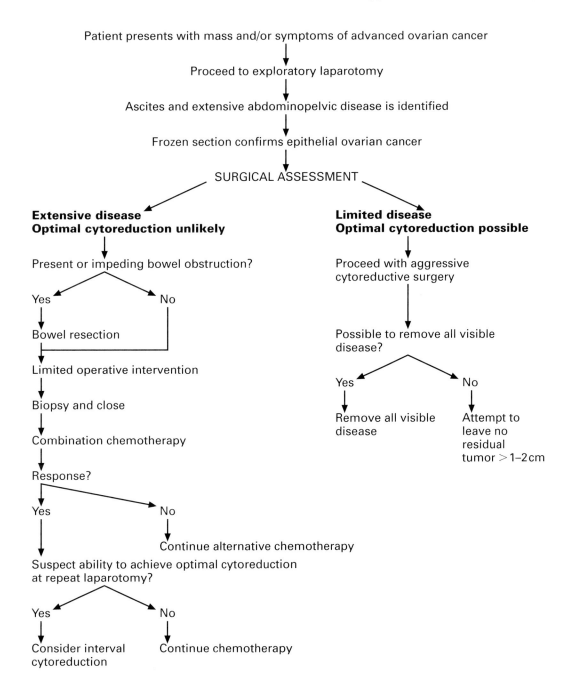

Figure 3.2
Schema for intraoperative decision-making in advanced ovarian cancer.

cytoreduction will be impossible, aggressive surgical procedures are not indicated. This situation may occur with unresectable and/or large masses involving the lesser sac, base of the mesentery, parenchyma of the liver, diaphragm, retroperitoneal lymph nodes, or multiple areas of the bowel. In such cases, a limited debulking is prudent, with aggressive maneuvers limited to palliation of present or impending bowel obstruction. Multiple studies indicate no significant difference in outcome among groups of patients with various degrees of residual tumor over 2 cm.[6,12,21,30] That is, there is no expected difference in survival between patients with 2 cm or 10 cm of residual disease.

Thus, with the exception of bowel resection for the relief of obstruction, aggressive cytoreductive surgical procedures should be limited to patients in whom optimal disease status is thought to be possible.

Techniques used in cytoreductive surgery

In patients with widespread disease, aggressive surgical procedures may be required to remove all visible tumor or achieve optimal cytoreduction. This may involve small bowel or colon resection, sometimes necessitating colostomy; resection of bladder or ureters, possibly requiring ureteroneocystotomy; extensive pelvic, para-aortic, or inguinal lymphadenectomy; stripping or resection of the diaphragm; or resection of the liver, spleen, pancreas, or kidney (Table 3.4).[2,9]

The operative approach to attaining optimal cytoreduction is a surgical challenge. The most prudent method in cases of widespread disease in the pelvis is to enter the retroperitoneal spaces: the prevesical, paravesical, pararectal, rectovaginal, and retrorectal spaces. The blood supply, namely the ovarian and uterine vessels, can be identified and controlled by ligating the infundibulopelvic ligament and uterine or hypogastric artery. The ureters and iliac vessels

Table 3.4   Aggressive surgical procedures used in cytoreductive surgery
Small bowel resection
Colon resection with or without colostomy
Resection of bladder or ureters
Extensive pelvic, para-aortic, or inguinal lymphadenectomy
Stripping or resection of the diaphragm
Resection of the liver, spleen, or kidney
Distal pancreatectomy
Supracolic omentectomy
Cytoreductive surgery using: Ultrasonic surgical aspiration Carbon dioxide laser surgery Argon beam coagulator

can be easily identified and protected. The central disease with the involved organs can then be swept to the midline and mobilized out of the pelvis (Figure 3.3). This approach often facilitates dissection of the bladder and rectum from the diseased uterus and adnexae, or facilitates resection of portions of the bladder or bowel if necessary. If a rectosigmoid resection is performed, a transanal/transabdominal end-to-end anastomosis can often be achieved with a stapling device, avoiding the need for a colostomy.

A 'retrograde hysterectomy' may be performed as initially described by Hudson,[81] with an anterior entrance to the vagina, dissection of the ureters from the parametria, and transection of the cardinal and uterosacral ligaments. The posterior cul-de-sac can then be inverted, facilitating removal of the tumor from the rectosigmoid.

The surgical procedure is continued with an infracolic omentectomy, in which the omentum is separated from the transverse colon, the lesser sac is entered, and the omentum is removed,

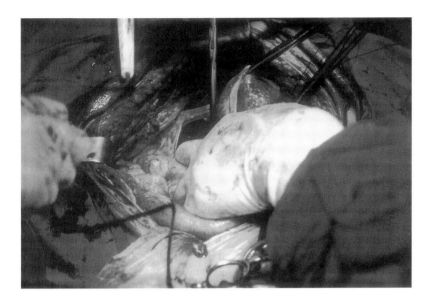

Figure 3.3
The retroperitoneum has been entered, the ureters and iliac vessels have been isolated and protected, and the tumor-involved pelvic organs have been mobilized out of the pelvis.

with attention being paid to preservation of the mesocolon and blood supply to the transverse colon. In some cases, the tumor may involve that portion of the omentum superior to the transverse colon. In cases where removal will affect an optimal cytoreduction, a supracolic omentectomy should be performed. The involved portion should be removed along the greater curvature of the stomach, and the short gastric arteries should be meticulously ligated.

Disease in the lesser sac presents a surgical challenge, but may necessitate a distal pancreatectomy if optimal cytoreduction is to be achieved. Likewise, a splenectomy may be required. If tumor is present on the hemidiaphragm, mobilization of the liver by division of the falciform ligament and ligamentum teres with gentle retraction of the liver may be required to gain access to the involved portion of the diaphragmatic surface.

Multiple small or large bowel resections may be indicated for the removal of large disease or for the relief of bowel obstruction. Resection and reanastomosis using a stapling device may obviate the need for a permanent colostomy or

stoma of more proximal small bowel. Diffuse peritoneal studding is not in itself an indication for bowel resection, and the decision to proceed with bowel resection should take into account the ability to achieve significant cytoreduction.

Newer methods of cytoreduction

The importance of cytoreduction has lead to a search for novel methods of removing tumor for patients in whom optimal cytoreduction would be otherwise impossible. Several instruments have been developed, including the ultrasonic surgical aspirator, carbon dioxide laser, and argon beam coagulator.

The ultrasonic surgical aspirator uses a high-frequency sound wave to fragment tissue through direct contact, and then to irrigate and aspirate the disrupted tissue. This method selectively spares connective tissue and blood vessels, and has been considered for debulking tumor from the diaphragm, spleen, liver, bowel, and bladder. Rose[82] found that ultrasonic surgical aspiration contributed to cytoreduction in 48% of patients with advanced ovarian cancer, and frequently avoided resection of the involved organs. Survival and outcome were not assessed. In a small, randomized study using ultrasonic surgical aspiration, van Dam et al[10] showed no effect on ability to achieve optimal cytoreduction or on survival, but did note a decrease in average blood loss, morbidity, and hospital stay with the use of ultrasonic surgical aspiration. One investigator reported disseminated intravascular coagulation with the use of ultrasonic surgical aspiration, but other investigators have not confirmed these findings.[83]

The carbon dioxide and neodynium–yttrium–aluminum–garnet (Nd-YAG) lasers have also been reported to be effective in the reduction of bulky ovarian tumors.[84]

Brand and Pearlman have investigated the argon beam coagulator for use in debulking surgery.[84] This electrosurgical device uses a beam of inert argon gas to conduct current to tissue. Seven patients with advanced ovarian cancer underwent optimal cytoreduction with the use of the argon beam coagulator, four of whom had no gross residual tumor at the completion of the procedure.[84]

Nomenclature and classification

Literature regarding the surgical treatment of ovarian cancer is replete with nonspecific surgical descriptions, such as 'conservative', 'radical', and 'ultraradical'. These terms have not been precisely defined, and have purposefully been avoided in this chapter. The degree of surgery and procedures performed for the diagnosis of advanced ovarian cancer can vary tremendously, and are separate from the designations of optimal or suboptimal residual disease. Currently no schema exists to describe the extent of the procedures performed.

We propose a classification of cytoreductive surgery to accurately describe the extent of surgery (Table 3.5). We suggest that procedures of types I and II represent more limited surgery,

and may be appropriate even in patients who would be unable to achieve optimal residual disease with more aggressive surgical procedures. Type III procedures are appropriate for patients who will achieve optimal disease status through these procedures, or for patients in whom a bowel obstruction can be alleviated or avoided. Procedures of types IV and V represent aggressive surgical procedures, and should be performed only if optimal disease status can be achieved. These categories of procedure should not be performed if optimal disease status will not result.

Morbidity and mortality of radical surgery

Regardless of the talent of the surgeon, cytoreductive surgery for the treatment of ovarian cancer does have attendant risks of morbidity and mortality. Previous studies have identified a 30–67% risk of at least one complication.[68,74] The most frequently reported complications include an intraoperative blood loss of greater than 1000 cm^3 (21%), urinary tract infection (8–23%), fever (2–53%), and ileus (2–17%) (Table 3.6).[74] The risk of fever, urinary tract infection, wound complication, or thromboembolic event is independent of the degree of cytoreduction achieved. In contrast, the risk of significant blood loss is higher in patients with advanced-stage ovarian cancer and in patients who undergo lymph node dissection. Patients with suboptimal tumor debulking have a higher risk of significant blood loss (37%) than patients with optimal tumor debulking (19%).[74] The risk of bowel complications, such as ileus, obstruction, or the need for colostomy, is higher in patients with suboptimal cytoreductive surgery. This may relate to tumor biology, since more aggressive neoplasms may be highly invasive and less amenable to optimal cytoreduction. Additionally, patients who have undergone bowel resection are 13 times more likely to require over 24 hours of postoperative intensive care.[85]

Table 3.5   Cytoreduction classification

Type I	Removal of uterus, adnexae, omentum
Type II	Type I procedure plus removal of pelvic peritoneum, and/or pelvic and para-aortic lymph node dissection
Type III	Type I or II procedure plus one large or small bowel resection, and/or simple bladder resection
Type IV	Type I or II or III procedure plus more than one large or small bowel resection, and/or complex bladder resection, and/or resection of diaphragmatic tumor
Type V	Type I or II or III or IV procedure plus resection of spleen, and/or distal pancreatectomy, and/or removal of tumor from the lesser sac, and/or resection of the liver, and/or removal of massive fixed or matted retroperitoneal lymph nodes

Table 3.6   Morbidity and mortality of cytoreductive surgery[a]

Complications	Total	Exploration only	Suboptimal reduction	Optimal reduction	p-value[b]
Blood loss > 1000 cm³	98 (21%)	2 (3%)	40 (37%)	56 (19%)	<0.001
Fever	20 (4%)	5 (8%)	6 (6%)	9 (3%)	<0.01
Urinary infection	86 (18%)	14 (21%)	22 (20%)	50 (17%)	<0.001
Bowel complication	34 (7%)	9 (14%)	11 (10%)	14 (5%)	NS
Wound complication	14 (3%)	3 (5%)	7 (7%)	4 (1%)	NS
Thromboembolism	10 (2%)	2 (3%)	3 (3%)	5 (2%)	<0.05
Mortality	5 (1%)	1 (2%)	3 (3%)	1 (0.3%)	NS

[a] Modified from Venesmaa P, Ylikorkala O, Morbidity and mortality associated with primary and repeat operations for ovarian cancer. *Obstet Gynecol* 1992; **79**: 168–72. Data are presented as numbers of patients, with percentages in parentheses.
[b] NS, not significant.

No significant increase in morbidity can be attributed to increasing patient age or the performance of lymphadenectomy.[74] Thus, optimal cytoreduction should be contemplated in every patient, regardless of age.

The mortality of primary cytoreductive surgery, defined as death within 30 days of the procedure,[74] has been reported as 1–3%.[9,74] Four out of five deaths in one series occurred in patients with advanced-stage disease.[74] The causes of death were pulmonary embolus, myocardial infarction, and three cases of progressive cancer with obstructive ileus. Resection of the bladder or ureters may also be a risk factor for mortality. Berek et al[86] reported a 12-month median survival in these patients and a 7-month median survival in patients with preoperative urinary tract obstruction.

What are the relative roles of initial surgery, interval surgery, and neoadjuvant chemotherapy in ovarian cancer?

Timing of radical surgery

Primary cytoreductive surgery

Surgical tumor debulking is a procedure whereby a surgically incurable malignant neoplasm is partially removed without curative intent, in order to make subsequent treatment with chemotherapy, radiation, or other adjunctive measures more effective, and thereby improve survival.[87] Primary cytoreductive surgery, or maximal tumor reduction at the time of the initial surgical exploration, is the standard initial approach for the patient with epithelial ovarian cancer. The vast majority of reviews that focus on surgical therapy address primary cytoreductive surgery, since this is appropriate for the majority of patients. Other alternatives in the timing of cytoreductive surgery have recently been investigated in order to improve the outcome of certain groups of patients with ovarian cancer.

Interval secondary cytoreduction

Following primary cytoreductive surgery, 50–70% of patients will be left with 'suboptimal' or bulky residual disease.[2,88] The median survival and progression-free interval are significantly worse in these patients with suboptimal cytoreduction than in patients who have been optimally cytoreduced. Subsequent optimal cytoreduction would theoretically remove tumor prior to the emergence of drug resistance, according to the Goldie–Coldman hypothesis, and, based on first-order cell kinetics, would allow chemotherapy to be more effective in eradicating disease.[11] Interval secondary cytoreduction, also known as 'chemosurgery', has been proposed for these patients with bulky advanced-stage ovarian cancer who have suboptimally debulked disease after primary cytoreductive surgery.[9] Patients who undergo interval cytoreduction receive a brief course of chemotherapy followed by a second attempt at achieving optimal cytoreduction before completing a prescribed chemotherapy regimen.[2]

Smith and Rutledge[89] first noted the ability of chemotherapy to decrease tumor burden and allow significant cytoreduction in 1970. Lawton subsequently determined that 75% of patients could be optimally cytoreduced at subsequent surgery.[90] Others have confirmed the success of interval cytoreduction in achieving optimal status, with percentages ranging from 45% to 89%.[91] One isolated report found only an 8% ability to successfully cytoreduce.[91]

Two groups of investigators have independently found an insignificant effect of interval cytoreduction on survival and progression-free interval. In 1983, Vogl et al[92] reported a minimal effect of a 'second-effort' surgical procedure performed six months after primary cytoreductive surgery. Redman et al performed a small prospective trial in 1994 evaluating patients with suboptimal primary cytoreduction.[93] The median survival was no different between patients who received chemotherapy alone and patients who underwent chemotherapy and interval debulking surgery, 73% of whom were left with less than 2 cm of residual disease.

Other investigators have reported an improvement in outcome of selected patients after interval cytoreductive surgery.[91] In 1985, Wiltshaw et al[94] evaluated patients who underwent interval cytoreduction five to seven months after primary cytoreductive surgery. Secondary cytoreduction had no impact on patients who had a complete response to chemotherapy, but a significant survival advantage was seen in patients who had only a partial response to chemotherapy. Lawton et al[90] have noted that interval cytoreduction should occur after no more than four cycles of chemotherapy, since nearly all responses to platinum occur within three cycles.

Three large studies have demonstrated a significant effect on outcome of interval cytoreductive surgery. Neijt evaluated 191 patients with advanced epithelial ovarian cancer.[45] Patients who were suboptimally cytoreduced at the initial surgical procedure and achieved optimal cytoreduction at interval surgery had the same survival as patients who were optimally cytoreduced at the initial surgical procedure. This implies an improvement in outcome of suboptimally cytoreduced patients directly related to interval cytoreduction.[95] Wils et al[33] had identical findings, in which the three-year survival rate for patients with optimal disease after primary cytoreductive surgery (60%) was not statistically different from that of patients with optimal disease after interval cytoreductive surgery (50%). Patients suboptimally cytoreduced after the primary surgery who did not undergo interval secondary cytoreduction had a worse outcome than either of the previous groups – again supporting the potential benefit of interval cytoreduction in patients with suboptimally cytoreduced disease.[33]

The European Organization for Research and Treatment of Cancer (EORTC) has performed a large, prospective trial in patients with suboptimal disease to determine the value of interval secondary cytoreduction following three cycles of cyclophosphamide and cisplatin.[34] Of the 278 patients, 65% had residual disease following three cycles of chemotherapy, and 45% of these patients achieved subsequent optimal cytoreduction through interval surgery. Patients with optimal cytoreduction after interval surgery had a significant improvement in median survival (26 months versus 20 months), two-year survival rate (56% versus 46%), and progression-free interval (18 months versus 13 months) over patients who received chemotherapy alone. These findings suggest a significant survival benefit for patients with suboptimal disease who undergo interval cytoreductive surgery. The morbidity and mortality rates are low (14% and 0% respectively) for repeat surgical exploration, and do not provide a contraindication for surgical therapy. Since the survival advantage for interval secondary cytoreduction is not uniformly evident but may represent a significant improvement in outcome for patients with initial suboptimal cytoreduction, there is a need for a large, prospective, randomized study to address this issue. Therefore, the GOG is currently conducting Protocol 152 and the UK Medical Research Council (MRC) is performing a similar study (OVO6). The results of these trials could influence the recommendations for therapy of patients with suboptimal cytoreduction of advanced ovarian cancer.

Neoadjuvant chemotherapy

The majority of patients who present with ovarian cancer are candidates for primary cytoreductive surgery followed by combination chemotherapy. In certain cases, however, it is not prudent for the patient to undergo cytoreductive surgery at the time of diagnosis secondary to increased surgical risk. Often, these patients will have massive reaccumulating effusions or severe medical problems that prevent major surgery.[84] In such patients, a presumptive diagnosis can be made by cytologic examination of pleural fluid or ascites, or by fine-needle aspiration of a soft tissue mass.[84] While in most cases of ovarian cancer, a diagnostic paracentesis is not recommended because of the risk of seeding the aspiration site with tumor, a pathologic diagnosis must be rendered before committing a patient to a chemotherapeutic regimen. Following diagnosis, these patients may benefit from two or three cycles of chemotherapy, during which time the effusions or medical contraindications to surgery may resolve, after which cytoreductive surgery and additional chemotherapy may be more feasible.

This technique, called neoadjuvant chemotherapy, has been evaluated in a retrospective, matched-control trial, in which patients underwent a biopsy without cytoreductive surgery at the time of laparotomy, followed by two to four cycles of chemotherapy, followed by cytoreductive surgery and additional chemotherapy. The matched patients underwent immediate re-exploration, cytoreductive surgery, and standard chemotherapy. The ability to achieve optimal cytoreduction was significantly increased in the patients who received neoadjuvant chemotherapy (77%) compared with standard therapy (39%), but no significant difference in survival was found.[96]

A second trial in Europe compared 88 patients who underwent neoadjuvant chemotherapy with 244 patients who underwent standard therapy, all of whom had advanced ovarian cancer.[97] The three- and five-year survival rates were no different between groups, but the percentage of patients cytoreduced to less than 2 cm of residual tumor, quality of life, and disease-free interval were improved in patients who underwent neoadjuvant chemotherapy (Table 3.7).[33,90,95–100]

Table 3.7   Outcomes in patients receiving neoadjuvant chemotherapy

Ref.	n	Significantly improved	No significant difference	% optimal cytoreduction
33	88	*	Complete response 3-years survival	75
94	36	% optimal cytoreduction	NP	75
95	44	% optimal cytoreduction	Median survival	77
96	332	Quality of life Disease-free interval	3-year survival 5-year survival	22
97	76	*	Survival	88
98	29	*	Time to progression Survival	NP
99	30	Median survival	*	82
100	285	Crude survival	*	NP

*, no variables in this category.
NP, not provided.

The utility of neoadjuvant chemotherapy for patients with advanced disease or severe medical illness is suggested by the above data. No randomized trials have yet been completed, but the EORTC is currently performing a trial (EORTC 55971) comparing neoadjuvant chemotherapy with interval debulking surgery and maximum debulking surgery prior to chemotherapy.

CONCLUSION

The last two decades have markedly increased the understanding of the surgical and chemotherapeutic management of epithelial ovarian cancer. A review of the literature regarding the benefit of aggressive cytoreductive surgery provides overwhelming indirect evidence that it is of benefit to the patient in many circumstances.

The volume of retrospective data regarding the role of cytoreductive surgery does define the role of aggressive cytoreduction versus conservative surgery in the treatment of epithelial ovarian cancer. If complete removal of all visible disease can be achieved, then extensive surgical procedures should be undertaken to accomplish this (e.g. type IV or V procedures). If visible disease will remain but optimal disease status will result (i.e. no nodule greater than 1–2 cm), then equally extensive surgical procedures are appropriate. If, however, the surgical assessment reveals that suboptimal disease status will result despite the most aggressive efforts (i.e. any residual tumor nodule greater than 2 cm), then aggressive surgery should not be performed. In this case, the surgeon should biopsy to ensure a definitive diagnosis and close the abdomen, or at the most perform a type I procedure.

The nuances of surgical therapy remain investigational, but the benefit of successful cytoreductive surgery in the treatment of epithelial ovarian cancer is clear.

LEARNING POINTS

✳ Survival and quality of life for patients with advanced ovarian cancer are improved by successful initial cytoreductive surgery.

✳ In selected cases, patients who have suboptimal cytoreductive surgery at their initial operation may benefit from interval cytoreductive surgery. The appropriate interval has not been well established, but appears to be after three or four courses of chemotherapy.

✳ Some patients with persistent or recurrent ovarian cancer will benefit from secondary cytoreductive surgery, either at the time of second-look surgery or as a separate surgical procedure for recurrent disease.

✳ Prospective clinical trials may establish the role of neoadjuvant chemotherapy in selected patients.

REFERENCES

1. Wharton JT, Edwards C, Cytoreductive surgery for common epithelial tumors of the ovary. *Clin Obstet Gynecol* 1983; **10**: 235–44.
2. Boente MP, Chi DS, Hoskins WJ, The role of surgery in the management of ovarian cancer: primary and interval cytoreductive surgery. *Semin Oncol* 1998; **25**: 326–34.
3. Long RTL, Johnson RE, Sala JM, Variations in survival among patients with carcinoma of the ovary. *Cancer* 1967; **20**: 1195–202.
4. Munnell EW, The changing prognosis and treatment in cancer of the ovary. *Am J Obstet Gynecol* 1968; **100**: 790–805.
5. Delclos L, Quinlan EJ, Malignant tumors of the ovary managed with postoperative megavoltage irradiation. *Radiology* 1969; **93**: 659–63.
6. Griffiths CT, Surgical resection of tumor bulk in the primary treatment of ovarian carcinoma. *Natl Cancer Inst Monogr* 1975; **42**: 101–4.
7. Griffiths CT, Fuller AF, Intensive surgical and chemotherapeutic management of advanced ovarian cancer. *Surg Clin North Am* 1978; **58**: 131–42.

8. Hoskins WJ, Surgical staging and cytoreductive surgery of epithelial ovarian cancer. *Cancer* 1993; **71**: 1534–40.

9. Clarke-Pearson DL, Kohler MF, Hurteau JA, Elbendary A, Surgery for advanced ovarian cancer. *Clin Obstet Gynecol* 1994; **37**: 439–60.

10. Van Dam PA, Tjalma W, Weyler J et al, Ultraradical debulking of epithelial ovarian cancer with the ultrasonic surgical aspirator: a prospective randomized trial. *Am J Obstet Gynecol* 1996; **174**: 943–50.

11. Goldie JH, Coldman JA, A mathematic model for relating the drug sensitivity of tumors to their spontaneous mutation rate. *Cancer Treat Rep* 1979; **63**: 1727–33.

12. Hoskins WJ, McGuire WP, Brady MF et al, The effect of diameter of largest residual disease on survival after primary cytoreductive surgery in patients with suboptimal residual epithelial ovarian carcinoma. *Am J Obstet Gynecol* 1994; **170**: 974–80.

13. Omura G, Blessing J, Ehrlich C et al, A randomized trial of cyclophosphamide and doxorubicin with or without cisplatin in advanced ovarian carcinoma. *Cancer* 1986; **57**: 1725–30.

14. Omura GA, Brady MF, Homesly HD et al, Long follow-up and prognostic factor analysis in advanced ovarian carcinoma: the Gynecologic Oncology Group experience. *J Clin Oncol* 1991; **9**: 1138–50.

15. Bertelsen K, Jakobsen A, Andersen JE et al, A randomized study of cyclophosphamide and *cis*-platin with or without doxorubicin in advanced ovarian carcinoma. *Gynecol Oncol* 1987; **28**: 161–9.

16. Baker TR, Piver MS, Hempling RE, Long term survival by cytoreductive surgery to less than 1 cm, induction weekly cisplatin and monthly cisplatin, doxorubicin, and cyclophosphamide therapy in advanced ovarian adenocarcinoma. *Cancer* 1994; **74**: 656–63.

17. Omura GA, Bundy BN, Berek JS et al, Randomized trial of cyclophosphamide plus cisplatin with or without doxorubicin in ovarian carcinoma: a Gynecologic Oncology Group study. *J Clin Oncol* 1989; **7**: 457–65.

18. Wharton JT, Herson J, Surgery for common epithelial tumors of the ovary. *Cancer* 1981; **48**: 582–9.

19. Potter ME, Partridge EE, Hatch KD et al, Primary surgical therapy of ovarian cancer: how much and when. *Gynecol Oncol* 1991; **40**: 195–200.

20. Williams CJ, Mead CM, Macbeth FR et al, Cisplatin combination chemotherapy versus chlorambucil in advanced ovarian carcinoma: mature results of a randomized trial. *J Clin Oncol* 1985; **3**: 1455–62.

21. Smith JP, Day TG, Review of ovarian cancer at the University of Texas Systems Cancer Center, M.D. Anderson Hospital and Tumor Institute. *Am J Obstet Gynecol* 1979; **135**: 984–93.

22. Malkasian GD, Melton LJ, O'Brien PC, Greene MH, Prognostic significance of histologic classification and grading of epithelial malignancies of the ovary. *Am J Obstet Gynecol* 1984; **149**: 274–84.

23. Carmichael JA, Shelley WE, Brown LB et al, A predictive index of cure versus no cure in advanced ovarian carcinoma patients – replacement of second-look laparotomy as a diagnostic test. *Gynecol Oncol* 1987; **27**: 269–78.

24. Curtin JP, Malik R, Venkatraman ES et al, Stage IV ovarian cancer: impact of surgical debulking. *Gynecol Oncol* 1997; **64**: 9–12.

25. Munkarah AR, Hallum AV, Morris M et al, Prognostic significance of residual disease in patients with stage IV epithelial ovarian cancer. *Gynecol Oncol* 1997; **64**: 13–17.

26. Bristow RE, Montz FJ, Lagasse LD et al, Survival impact of surgical cytoreduction on stage IV epithelial ovarian cancer. *Gynecol Oncol* 1999; **72**: 278–87.

27. Griffiths CTH, in: Allen DG, Heintz APM, Touw FWMM, A meta-analysis of residual disease and survival in stage III and IV carcinoma of the ovary. *Eur J Gynaecol Oncol* 1995; **16**: 349–56.

28. Lambert HE, Berry RJ, High dose cisplatin compared with high dose cyclophosphamide in the management of advanced epithelial ovarian cancer (FIGO stages III and IV): report from the North Thames Cooperative Group. *BMJ* 1985; **190**: 889–93.

29. Gynaecological Group, Clinical Oncological Society of Australia, and the Sydney Branch, Ludwig Institute for Cancer Research, Chemotherapy of advanced ovarian adenocarcinoma: a randomized comparison of combination versus sequential therapy using chlorambucil and cisplatin. *Gynecol Oncol* 1986; **23**: 1–13.

30. Neijt JP, Van der Burg MEL, Vriesendorp R et al, Randomised trial comparing two combination chemotherapy regimens (Hexa-CAF vs CHAP-5) in advanced ovarian carcinoma. *Lancet* 1984; **ii**: 594–600.

31. Louie KG, Ozols RF, Myers CE et al, Long-term results of a cisplatin-containing chemotherapy regimen for the treatment of advanced ovarian carcinoma. *J Clin Oncol* 1986; **4**: 1579–85.

32. Redman JR, Petroni GR, Saigo PE et al, Prognostic factors in advanced ovarian carcinoma. *J Clin Oncol* 1986; **4**: 515–23.

33. Wils J, Blijhma G, Naus A et al, Primary or delayed debulking surgery and chemotherapy consisting of cisplatin, doxorubicin, and cyclophosphamide in stage III–IV epithelial ovarian carcinoma. *J Clin Oncol* 1986; **4**: 1068–73.

34. Van der Burg MEL, Van Lent M, Buyse M et al, The effect of debulking surgery after induction chemotherapy on the prognosis in advanced epithelial ovarian cancer. *N Engl J Med* 1995; **332**: 629–34.

35. Hainsworth JD, Grosh WW, Burnett LS et al, Advanced ovarian cancer: long-term results of treatment with intensive cisplatin-based chemotherapy of brief duration. *Ann Intern Med* 1988; **108**: 165–70.

36. Delgado G, Oram DH, Petrilli ES, Stage III epithelial ovarian cancer: the role of maximal surgical reduction. *Gynecol Oncol* 1984; **18**: 293–8.

37. Ehrlich CE, Einhorn L, Stehman FB, Blessing J, Treatment of advanced epithelial ovarian cancer using cisplatin, Adriamycin and Cytoxan – the Indiana University experience. *Clin Obstet Gynecol* 1983; **10**: 325–35.

38. Petru E, Lahousen M, Tamussino K et al, Prognostic implications of residual tumor volume in stage III ovarian cancer patients undergoing adjuvant cytotoxic chemotherapy. *Baillière's Clin Obstet Gynecol* 1989; **3**: 109–17.

39. Pfleiderer A, Tumor reduction and chemotherapy in ovarian cancer. *Baillière's Clin Obstet Gynecol* 1989; **3**: 119–78.

40. Unzelman RF, Advanced epithelial ovarian carcinoma: long-term survival experience at the community hospital. *Am J Obstet Gynecol* 1992; **166**: 1663–71.

41. Neijt JP, in: Allen DG, Heintz APM, Touw FWMM, A meta-analysis of residual disease and survival in stage III and IV carcinoma of the ovary. *Eur J Gynaecol Oncol* 1995; **16**: 349–56.

42. Einhorn N, Nilsson B, Sjovall K, Factors influencing survival in carcinoma of the ovary. *Cancer* 1985; **55**: 2019–25.

43. Sigurdsson K, Alm P, Gullberg B, Prognostic factors in malignant epithelial ovarian tumors. *Gynecol Oncol* 1983; **15**: 370–80.

44. Michel G, DeIaco P, Castaigne D et al, Extensive cytoreductive surgery in advanced ovarian carcinoma. *Eur J Gynaecol Oncol* 1997; **18**: 9–15.

45. Neijt JP, ten Bokkel Huinink WW, Van Der Burg MEL et al, Long-term survival in ovarian cancer. *Eur J Cancer* 1991; **27**: 1367–72.

46. Conte PF, Bruzzone M, Chiara S et al, A randomized trial comparing cisplatin plus cyclophosphamide versus cisplatin, doxorubicin, and cyclophosphamide in advanced ovarian cancer. *J Clin Oncol* 1986; **4**: 965–71.

47. Makar AP, Baekelandt M, Trope CG, Kristensen GB, The prognostic significance of residual disease, FIGO substage, tumor histol-

ogy, and grade in patients with FIGO stage III ovarian cancer. *Gynecol Oncol* 1995; **56**: 175–80.

48. Del Campo JM, Felip E, Rubio D et al, Long-term survival in advanced ovarian cancer after cytoreduction and chemotherapy treatment. *Gynecol Oncol* 1994; **53**: 27–32.

49. Aure JC, Hoeg K, Kolstad P, Clinical and histologic studies of ovarian carcinoma. *Obstet Gynecol* 1971; **37**: 1–9.

50. Pohl R, Dallenbach-Hellweg G, Plugge T, Czernobilinsky B, Prognostic parameters in patients with advanced ovarian malignant tumors. *Eur J Gynaecol Oncol* 1984; **5**: 160–9.

51. Eisenkop SM, Friedman RL, Wang HJ, Complete cytoreductive surgery is feasible and maximized survival in patients with advanced epithelial ovarian cancer: a prospective study. *Gynecol Oncol* 1998; **69**: 103–8.

52. Heintz APM, Van Oosterom AT, Baptist J et al, The treatment of advanced ovarian carcinoma (I): Clinical variables associated with prognosis. *Gynecol Oncol* 1988; **30**: 347–58.

53. Gershenson DM, Wharton JT, Copeland LJ et al, Treatment of advanced epithelial ovarian cancer with cisplatin and cyclophosphamide. *Gynecol Oncol* 1989; **32**: 336–41.

54. Edwards CL, Herson J, Gershenson DM et al, A prospective randomized clinical trial of melphalan and *cis*-platinum versus hexamethylmelamine, Adriamycin, and cyclophosphamide in advanced ovarian cancer. *Gynecol Oncol* 1983; **15**: 267–77.

55. Shelley WE, Carmichael JC, Brown LB et al, Adriamycin and cisplatin in the treatment of stage III and IV epithelial ovarian carcinoma. *Gynecol Oncol* 1988; **29**: 208–21.

56. Farias-Eisner R, Teng F, Oliveira M et al, The influence of tumor grade, distribution, and extent of carcinomatosis in minimal residual stage III epithelial ovarian cancer after optimal primary cytoreductive surgery. *Gynecol Oncol* 1994; **55**: 108–10.

57. Schwartz PE, Chambers JT, Kohorn EI et al, Tamoxifen in combination with cytotoxic chemotherapy in advanced epithelial ovarian cancer. *Cancer* 1989; **63**: 1074–8.

58. Wharton JT, Rutledge F, Smith JP et al, Hexamethylmelamine: an evaluation of its role in the treatment of ovarian cancer. *Am J Obstet Gynecol* 1979; **133**: 833–44.

59. Bruckner HW, Cohen CJ, Goldberg JD et al, Cisplatin regimens and improved prognosis of patients with poorly differentiated ovarian cancer. *Am J Obstet Gynecol* 1983; **145**: 653–8.

60. Gruppo Interegionale Cooperativo Oncologico Ginecologia, Randomised comparison of cisplatin with cyclophosphamide/cisplatin and with cyclophosphamide/doxorubicin/cisplatin in advanced ovarian cancer. *Lancet* 1987; **ii**: 353–9.

61. Piccart MJ, Speyer JL, Wernz JC et al, Advanced ovarian cancer: three-year results of a 6–8 month, 2-drug cisplatin-containing regimen. *Eur J Cancer Clin Oncol* 1987; **23**: 631–41.

62. Leonard RCF, Smart GE, Livingstone JRB et al, Randomised trial comparing prednimustine with combination chemotherapy in advanced ovarian carcinoma. *Cancer Chemother Pharmacol* 1989; **23**: 105–10.

63. Edmonson JH, McCormack GW, Fleming TR et al, Comparison of cyclophosphamide plus cisplatin versus hexamethylmelamine, cyclophosphamide, doxorubicin, and cisplatin in combination as initial chemotherapy for stage III and IV ovarian carcinomas. *Cancer Treat Rep* 1985; **69**: 1243–8.

64. Sessa C, Bolis G, Colombo N et al, Hexamethylmelamine, Adriamycin, and cyclophosphamide (HAC) versus *cis*-dichlorodiamineplatinum, Adriamycin, and cyclophosphamide (PAC) in advanced ovarian cancer: a randomized clinical trial. *Cancer Chemother Pharmacol* 1985; **14**: 222–8.

65. Sutton GP, Stehman FB, Einhorn LH et al, Ten-year follow-up of patients receiving cisplatin, doxorubicin, and cyclophosphamide chemotherapy for advanced epithelial ovarian carcinoma. *J Clin Oncol* 1989; **7**: 223–9.

66. Young RC, Chabner BA, Hubbard SP et al, Advanced ovarian adenocarcinoma: a prospective clinical trial of melphalan (L-PAM) versus combination chemotherapy. *N Engl J Med* 1978; **299**: 1261–6.

67. Neijt JP, ten Bokkel Huinink WW, Van der Burg MEL et al, Randomized trial comparing two combination chemotherapy regimens (CHAP-5 v CP) in advanced ovarian carcinoma. *J Clin Oncol* 1987; **5**: 1157–68.

68. Venesmaa P, Epithelial ovarian cancer: impact of surgery and chemotherapy on survival during 1977–1990. *Obstet Gynecol* 1994; **84**: 8–11.

69. Hacker NF, Van der Burg MEL, Debulking and intervention surgery. *Ann Oncol* 1993; **4**(S4): S17–22.

70. Hogberg T, Primary surgery in ovarian cancer: current opinions. *Ann Med* 1995; **27**: 95–100.

71. Burghardt E, Lahousen M, Stettner H, The role of lymphadenectomy in ovarian cancer. In: *Ovarian Cancer: Biological and Therapeutic Challenges* (Sharp F, Mason WP, Leake RE, eds). London: Chapman & Hall, 1989: 425–33.

72. Allen DG, Heintz APM, Touw FWMM, A meta-analysis of residual disease and survival in stage III and IV carcinoma of the ovary. *Eur J Gynaecol Oncol* 1995; **16**: 349–56.

73. Hunter RW, Alexander NDE, Soutter WP, Meta-analysis of surgery in advanced ovarian carcinoma: Is maximum cytoreductive surgery an independent determinant of prognosis? *Am J Obstet Gynecol* 1992; **166**: 504–11.

74. Venesmaa P, Ylikorkala O, Morbidity and mortality associated with primary and repeat operations for ovarian cancer. *Obstet Gynecol* 1992; **79**: 168–72.

75. Ozols RF, Treatment of ovarian cancer: current status. *Semin Oncol* 1994; **21**(S2): 1–9.

76. Hoskins WJ, Bundy BN, Thigpen JT, Omura GA, The influence of cytoreductive surgery on recurrence-free interval and survival in small-volume stage III epithelial ovarian cancer: a Gynecologic Oncology Group study. *Gynecol Oncol* 1992; **47**: 159–66.

77. Goodman HM, Harlow BL, Sheets EE et al, The role of cytoreductive surgery in the management of stage IV epithelial ovarian cancer. *Gynecol Oncol* 1992; **46**: 367–71.

78. Liu PC, Benjamin I, Morgan MA et al, Effect of surgical debulking on survival in stage IV ovarian cancer. *Gynecol Oncol* 1997; **64**: 4–8.

79. Blythe JG, Wahl TP, Debulking surgery: Does it increase the quality of survival? *Gynecol Oncol* 1982; **14**: 396–408.

80. National Institutes of Health Consensus Development Conference Statement, Ovarian cancer: screening, treatment, and follow-up. April 5–7, 1994. *Gynecol Oncol* 1994; **55**: S4–14.

81. Hudson CN, Surgical treatment of ovarian cancer. *Gynecol Oncol* 1973; **1**: 370.

82. Rose PG, The cavitational ultrasonic surgical aspirator for cytoreduction in advanced ovarian cancer. *Am J Obstet Gynecol* 1992; **166**: 843–6.

83. Donovan JT, Veronikis DK, Powell JL et al, Cytoreductive surgery for ovarian cancer with the Cavitron ultrasonic surgical aspirator and the development of disseminated intravascular coagulation. *Obstet Gynecol* 1994; **83**: 1011–14.

84. Braid E, Pearlman N, Electrosurgical debulking of ovarian cancer: A new technique using the argon beam coagulator. *Gynecol Oncol* 1990; **39**: 115–18.

85. Amir A, Shabot MM, Karlan BY, Surgical intensive care unit care after ovarian cancer surgery: an analysis of indications. *Am J Obstet Gynecol* 1997; **176**: 1389–93.

86. Berek JS, Hacker NF, Lagasse LD et al, Survival of patients following secondary cytoreductive surgery in ovarian cancer. *Obstet Gynecol* 1983; **61**: 189–93.

87. Silberman AW, Surgical debulking of tumors. *Surg Gynecol Obstet* 1982; **155**: 577–85.

88. Hoskins WJ, The influence of cytoreductive surgery on progression-free interval and survival in epithelial ovarian cancer. *Baillière's*

Clin Obstet Gynaecol 1989; **3**: 59–71.

89. Smith JP, Rutledge F, Chemotherapy in the treatment of cancer of the ovary. *Am J Obstet Gynecol* 1970; **107**: 691–703.

90. Lawton FG, Redman CWE, Luesley DM et al, Neoadjuvant (cytoreductive) chemotherapy combined with intervention debulking surgery in advanced, unresected epithelial ovarian cancer. *Obstet Gynecol* 1989; **73**: 61–5.

91. Bristow RE, Lagasse LD, Karlan BY, Secondary surgical cytoreduction for advanced epithelial ovarian cancer. *Cancer* 1996; **78**: 2049–62.

92. Vogl SE, Pagano M, Kaplan BH et al, Cis-platin based combination chemotherapy for advanced ovarian cancer. *Cancer* 1983; **51**: 2024–30.

93. Redman CWE, Warwick J, Luesley DM et al, Intervention debulking surgery in advanced epithelial ovarian cancer. *Br J Obstet Gynaecol* 1994; **101**: 142–6.

94. Wiltshaw E, Raju KS, Dawson I, The role of cytoreductive surgery in advanced carcinoma of the ovary: an analysis of primary and secondary surgery. *Br J Obstet Gynaecol* 1985; **92**: 522–7.

95. Jacob JH, Gershenson DM, Morris M et al, Neoadjuvant chemotherapy and interval debulking for advanced epithelial ovarian cancer. *Gynecol Oncol* 1991; **42**: 146–50.

96. Onnis A, Marchetti M, Padovan P, Castellan L, Neoadjuvant chemotherapy in advanced ovarian cancer. *Eur J Gynaecol Oncol* 1996; **17**: 393–6.

97. Chambers JT, Chambers SK, Voynick IM, Schwartz PE, Neoadjuvant chemotherapy in stage X ovarian carcinoma. *Gynecol Oncol* 1990; **37**: 327–31.

98. Schwartz PE, Chambers JT, Makuch R, Neoadjuvant chemotherapy for advanced ovarian cancer. *Gynecol Oncol* 1994; **53**: 33–7.

99. Lim JT, Green JA, Neoadjuvant carboplatin and ifosfamide chemotherapy for inoperable FIGO stage III and IV ovarian carcinoma. *Clin Oncol (R Coll Radiol)* 1993; **5**: 198–202.

100. Vergote I, DeWever I, Tjalma W et al, Neoadjuvant chemotherapy or primary debulking surgery in advanced ovarian carcinoma: a retrospective analysis of 295 patients. *Gynecol Oncol* 1998; **71**: 431–6.

APPENDIX

Outcome of patients with advanced epithelial ovarian cancer as a function of residual disease

Ref.	Endpoints[a]	Division of residual disease	n	p-value[b]	Stages	Significant?
4	24-m survival	Biopsy; partial removal; complete	108	NP	III and IV	Appears to be
6	Median survival	Microscopic; 0–0.5 cm; 0.6–1.5 cm; 1.5 cm	102	<0.05	II and III	Yes
7	24-m survival	1.5 cm	89	NP	III	Trend
12	RR death	2 cm	294	<0.01	III	Yes
15	Median survival	1 cm	255	<0.001	III and IV	Yes
16	5-y survival	1 cm	136	<0.001	III and IV	Yes
	8-y survival		136	<0.001	III and IV	Yes
	5-y DFI		136	<0.001	III and IV	Yes
	8-y DFI		136	<0.001	III and IV	Yes
17	DFI	Microscopic; macroscopic; <1 cm	349	0.0001	III	Yes
18	Median survival	2 cm	104	0.0057	III and IV	Yes
	Any response		104	0.65	III and IV	No
19c	Median survival	Microscopic; <1 cm; 1–2 cm; 2–5 cm; >5 cm	163	0.0382	III and IV	Trend
20	Response rate	2 cm	83	NP	III and IV	Appears to be
21	24-m survival	Microscopic; <1 cm; 1–2 cm; 2 cm	614	NP	III	Yes
	5-y survival		614	NP	III	Yes
	24-m survival		178	NP	IV	Yes
	5-y survival		178	NP	IV	Yes
22	24-m survival	2 cm	730	<0.001	III	Yes
	5-y survival		730	<0.001	III	Yes
	24-m survival		195	<0.001	IV	Yes[d]
	5-y survival		195	<0.001	IV	Yes
23	24-m NED	Micro/macroscopic	146	0.006	III and IV	Yes
24	Median survival	2 cm	92	0.0136	IV	Yes
25	Median survival	2 cm	92	<0.02	IV	Yes
	DFI		92	0.1	IV	No
26	Median survival	1 cm	84	0.0004	IV	Yes
27	24-m survival	Microscopic; <2 cm; >2 cm	60	NP	III and IV	Appears to be
	5-y survival		60	NP	III and IV	Appears to be
28	Median survival	Biopsy; debulking surgery	86	0.006	III and IV	Yes
29	Median survival	2 cm	284	<0.03	III and IV	Trend only
30	Survival	1 cm	186	0.03	III and IV	Yes
	CR		186	<0.001	III and IV	Yes
31	Median survival	Microscopic; <2 cm; 2–10 cm; >10 cm	62	NS	III and IV	No
32	DFI	<1 cm; 1–2 cm; >2 cm	86	0.003	III and IV	Yes
	Median survival		86	0.00085	III and IV	Yes
33	CR	1.5 cm	88	<0.0005	III and IV	Yes
	3-y survival		88	<0.0005	III and IV	Yes
	Median survival		88	<0.0005	III and IV	Yes
34	Median survival	1 cm	127	0.04	IIB–IV	Trend
35	Median survival	3 cm	55	<0.001	III and IV	Yes
	CR		47	<0.05	III and IV	Yes
36	Median survival	Micro/macroscopic	75	NP	III	No
	Median survival	2 cm	75	NP	III	Yes
37	Median survival	3 cm	56	0.04	III and IV	Trend
38	24-m survival	Microscopic; <2 cm; >2 cm	75	<0.05	III and IV	Yes
	5-y survival		75	<0.05	III and IV	Yes
	Median survival		75	<0.05	III and IV	Yes

Ref.	Endpoints[a]	Division of residual disease	n	p-value[b]	Stages	Significant?
39	24-m survival		175	NP	III	Yes
	5-y survival	Microscopic; <2 cm; >2 cm	175	NP	III	Yes
	Median survival		175	NP	III	Yes
40	24-m survival		90	NP	III and IV	Appears to be
	5-y survival	Microscopic; <2 cm; >2 cm	90	NP	III and IV	Appears to be
	Median survival		90	NP	III and IV	Appears to be
41	24-m survival		265	NP	III and IV	Appears to be
	5-y survival	2 cm	265	NP	III and IV	Appears to be
42	5-y survival	<2 cm; 2–5 cm; >5 cm	574	NP	IIB–IV	Appears to be
43	Survival	2 cm	239	<0.01	III	Yes
44	24-m survival	Microscopic; <2 cm; >2 cm	152	0.0001	III and IV	Yes
45[c]	5-y survival		186	0.0119	III and IV	Yes
	10-y survival		186	0.0119	III and IV	Yes
	5-y survival, no. 2		189	0.0007	III and IV	Yes
	8-y survival, no. 2	1 cm	189	0.0001	III and IV	Yes
	Median survival		186	0.0119	III and IV	Yes
	Median survival, no. 2		189	0.0001	III and IV	Yes
46	Median survival	2 cm	125	0.001	I–IV	Yes
47	24-m survival	2 cm	455	<0.001	III	Yes
	24-m survival	Micro/macroscopic	139	0.04	IIIA–B	Yes
48	Median survival	Microscopic; 2 cm	91	<0.0001	III and IV	Yes
49	5-y survival	Micro/macroscopic	225	<0.025	III	Yes
50	Median survival		94	0.0002	II–IV	Yes
	3-y survival	2 cm	94	0.0002	II–IV	Yes
	5-y survival		94	0.0002	II–IV	Yes
51	Median survival	Micro/macroscopic	163	0.001	III and IV	Yes
52	Median survival		65	0.05	IIB–IV	Yes
	DFI	1.5 cm	65	0.03	IIB–IV	Yes
53	Median survival		50	0.03	III and IV	No
	DFI	2 cm	50	0.03	III and IV	No
54	Response rate		153	0.004	III and IV	Yes
	Median survival	2 cm	158	0.0006	III and IV	Yes
55	Response rate		319	<0.0001	III and IV	Yes
	3-y survival	Microscopic; <2 cm; 2–10 cm; >10 cm	340	0.0022	III and IV	Yes
56	Actuarial survival	Micro/macroscopic	78	<0.001	III	Yes
57	Cumulative survival	Microscopic; macroscopic; <2 cm	117	0.0024	III and IV	Yes
	Cumulative survival	Microscopic; macroscopic; >2 cm	117	0.0003	III and IV	Yes
58	CR		54	0.926	III and IV	No
	Any response	2 cm	54	0.926	III and IV	No
	Median survival		54	0.005	III and IV	Yes
59	RR progression		55	[f]	III and IV	No
	RR death	6 cm	55	[f]	III and IV	No
60	RR CR		531	[f]	III and IV	Yes
	RR response		531	[f]	III and IV	Yes
	RR survival	<2 cm; 2–5 cm; 5–10 cm; >10 cm	531	[f]	III and IV	Yes
	RR PFS		531	[f]	III and IV	Yes
	RR DFS		531	[f]	III and IV	Yes
61	Median survival	2 cm	52	0.02	III and IV	Trend
62	Survival	2 cm	73	0.04/NS	III and IV	[g]
63	24-m survival		181	<0.0001	III and IV	Yes
	36-m survival	Microscopic; <2 cm; >2 cm; </>250 g	158	<0.0001	III and IV	Yes

Ref.	Endpoints[a]	Division of residual disease	n	p-value[b]	Stages	Significant?
64	Median survival	<2 cm; 2–5 cm; >5 cm	120	<0.00005	III and IV	Yes
65	Median survival		56	NS	III and IV	No
	CR		56	NS	III and IV	No
	Any response	3 cm	56	NS	III and IV	No
	Median DFI		56	<0.02	III and IV	Yes
66	Response rate	2 cm	77	0.05	III and IV	Yes
67	Median survival		307	0.0001	II–IV	Yes
	45-m survival	1 cm	191	0.0001	IIB–IV	Yes
68	5-y survival	2 cm	244	<0.001	I–IV	Yes
	Median survival	Microscopic; <1 cm; >1 cm	175	NP	III and IV	Trend
69	Median survival	Microscopic; <2 cm; >2 cm	59	0.05	III and IV	Trend
70	5-y survival	Microscopic; <1 cm; 1–3 cm; >3 cm	175	NP	III and IV	Trend
	Median survival	Microscopic; <1 cm; >1 cm	175	NP	III and IV	Trend
71	Actuarial survival	Microscopic; <2 cm; >2 cm	119	NP	III and IV	Appears to be

[a] m, month; y, year; RR, relative risk; DFI, disease-free interval; NED, no evidence of disease; CR, complete response; PFS, progression-free survival.

[b] NP, not provided; NS, not significant.

[c] Trend for all groups except microscopic disease.

[d] Significant for grades 1 and 4.

[e] Significant in only one of two treatment groups evaluated.

[f] Confidence intervals.

[g] Two treatment groups evaluated separately.

4

Mucinous tumours of the ovary: primary or secondary?

Timothy J Perren, Nafisa Wilkinson

INTRODUCTION

Approximately 20% of primary epithelial ovarian carcinomas are of the mucinous subtype, and may be subdivided into benign mucinous adenomas, borderline tumours (which are also known as tumours of low malignant potential) and invasive mucinous carcinomas. Concealed within this apparently simple classification is a range of diseases with marked differences in behaviour and outcome.

The ovary is not infrequently involved by metastatic carcinoma from a range of primary sites, and clinically and pathologically it can be extremely difficult to distinguish between these two diagnoses. The distinction is crucial, however, since management of primary ovarian carcinoma may be completely different to the management of a tumour metastatic to the ovary.

In this chapter, we use the first case history to illustrate some of the contentious areas that lie around the classification of borderline mucinous ovarian tumours, the nature and management of pseudomyxoma peritonei, and the significance of the appendiceal tumour that is sometimes found in association with mucinous ovarian tumours. In the second case history, we explore the issue of ovarian involvement by metastatic mucinous carcinoma, and how it may be distinguished from primary mucinous ovarian carcinoma.

CASE HISTORY 1

A 49-year-old woman presented with a nine-month history of menstrual irregularity and a three-month history of abdominal distension and discomfort. She had a large cystic mass arising from the right ovary, which ruptured during surgery, releasing mucoid contents. There was a similar cyst in the left ovary measuring only 4 cm. Pockets of mucinous material were noted throughout the peritoneal cavity. The upper surface of the liver was granular, but no large metastases were noted. All peritoneal surfaces appeared inflamed and were involved by tiny deposits. There was a solid appendiceal mass measuring 6 cm by 3 cm, which invaded the caecum. A partial caecectomy and appendicectomy were performed, together with total abdominal hysterectomy and bilateral salpingo-oophorectomy.

What is the likely diagnosis?

The patient clearly has widespread abdomino-pelvic malignancy. The mucinous cyst content and the pockets of mucinous material throughout the peritoneal cavity strongly suggest the diagnosis of a mucinous tumour with pseudomyxoma peritonei. This was confirmed by pathological examination, which showed a well-differentiated invasive mucinous adenocarcinoma involving both ovaries. The appendix was involved by similar tumour, and there was full-thickness infiltration of its wall. There was also evidence of pseudomyxoma peritonei in the surrounding peritoneum. Within the ovaries, the histological appearances of the tumour appeared quite bland in many areas.

Classification of mucinous ovarian tumours

Approximately 75% of mucinous ovarian tumours are benign, 10% are of borderline malignancy and 15% are frankly malignant.[1] Tumours of borderline malignancy are also referred to as tumours of low malignant potential, or atypically proliferating tumours. In this chapter, the term 'borderline' is used. Benign mucinous tumours tend to occur during the third to the fifth decades, but may be seen in younger women, and in pregnancy; borderline tumours have a peak incidence in the middle of the fourth decade, but may rarely occur in young girls; invasive mucinous tumours occur mostly in women in their fourth to seventh decades.[2]

The epithelial lining of mucinous neoplasms may be composed either of intestinal-type mucinous epithelium or of endocervical-type (Müllerian) mucinous epithelium. Benign mucinous tumours tend to be divided approximately equally between the endocervical-type and the intestinal-type mucinous epithelium, and are bilateral in only 2–3% of cases.[2] The vast majority of mucinous borderline tumours have intestinal-type mucinous differentiation, and only 15% have endocervical-type epithelial differentiation.[3] Of those with intestinal differentiation, only 6–8% are bilateral, as opposed to 40% of those with Müllerian differentiation.[2] Invasive mucinous carcinomas

are bilateral in around 15–20% of cases. Histologically, they may be of pure endocervical type or of pure intestinal type, or may contain a combination of the two cell types.

Clinical features of mucinous ovarian tumours

The presenting features of mucinous ovarian carcinoma are not different to those of ovarian carcinoma in general. Patients usually present with abdominal distension, which may be due to the presence of a cystic tumour, or due to the presence of ascites. Other presenting features include abdominal discomfort and vague gastrointestinal symptoms. Mucinous ovarian cysts may reach a considerable size. The ascitic fluid may be thick and mucinous, especially in patients with pseudomyxoma peritonei, who may present with huge abdominal distension.

The vast majority of patients with mucinous borderline tumours present with stage 1 disease. In a large series from the Norwegian Radium Hospital, 83% had FIGO stage I disease, 3% stage II disease and 14% stage III disease.[4] Extra ovarian implants are usually due to deposits of pseudomyxoma peritonei. However, Rutgers and Scully[3] have described extra ovarian implants analogous to those seen in serous tumours, which may be of borderline or invasive malignancy.

Pseudomyxoma peritonei

Pseudomyxoma peritonei has been reported as a complication of mucinous tumours involving the ovary. It is, however, an ambiguous term in that it is often used to encompass all types of extra-ovarian intraabdominal mucus associated with mucinous ovarian tumours. These types comprise free mucin in the abdominal cavity (mucinous ascites); small or large deposits of mucin adherent to peritoneal surfaces, containing inflammatory and mesothelial cells and sometimes organizing capillaries and fibroblasts, but usually lacking neoplastic epithelial cells; and masses composed of pools of mucin, which may or may not contain neoplastic cells, surrounded by dense collagenous tissue (dissecting mucin). The presence of pools and tracts of mucin dissecting through the ovarian stroma is designated as pseudomyxoma ovarii, and, when present, is almost always associated with pseudomyxoma peritonei.

There is no consensus in the literature as to how many of these types of intraabdominal mucus warrant the designation pseudomyxoma peritonei. Ronnett et al,[5] in a review of 109 cases of multifocal mucinous tumours of various origins, have proposed two distinct diagnostic categories: disseminated peritoneal adenomucinosis and peritoneal mucinous carcinomatosis. Cases classified as disseminated peritoneal adenomucinosis were characterized by peritoneal lesions composed of abundant extracellular mucin containing scant simple to focally proliferative mucinous epithelium with little cytological atypia or mitotic activity, with or without an associated appendiceal mucinous adenoma. Cases classified as peritoneal mucinous carcinomatosis were characterized by peritoneal lesions composed of more abundant mucinous epithelium with the architectural and cytological features of carcinoma, with or without an associated primary mucinous adenocarcinoma. Fourteen of the cases described by Ronnett et al[5] could not be classified, since they had intermediate or discordant features. Of the cases described, 44 occurred in women. Of these, only 23 had mucinous tumours involving the ovary. According to the criteria of Ronnett and her colleagues, none of these cases was of unequivocal ovarian origin.

Pseudomyxoma peritonei tends to be associated with tumours at the lower end of the malignant spectrum; however, this association is not invariable. When it occurs in association with borderline tumours, it tends to be associated with tumours showing intestinal, rather than müllerian, differentiation.[3] There is a correlation between prognosis and the presence or absence of tumour cells in the peritoneal mucin and the cytological features of those cells.[6–8] These features should therefore be carefully documented.

The diagnosis of pseudomyxoma peritonei is often made unexpectedly during the course of surgery for an ovarian tumour. The patient is found to have varying volumes of mucinous ascites. Sugarbaker[9] has elegantly described a characteristic pattern of 'completely redistributed peritoneal carcinomatosis', where there is involvement of the greater omentum, the undersurface of the hemidiaphragms, and the pelvic peritoneum. Other sites of involvement are areas where tumour-containing fluid may pool: in addition to the pelvis, these include the right retrohepatic space, the ligament of Treitz, and the paracolic abdominal gutters. Characteristically, tumour is present in the form of soft gelatinous masses (Figure 4.1). Tumour implants rarely occur on the serosal aspect of bowel that is actively involved in peristalsis. Serosal implants may, however, occur at immobile intestinal sites such as the pyloric antrum, ileocaecal valve, ligament of Treitz, and rectosigmoid colon. There is characteristically an absence of lymph node or liver metastases throughout the course of the disease.[9]

The diagnosis of pseudomyxoma peritonei may be made preoperatively by modern imaging techniques such as computed tomography (CT) or ultrasound; there is currently little data on magnetic resonance imaging (MRI).[10] CT characteristically shows the mucinous material, which is similar in density to fat, and may appear heterogeneous. Serosal involvement of the liver and spleen gives rise to a typical scalloped appearance (Figure 4.2). Occasionally, calcifications may be seen. Tumour masses may also be

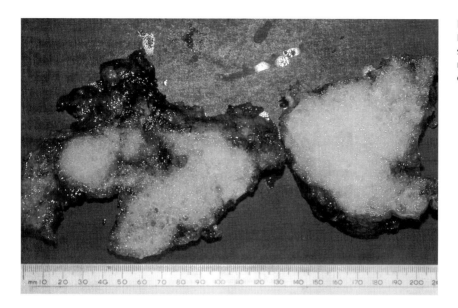

Figure 4.1
Pseudomyxoma peritonei: soft gelatinous material removed from the peritoneal cavity.

seen, as may narrowing of small bowel loops with segmental obstruction. Ultrasound typically shows non-mobile echogenic ascites. Scalloping of the liver and spleen may again also be seen.[10]

What is the significance of the appendiceal tumour?

The synchronous presence of tumours in both the ovary and appendix in the presence of pseudomyxoma peritonei is unusual. When mucinous lesions of both the ovary and appendix are present, there is considerable controversy as to whether they should be regarded as independent, synchronous primary tumours or whether the ovarian tumour is metastatic from the appendix.

Proponents of the hypothesis that the ovarian tumour represents a metastasis from the appendix have marshalled the following arguments in support of their position:[6,7,11,12]

1. Ovarian and appendiceal tumours often present simultaneously in cases of pseudomyxoma peritonei, and are histologically similar.
2. Ovarian tumours are commonly bilateral, yet where a unilateral tumour occurs, there is a distinct right-sided predominance, which supports a hypothesis of direct or transperitoneal spread of the tumour from the appendix to the ovary.
3. In cases where appendiceal and peritoneal involvement occur synchronously, there is often evidence within the ovary of pseudomyxoma ovarii, which is a rare finding in primary mucinous ovarian tumours.
4. The mucinous epithelium of the ovarian tumours is often unusually tall in such cases.
5. The appendiceal tumour always shows the histological features of a primary tumour, being either an adenoma or adenocarcinoma.

These authors go on to state that the appendiceal source of the pseudomyxoma can only be excluded after adequate sampling and microscopic examination of the appendix,[11] which has not been carried out in most of the cases of pseudomyxoma peritonei described as being associated with primary mucinous ovarian carcinoma in the literature.

Proponents of the dual primary tumour hypothesis marshal the following arguments in support of their position:[13]

1. The ovarian tumour is commonly of large size and often contains a benign-looking epithelial component, whereas the appendiceal tumour is commonly of small size, low grade or benign histological appearance.
2. The appendiceal wall is usually intact on gross inspection or even microscopic examination.
3. The appendiceal tumour may occasionally present months to years after the discovery of the ovarian tumour.
4. There are sometimes differences in the histological grade of the ovarian and appendiceal tumours, and there may be discordant epithelial immunohistochemical staining of the two tumours.
5. The disease course in patients with synchronous ovarian and appendiceal tumours is more favourable than would be expected for patients who present with metastatic carcinoma in other situations.

Several molecular genetic studies have been done in an attempt to clarify this issue.[14,15] An analysis of loss of heterozygosity (LOH) on chromosomes 17q (*nm23* gene), 3p (*VHL* gene), and 5q in 12 cases disclose divergent findings in the ovarian and appendiceal tumours in three cases (supporting two separate primaries) and similar findings in another three (supporting a single primary tumour with metastatic spread).[14] However, despite such studies, the relationship of the ovarian and appendiceal tumours in cases of pseudomyxoma peritonei has not been resolved.

Some investigators who support the hypothesis that the primary appendiceal and ovarian tumours arise independently also believe that the peritoneal tumour seen in cases of pseudomyxoma peritonei is a further independent site of neoplastic origin. They believe that these cases may represent examples of multifocal neoplasia of the peritoneum, ovary, and appendix.[13] Future studies involving extensive sampling of the various tumour sites, together with histological examination and molecular biological techniques, may help to resolve these unanswered issues.

It is currently recommended that cystic ovarian tumours associated with pseudomyxoma peritonei be staged as ovarian tumours. However, it should be remembered that in this situation, the clinical course is likely to be different to that of mucinous tumours of unquestionable ovarian origin.

What is the clinical course of mucinous ovarian neoplasms?

The most important determinant of prognosis for patients presenting with mucinous ovarian malignancy appears to be the FIGO stage at diagnosis. Two series from the MD Anderson Hospital, Texas, which included patients with all histological subtypes of mucinous ovarian malignancy, have shown that patients who present with advanced-stage disease, of whatever histological subtype, have a poor prognosis.[16,17] In one of these series 14 of 16 patients presenting with stage III or IV disease died. Five of these 14 had non-invasive mucinous carcinoma, which was stage III in 4 cases and stage I in the other.[17] Other series have been restricted to patients with borderline tumours. The largest of these is from the Norwegian Radium Hospital,[4] and included 178 patients with mucinous tumours. Again survival was related to stage; the corrected 15-year survival rates for patients with FIGO stage I, II, and III disease were 95%, 67%, and 57%, respectively.

There is no doubt that patients who present with a FIGO stage I mucinous ovarian tumour of either borderline or invasive subtype will have an excellent prognosis, whereas in those with more widespread disease, the prognosis will be substantially worse even if the tumour is borderline. One of the problems in interpreting published historical series is that, in many of these, surgical staging was suboptimal in at least a proportion of cases. This is important to recognize, since poor outcome in a proportion of those patients with apparent stage I disease may be due to failure to recognize, or sample, areas of possible disease that may have been present beyond the ovary. The presence of disease in extra ovarian sites would of course upstage the patient and lead to a significantly worse prognosis.

Equally, pathological criteria have changed and developed over the years. There has been controversy concerning the features required to make a diagnosis of invasive carcinoma, and different authors have used differing criteria. Rutgers and Scully,[3] in 1988, described the morphological differentiation of mucinous borderline tumours into those showing intestinal differentiation and those showing endocervical (Müllerian) differentiation. This differentiation is of importance because it appears to be of prognostic significance. In their original report, Rutgers and Scully[3] noted that none of 30 patients whose tumours showed Müllerian differentiation developed pseudomyxoma peritonei or died from their disease, whereas 17% of those with intestinal differentiation developed pseudomyxoma peritonei and 14% had tumour-related death. Siriaunkgul et al[18] subsequently confirmed these findings.

The importance of thorough surgical staging and expert pathological examination cannot be overemphasized. This is particularly so in patients with apparent early-stage disease, where a decision between observation alone and systemic adjuvant chemotherapy must be made. In the absence of such data, it may be necessary to perform a further surgical procedure to complete the staging.

How should this patient be managed?

Because of the widespread abdomino-pelvic malignancy and the uncertainty as to whether this was a primary ovarian carcinoma with metastases in the appendix or vice versa, the patient was treated with four cycles of systemic chemotherapy with cisplatin and continuous ambulatory infusion of 5-fluorouracil (5-FU). There was some initial improvement in CA125 levels and in the CT scan after two cycles of treatment, but after four cycles of treatment, the CT scan showed new nodules of disease in anterior peritoneal fat, and chemotherapy was discontinued.

What is the role of chemotherapy in invasive mucinous ovarian malignancy?

Chemotherapy was used in this case because of the invasive nature of the malignancy, and because there was widespread residual disease. However, as illustrated, the efficacy of systemic chemotherapy in low-grade invasive mucinous carcinoma with pseudomyxoma peritonei is extremely disappointing. Although there was some initial improvement, it proved extremely short-lived, and the disease started to progress whilst the patient was still receiving treatment.

Patients who present with a clear diagnosis of advanced-stage invasive mucinous ovarian carcinoma are routinely treated with systemic chemotherapy. The current standard of care in the USA and Europe comprises a combination of a platinum drug, either cisplatin or carboplatin, with paclitaxel.[19]

It has been suggested that the poor outcome reported for patients with advanced-stage invasive mucinous ovarian carcinoma comes about because the disease is intrinsically resistant to chemotherapy.[20] Formal analyses of prognostic factors conducted by the Gynaecologic Oncology

Group (GOG)[21] in 726 patients with suboptimal stage III or stage IV ovarian cancer showed that in 726 patients, factors predicting for a poor prognosis were mucinous or clear cell histology, non-cisplatin-containing chemotherapy, poor performance status, older age, FIGO stage IV disease, significant bulk of residual disease, and the presence of ascites. In this study, patients with borderline tumours were excluded. The adverse prognostic effect of mucinous histology was apparent despite the fact that there was a significant association between cell type and histological grade: 16 (49%) of the 33 mucinous tumours were grade I, and only 4 (12%) were grade III. In this study, there was a strong suggestion that the reason that patients with mucinous or clear cell histology had a poor prognosis was that they responded poorly to chemotherapy: none of 32 patients with mucinous (14 patients) or clear cell (18 patients) histology subjected to second-look laparotomy achieved a pathological complete response, whereas such responses were seen in 4.3% of those with serous histology, 16.7% of those with endometrioid histology, and 7.2% of those with undifferentiated, mixed or unspecified histological subtypes. However, despite their apparently poor prognosis, these patients are not currently routinely excluded from phase III randomized clinical trials in ovarian cancer.[19]

What is the role of chemotherapy in low-grade mucinous ovarian malignancy?

There are no data from randomized clinical trials specifically concerning the use of chemotherapy in patients with low-grade mucinous carcinoma, or pseudomyxoma peritonei. Those data that do exist are from small phase II studies or individual case reports. These studies often combine together pseudomyxoma peritonei arising from ovary with those from appendiceal, colorectal and other primary sites.

Approaches that have been tried include intraperitoneal chemotherapy with drugs such as 5-FU, mitomycin C and cisplatin, either alone or in combination. Hyperthermic intraperitoneal chemotherapy has also been tried.[22] There is no doubt that responses are seen in selected patients; however, some of the novel intraperitoneal approaches to treatment have been associated with unexpected fatal toxicities.[23,24]

There is considerable scope for the development of new and improved treatments for mucinous ovarian neoplasms of all histological subtypes.

What is the optimal management of pseudomyxoma peritonei?

The patient remained well for eight months, but then re-presented with abdominal bloating and a sensation of dragging. She was found to have a mass in her lower abdomen. CT showed scalloping around the liver and spleen, together with an omental 'cake' (Figure 4.2). A cystic mass anterior to the lower end of the inferior vena cava had also enlarged. It was felt that her chances of response to further chemotherapy were remote, and, following multidisciplinary discussion and review, she was referred for palliative surgery, which was performed two months later. At operation, there was a large omental 'cake' and multiple deposits of pseudomyxoma in the pelvis. The bulk of disease was in the upper abdomen around the stomach, spleen, liver, and portahepatis. The lesser sac was also involved. An omentectomy was performed, and all other areas of pseudomyxoma were debulked where possible (Figure 4.1). The upper abdominal disease was non-resectable.

Histological examination showed the omentum to be extensively replaced by pseudomyxoma peritonei. Where epithelium was seen, it appeared markedly bland.

She made a good recovery from surgery, but within six months had symptoms of increasing

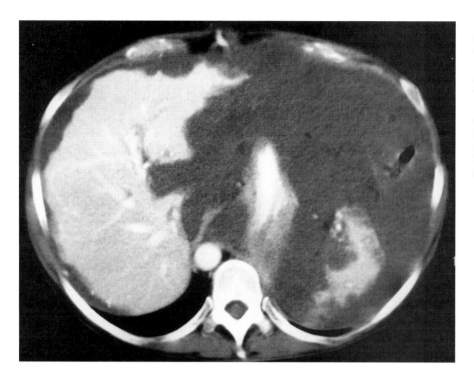

Figure 4.2
CT-scan slice through the upper abdomen in a patient with pseudomyxoma peritonei, showing the characteristic scalloping of the liver and spleen, together with large volumes of mucinous material surrounding and compressing the stomach.

bloating, nausea, and intermittent vomiting. CT scan confirmed progressive disease within the upper abdomen, causing pressure on the stomach. There was an increase in the volume of free fluid within the pelvis. She was treated with metoclopromide and spironolactone with good effect. However, a year later she developed vaginal discharge and postcoital bleeding. She was found to have a mass of pseudomyxoma peritonei eroding the vaginal vault. After a further eight months, there was a marked deterioration in her general condition, and the vaginal bleeding was also worse.

The gynaecological oncologist and a gastrointestinal surgeon jointly performed a laparotomy. Substantial tumour was found in the supracolic compartment and also in the pelvis, involving the vagina and rectum. Other disease affected the right colon, and there were multiple peritoneal small bowel deposits. The supracolic compartment was debulked, but substantial tumour remained. The

disease involving the posterior wall of the vagina was debulked, but tumour involving the rectum was left. Multiple areas of disease on the abdominal wall were debulked.

Eighteen hundred grams of tissue were submitted for pathological examination, which confirmed the previous diagnosis of pseudomyxoma peritonei. Postoperative recovery was complicated by faecal peritonitis, from which she could not be resuscitated, and she died three and a half years after her initial presentation.

What is the role of surgery in the management of pseudomyxoma peritonei?

Surgery remains the mainstay of treatment. The aim of surgery should be to remove all evidence of gross disease. Unfortunately, surgery is rarely curative, and, as illustrated by this case report, some patients may require multiple operations. Surgery is often difficult because of adhesions and fibrosis. This leads to a greatly increased risk of unintentional enterotomies and subsequent leaks and fistulae. Salvage surgery can be very worthwhile, and many patients will enjoy substantial additional survival with good quality of life.[10]

Sugarbaker and his colleagues have developed an ultraradical approach to surgery in which they attempt up to six peritonectomy procedures using diathermy. The peritoneum is stripped from the left upper quadrant, right upper quadrant, and pelvis, where a sleeve resection of the sigmoid colon is also performed. A lesser omentectomy–cholecystectomy is performed, with the stripping of the omental bursa. An antrectomy is also performed.[25] This procedure is commonly accompanied by a perioperative chemotherapy wash of the peritoneal cavity. Using this combination of treatment, Sugarbaker and colleagues report an overall five-year survival rate of 69% in 288 patients. In patients in whom a complete resection was achieved, the eight-year survival rate was 72%, compared to 0% after incomplete resection.

CASE HISTORY 2

A 62-year-old woman was referred for a second opinion regarding the management of her 'stage IV ovarian carcinoma'. She initially presented with frequent bouts of vomiting, epigastric pain and abdominal distension, together with increased bowel sounds and constipation. At laparotomy, she was found to have a moderate to poorly differentiated adenocarcinoma of the caecum. There was evidence of lymphatic invasion within the tumour, but no nodal involvement – Dukes stage B. She received no postoperative therapy.

A year later, she developed acute abdominal pain, and was found to have a large abdominal mass and ascites; these findings were confirmed by ultrasound. At laparotomy, there was a 20 cm right

ovarian tumour. A bilateral salpingo-oophrectomy was performed. A nodule from the small bowel mesentery was also excised, together with a fibroid from the uterine wall.

Histological examination showed mucinous adenocarcinoma involving the ovaries. The uterine fibroid was also involved, but the peritoneal nodule was not. Preoperative serum CA125 was 239 U/ml (normal range <23 U/ml), but normalized rapidly after surgery; carcinoembryonic antigen (CEA) was normal.

A diagnosis of a second primary malignancy arising in the ovary was made. She was treated with six courses of carboplatin chemotherapy without evidence of response. Within a few months, she developed a tender nodule in the right upper quadrant of the abdomen at the site of a previous drain. Further CT scan showed the right pelvic mass now to be involving the right ureter and causing hydronephrosis. The CA125 was 11 U/ml and the CEA 22 ng/ml.

She then received altretamine chemotherapy, but severe nausea, vomiting, constipation, and pain complicated this. The right upper quadrant nodule increased further in size, and altretamine was discontinued after a single course. She was next treated with 10 fractions of palliative pelvic radiotherapy.

She was referred for review at this stage. She had symptoms of abdominal pain. The subcutaneous metastasis in the right upper quadrant of the abdomen measured 4.5 cm by 3 cm. There were two other subcutaneous deposits on either side of the lower midline incision scar, and there was a 10 cm mass arising from the pelvis.

Review of the sequential CT confirmed that there had been no response to any of the treatment given since diagnosis of the ovarian tumour.

What is the likely diagnosis in this case?

The differential diagnosis is between a primary ovarian carcinoma occurring in a patient with a history of mucinous adenocarcinoma of the caecum, and a metastasis from the previous caecal carcinoma involving the ovary.

How frequent are metastatic tumours in the ovary and from which primary sites?

Metastatic tumours are an important group of ovarian neoplasms because treatment may differ significantly from that of primary ovarian carcinoma. Metastasis to the ovaries may occur regardless of the location of the primary tumour.[26] The frequency with which the ovaries are involved in metastatic disease is difficult to assess from the literature because of the differing methods of pathological examination and analysis. There is also a wide geographical variation in the incidence of the common gastric, breast, and colonic carcinomas, as well as changing incidences in many population groups over recent decades. Gastric carcinoma has become less common, whereas breast and colorectal malignancy have become more common. Metastatic carcinoma was reported to account for approximately 40% of all ovarian cancers in one series from Japan where gastric carcinoma is common, but for fewer than 3% in a series from Uganda, where this form of cancer is relatively rare.[27]

Approximately 4% of women with intestinal carcinoma have ovarian metastasis at some time during the course of their disease.[28–31] In one detailed pathological study this figure was as high as 10% when the ovaries were cut into 2 mm slices.[32] In a study of secondary ovarian tumours by Ulbright et al,[33] more than two-thirds of their cases of metastatic colonic carcinomas were initially interpreted as primary ovarian carcinoma.

What is the pathogenesis of ovarian metastases?

Tumours can spread to the ovary by several routes. The lymphatic route is the most important, and accounts for many metastases from the genitourinary tract as well as from the colon, stomach and breast. Lymphatic permeation is most recognized in the ovarian hilus, and may be conspicuous in the submucosal lymphatics of the fallopian tube. Haematogenous dissemination is most often seen in patients with advanced disease, and other bloodborne metastases are usually apparent. The well-vascularized ovaries of premenopausal women are said to be particularly receptive to seeding in this way.[34–36] Transcoelomic spread is associated principally with primary tumours of the abdominal viscera. A transluminal route may be utilized by endometrial and tubal carcinomas. Clusters of carcinoma cells can be identified in the lumen of the fallopian tube in these cases, and it is feasible that cells shed from the ostea could implant in the ovary. This route is said to be common with adenosquamous carcinomas of the endometrium.[35] Direct infiltration of the ovary by tumours arising in pelvic organs is also an important mechanism, especially in advanced disease. Uterine, tubal, colonic, bladder, mesothelial and retroperitoneal tumours may involve the ovaries in this way, as well as metastasizing to the ovarian parenchyma. Spread to pre-existing primary ovarian neoplasms has also been reported: for example, breast tumours may metastasize to Brenner tumours,[37] and melanoma or colonic adenocarcinoma to mature cystic teratoma.

How may metastatic involvement of the ovary be distinguished from primary mucinous carcinoma?
Histological features and immunohistochemical examination

Pathological review of the right hemicolectomy specimen revealed a moderately differentiated mucinous adenocarcinoma within the caecum, infiltrating through the muscularis propria into the surrounding pericaecal fat (Figure 4.3). Resected mesenteric lymph nodes were negative. The serosal

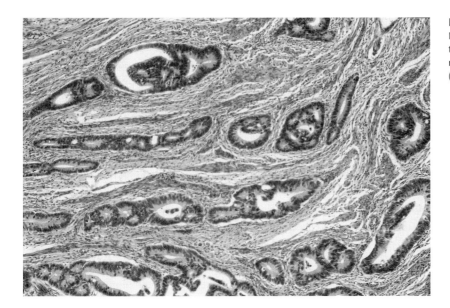

Figure 4.3
Moderately to well-differentiated invasive mucinous adenocarcinoma of large bowel (×200).

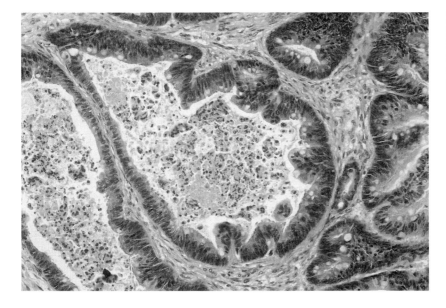

Figure 4.4
Colonic *metastasis* to ovary: the adenocarcinoma consists of cystically dilated glands showing 'dirty necrotic debris' (×500).

surface of the caecum was not involved. Review of the ovarian mass that was subsequently removed revealed numerous cystically dilated glandular structures. A mixture of goblet cells and mucin-free cells lined these. The glands were arranged at the edge of the necrotic material in a garland-like fashion. Within the cystic structures, there was extensive necrotic eosinophilic and coarsely granular material. There was also evidence of segmental necrosis of crypts. These features are known as 'dirty' necrosis[38] (Figure 4.4). Immunohistochemical examination showed both the primary caecal

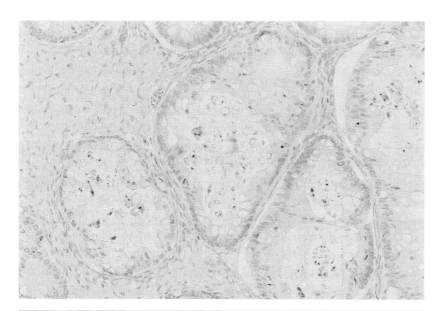

Figure 4.5
Colonic *metastasis* to ovary, showing negative immunoreactivity for CA125 (×500).

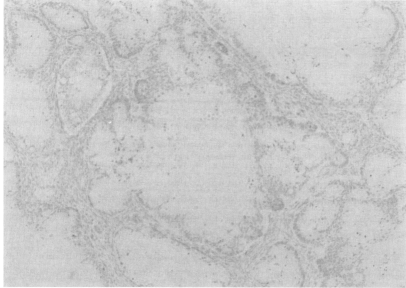

Figure 4.6
Colonic *metastasis* to ovary, showing negative immunoreactivity for cytokeratin 7 (×200).

carcinoma and the ovarian tumour to show strong patchy positive immunoreactivity with cytokeratin 20 and CEA-M. Cytokeratin 7 and CA125 were negative in both the tumours (Figures 4.5–4.8). The morphological features, together with the immunohistochemical findings, strongly suggested that the disease in the ovary was in fact metastatic from the previous colonic carcinoma.

Approximately 70% of ovarian metastases from mucinous colorectal carcinoma are bilateral, and may be very large. Solid areas may be present, but they are predominantly cystic. On gross examination, the cystic components frequently contain necrotic tumour, mucinous or clear fluid, or altered blood.

The neoplastic cells morphologically resemble

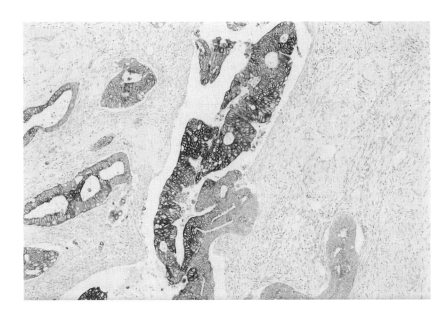

Figure 4.7
Colonic adenocarcinoma, exhibiting strong positive immunoreactivity for cytokeratin 20 (top) and CEA-M (below) (×200).

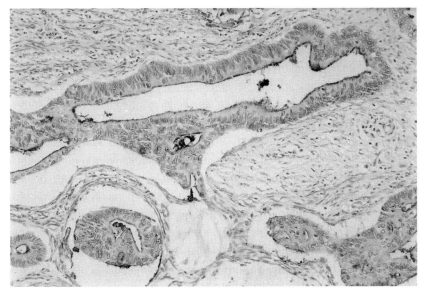

the corresponding primary colorectal carcinoma and show pseudocystic change, which results from central necrosis of tumour nodules leaving a rim of viable epithelium, a so-called 'garland' pattern.[38] Necrosis is common and often extensive, forming central eosinophilic masses of nuclear debris within glandular lumina; this feature has been referred to as 'dirty' necrosis (Figure 4.4). Individual glands may also show segmental necrosis of their epithelial lining. Bilaterality of tumour, multinodular pattern, extensive necrosis, lack of a fibrous capsule or of a true cystic component, and prominent stromal luteinization favour metastatic over primary carcinoma.[39] Ovarian metastases from colorectal carcinomas often simulate endometrioid carcinomas.

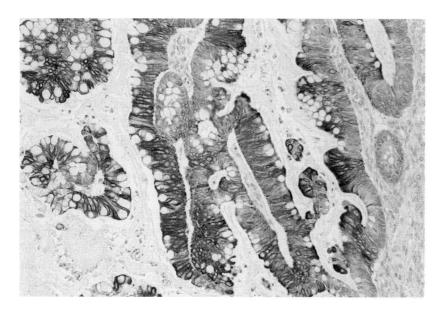

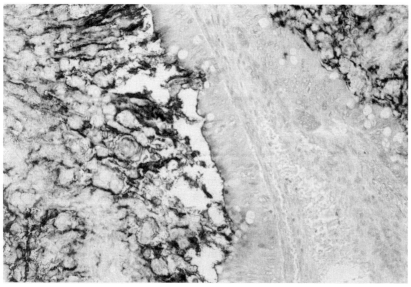

Figure 4.8
Colonic metastasis to ovary, showing positive immunoreactivity for cytokeratin 20 (top) and CEA-M (below).

The use of immunohistochemistry may be helpful in differentiating between ovarian metastasis from colonic carcinomas and primary ovarian carcinomas. Colonic metastases tend to be negative for cytokeratin 7 (Figure 4.6) and positive for cytokeratin 20 (Figure 4.8), whereas primary carcinomas of the ovary are generally positive for cytokeratin 7 and negative for cytokeratin 20.[40,41] An exception to this is a small proportion of mucinous cystadenocarcinomas of the ovary that are also positive for cytokeratin 20, potentially leading to confusion with the colorectal carcinoma immunophenotype. However, unlike colorectal carcinomas, these tumours also tend to be positive for cytokeratin 7. Immunohistochemistry for CEA and CA125 may also be useful, and will provide additional clarity in some cases (Figures 4.5 and 4.8).[42–45] However, none of these tests are 100% specific, and the final diagnosis can only be reached by expert multidisciplinary review of all the clinical, radiological and pathological information.

Differences in clinical features between metastases and primary ovarian carcinoma

In general, patients presenting with metastatic disease involving the ovary report exactly the same vague constellation of symptoms as any patient presenting with a primary ovarian carcinoma. Most patients will have evidence of an abdomino-pelvic mass or ascites; however, other sites of metastatic disease less commonly seen in patients with primary ovarian cancer, such as liver or lung, may also be found. In other patients, ovarian involvement may be discovered incidentally by CT or ultrasound examination during more detailed investigation of patients presenting in other ways, for instance with liver metastases.

In many cases, the diagnosis is not made pre-operatively, and sometimes, as illustrated by the case history, not at surgery.

Recognition of the metastatic nature of an ovarian tumour depends on several factors: an awareness of the frequency with which ovarian metastases occur and simulate a variety of primary tumours; a detailed clinical history, particularly of previous malignancy; a thorough clinical and operative search by the gynaecologist for a primary tumour outside the ovary and for other sites of tumour spread; and a careful evaluation of the gross and microscopic features of the ovarian tumour by the pathologist.

A diagnosis of ovarian metastasis must be strongly considered if the distribution of metastatic disease is atypical for primary ovarian cancer, or if the histological examination is suggestive of metastasis. For example, in a patient with

ovarian cancer, it would be unusual to find liver metastases, without evidence of extensive peritoneal involvement and an omental cake; but this would not be unusual in a patient with colonic carcinoma that had metastasized to the ovary.

Some patients may present with clinical or pathological evidence of excessive female steroid hormone production. This, however, does not exclude the diagnosis of a metastatic tumour, which may have a functioning stroma.

Investigation of ovarian disease in a patient with previous malignancy

Specific investigations that should be carried out in any patient where metastatic disease is being considered include radiological investigations such as CT scan of the abdomen and pelvis. This will provide detailed staging of sites of disease, and may also reveal sites of disease not already suspected, such as parenchymal liver metastases. A good-quality CT scan of the abdomen and pelvis with adequate gastric distension may also give useful information about the gastrointestinal (GI) tract. It may show a filling defect within the stomach suggestive of an intrinsic lesion, or thickening or distortion of the gastric wall suggestive of intrinsic or extrinsic disease. It may also give information concerning the colon, perhaps revealing a mass lesion or showing radiological evidence of intrinsic or extrinsic involvement, with or without evidence of obstruction. CT is not, however, the investigation of choice for detailing GI lesions, and further investigation of specific GI abnormalities such as upper or lower GI endoscopy may be required. CT will also show anatomical sites of potential primary disease such as the pancreas, which cannot easily be evaluated by other means.

A chest X-ray should also be performed to exclude a possible primary carcinoma of the lung, or pulmonary metastases. It may also give information concerning any mediastinal disease.

A CT scan of the chest may also be required for more detailed evaluation.

If histological information is not already available, for instance in a patient under follow-up for another malignancy who develops symptoms of abdomino-pelvic disease, we have found that a CT- or ultrasound-guided core biopsy of an accessible lesion such as an omental cake is extremely useful if followed by expert histopathological evaluation including immuno-histochemistry, as described above.

In a patient where metastasis from breast cancer is a possible diagnosis, specific clinical examination of the breast, including mammography and breast ultrasound, may also be helpful. Fine-needle aspiration cytology or core biopsy should be carried out to further investigate any suspicious breast lesion detected.

A range of serum of tumour markers may give further guidance.[46,47] CA125 is widely used as an ovarian cancer tumour marker. It is, however, not specific for ovarian cancer, and may be raised in a range of conditions where there is diffuse peritoneal involvement or inflammation. It is also raised in conditions such as cirrhosis or pregnancy. CEA is widely used as a marker in patients with colonic cancer; however, it is also raised in many other malignant conditions, including breast cancer. It may also be raised in smokers. CA15.3 is used as a breast cancer marker, but again it is not completely specific. CA19.9 is used as a marker for upper gastrointestinal malignancy, including oesophagus, stomach, pancreas and hepatobiliary malignancy; however, it may also be raised in some patients with epithelial ovarian cancer. α-Fetoprotein (AFP) and β human chorionic gonadotropin (βhCG) may also be helpful. Both markers are raised in patients with germ cell malignancies, although this is unlikely to be a cause of confusion in this instance. AFP is also raised in patients with hepatocellular carcinoma, and can be raised in patients with diffuse metastatic involvement of the liver. βhCG may also be raised non-specifically in many patients with diffuse malignancy. Some extremely poorly differentiated carcinomas may produce high levels of βhCG, leading to a potential confusion with gestational trophoblastic disease.

How should metastatic disease involving the ovary be managed?

The management of a patient shown to have metastatic disease involving the ovary depends upon the primary site of the malignancy.

As illustrated in the case history, many patients only have the diagnosis of metastatic disease made following debulking surgery. Surgery can never be curative in this situation, and in most cases is not the treatment of choice. It can be avoided in many cases by careful preoperative multidisciplinary review and discussion, together with appropriate imaging investigations and guided biopsy. Surgery may on occasions, however, be appropriate to palliate symptoms such as extensive bulk disease or disease causing intestinal obstruction.

For most patients, systemic treatment with palliative chemotherapy will need to be considered. Where appropriate, patients with a mucinous carcinoma arising from a colorectal primary site may be treated with a 5-FU-based regimen. The addition of new drugs such as irinotecan or oxaliplatin is increasingly being investigated, with encouraging results.

Patients with a tumour arising from a gastric primary should be considered for treatment based around combinations of cisplatin, 5-FU and anthracyclines. Patients with breast carcinoma should be considered for one of a range of chemotherapy treatments, usually based around anthracyclines and increasingly taxanes. Hormonal therapy with a drug such as tamoxifen, a progestogen or an aromatase inhibitor may also be useful in patients with breast carcinoma that expresses hormone receptors.

It should constantly be remembered that even despite therapy, the long-term outlook is, unfortunately, likely to be poor for many of these patients. The focus of treatment must therefore be based around effective palliation and symptom control. The results of chemotherapy need to be carefully monitored so that those patients who will achieve good palliative responses to systemic chemotherapy can be identified and appropriately treated, whilst those with drug-resistant disease can be identified early, and exposure to ineffective and potentially toxic therapy minimized. The role of specialists in palliative medicine should be remembered, and they should be involved in the management of the patient with metastatic disease from an early stage.

LEARNING POINTS

- Approximately 75% of primary mucinous ovarian tumours are benign, 10% are of borderline malignancy and 15% are frankly malignant.
- Approximately 20% of primary epithelial ovarian carcinomas are of the mucinous subtype.
- The frequency with which the ovaries are involved in metastatic disease is difficult to assess from the literature, and varies according to methods used for its analysis. The range reported in the literature is 3–40% of all ovarian malignancies.
- Patients with stage I mucinous ovarian neoplasms of whatever subtype tend to have an extremely good prognosis.
- The epithelial lining of mucinous neoplasms may be composed either of intestinal-type mucinous epithelium or of endocervical-type (müllerian) mucinous epithelium. In contrast to patients with tumours showing intestinal differentiation, those with tumours showing müllerian differentiation rarely develop pseudomyxoma peritonei or die from their disease.
- Primary mucinous ovarian carcinoma is relatively resistant to chemotherapy, and patients with widespread disease have a poor prognosis in comparison with those with the more common serous or endometrioid carcinoma.
- Mucinous ovarian malignancies may be associated with pseudomyxoma peritonei. In this situation, the ovarian tumour is often associated with an appendiceal neoplasm. There is controversy as to whether the two neoplasms are independent primary tumours or whether one is metastatic from the other.
- Immunohistochemistry may be helpful in differentiating between ovarian metastasis from colonic carcinomas and primary ovarian carcinomas. Colonic metastases tend to be negative for cytokeratin 7 and positive for cytokeratin 20, whereas the reverse is found in primary carcinomas of the ovary.
- In patients where the diagnosis of metastatic ovarian involvement is considered possible, an imaging-guided core biopsy with immunohistochemical evaluation of the tumour may provide the diagnosis, and avoid unnecessary surgery.

REFERENCES

1. Koonings PP, Campbell K, Mishell DR Jr, Grimes DA, Relative frequency of primary ovarian neoplasms: a 10-year review. *Obstet Gynecol* 1989; 74: 921–6.
2. Russell P, Farnsworth A, Mucinous tumours. In: *Surgical Pathology of the Ovaries* (Russell P, Farnsworth A, eds). Edinburgh: Churchill Livingstone, 1997: 273–98.
3. Rutgers JL, Scully RE, Ovarian müllerian mucinous papillary cystadenomas of border-

line malignancy. A clinicopathologic analysis. *Cancer* 1988; **61**: 340–8.

4. Kaern J, Trope CG, Abeler VM, A retrospective study of 370 borderline tumors of the ovary treated at the Norwegian Radium Hospital from 1970 to 1982. A review of clinicopathologic features and treatment modalities. *Cancer* 1993; **71**: 1810–20.

5. Ronnett BM, Zahn CM, Kurman RJ et al, Disseminated peritoneal adenomucinosis and peritoneal mucinous carcinomatosis. A clinicopathologic analysis of 109 cases with emphasis on distinguishing pathologic features, site of origin, prognosis, and relationship to 'pseudomyxoma peritonei'. *Am J Surg Pathol* 1995; **19**: 1390–408.

6. Prayson RA, Hart WR, Petras RE, Pseudomyxoma peritonei. A clinicopathologic study of 19 cases with emphasis on site of origin and nature of associated ovarian tumors. *Am J Surg Pathol* 1994; **18**: 591–603.

7. Ronnett BM, Kurman RJ, Zahn CM et al, Pseudomyxoma peritonei in women: a clinicopathologic analysis of 30 cases with emphasis on site of origin, prognosis, and relationship to ovarian mucinous tumors of low malignant potential. *Hum Pathol* 1995; **26**: 509–24.

8. Costa MJ, Pseudomyxoma peritonei. Histologic predictors of patient survival. *Arch Pathol Lab Med* 1994; **118**: 1215–19.

9. Sugarbaker PH, Observations concerning cancer spread within the peritoneal cavity and concepts supporting an ordered pathophysiology. *Cancer Treat Res* 1996; **82**: 79–100.

10. Hinson FL, Ambrose NS, Pseudomyxoma peritonei. *Br J Surg* 1998; **85**: 1332–9.

11. Young RH, Gilks CB, Scully RE, Mucinous tumors of the appendix associated with mucinous tumors of the ovary and pseudomyxoma peritonei. A clinicopathological analysis of 22 cases supporting an origin in the appendix. *Am J Surg Pathol* 1991; **15**: 415–29.

12. Prat J, Ovarian tumors of borderline malignancy (tumors of low malignant potential): a critical appraisal. *Adv Anat Pathol* 1999; **6**: 247–74.

13. Seidman JD, Elsayed AM, Sobin LH, Tavassoli FA, Association of mucinous tumors of the ovary and appendix. A clinicopathologic study of 25 cases. *Am J Surg Pathol* 1993; **17**: 22–34.

14. Chuaqui RF, Zhuang Z, Emmert-Buck MR et al, Genetic analysis of synchronous mucinous tumors of the ovary and appendix. *Hum Pathol* 1996; **27**: 165–71.

15. Cuatrecasas M, Matias-Guiu X, Prat J, Synchronous mucinous tumors of the appendix and the ovary associated with pseudomyxoma peritonei. A clinicopathologic study of six cases with comparative analysis of c-Ki-ras mutations. *Am J Surg Pathol* 1996; **20**: 739–46.

16. Chaitin BA, Gershenson DM, Evans HL, Mucinous tumors of the ovary. A clinicopathologic study of 70 cases. *Cancer* 1985; **55**: 1958–62.

17. Watkin W, Silva EG, Gershenson DM, Mucinous carcinoma of the ovary. Pathologic prognostic factors. *Cancer* 1992; **69**: 208–12.

18. Siriaunkgul S, Robbins KM, McGowan L, Silverberg SG, Ovarian mucinous tumors of low malignant potential: a clinicopathologic study of 54 tumors of intestinal and müllerian type. *Int J Gynecol Pathol* 1995; **14**: 198–208.

19. McGuire WP, Hoskins WJ, Brady MF et al, Cyclophosphamide and cisplatin compared with paclitaxel and cisplatin in patients with stage III and stage IV ovarian cancer. *N Engl J Med* 1996; **334**: 1–6.

20. Shimizu Y, Nagata H, Kikuchi Y et al, Cytotoxic agents active against mucinous adenocarcinoma of the ovary. *Oncol Rep* 1998; **5**: 99–101.

21. Omura G, Brady M, Homesley H et al, Long-term follow-up and prognostic factor analysis in advanced ovarian carcinoma: the Gynecologic Oncology Group experience. *J Clin Oncol* 1991; **9**: 1138–50.

22. Zoetmulder FA, van der Vange N, Witkamp AJ et al, Hyperthermic intra-peritoneal chemotherapy (HIPEC) in patients with peritoneal pseudomyxoma or peritoneal metastases of colorectal carcinoma; good preliminary results

from the Netherlands Cancer Institute. *Ned Tijdschr Geneeskd* 1999; **143**: 1863–8.

23. El-Attar AF, Skeel RT, Howard JM, Pseudomyxoma peritonei: sudden cardiac death complicating post operative intraperitoneal treatment with 5-fluorouracil. *Dig Surg* 1999; **16**: 80–2.

24. Ubhi SS, McCulloch P, Veitch PS, Preliminary results of the use of intraperitoneal carbon-adsorbed mitomycin C in intra-abdominal malignancy. *Br J Cancer* 1997; **76**: 1667–9.

25. Sugarbaker PH, Peritonectomy procedures. *Ann Surg* 1995; **221**: 29–42.

26. Mazur MT, Hsueh S, Gersell DJ, Metastases to the female genital tract. Analysis of 325 cases. *Cancer* 1984; **53**: 1978–84.

27. James PD, Taylor CW, Templeton AC, Tumours of the female genitalia. In: *Tumours in a Tropical Country: A Survey of Uganda 1964–1968* (Templeton AC, ed). New York: Springer-Verlag, 1973.

28. Birnkrant A, Sampson J, Sugarbaker PH, Ovarian metastasis from colorectal cancer. *Dis Colon Rectum* 1986; **29**: 767–71.

29. Birt CAV, Prophylactic oophorectomy with resection of the large bowel for cancer. *Am J Surg* 1951; **82**: 572–7.

30. Cutait R, Lesser ML, Enker WE, Prophylactic oophorectomy in surgery for large-bowel cancer. *Dis Colon Rectum* 1983; **26**: 6–11.

31. O'Brien PH, Newton BB, Metcalf JS, Rittenbury MS, Oophorectomy in women with carcinoma of the colon and rectum. *Surg Gynecol Obstet* 1981; **153**: 827–30.

32. Graffner HO, Alm PO, Oscarson JE, Prophylactic oophorectomy in colorectal carcinoma. *Am J Surg* 1983; **146**: 233–5.

33. Ulbright TM, Roth LM, Stehman FB, Secondary ovarian neoplasia. A clinicopathologic study of 35 cases. *Cancer* 1984; **53**: 1164–74.

34. MacKeigan JM, Ferguson JA, Prophylactic oophorectomy and colorectal cancer in premenopausal patients. *Dis Colon Rectum* 1979; **22**: 401–5.

35. Scully RE, Tumors of the ovary and maldeveloped gonads. In: *Atlas of Tumour Pathology*. Washington, DC: Armed Forces Institute of Pathology, 1979: 323–63.

36. Parker RT, Currie JL, Metastatic tumours of ovary. In: *Gynecologic Oncology* (Coppleson M, ed). Edinburgh: Churchill Livingstone, 1992: 987–1000.

37. Hines JR, Gordon RT, Widger C, Kolb T, Cystosarcoma phyllodes metastatic to a Brenner tumor of the ovary. *Arch Surg* 1976; **111**: 299–300.

38. Lash RH, Hart WR, Intestinal adenocarcinomas metastatic to the ovaries. A clinicopathologic evaluation of 22 cases. *Am J Surg Pathol* 1987; **11**: 114–21.

39. Russell P, Farnsworth A, Metastatic gastrointestinal carcinomas and carcinoids. In: *Haines and Taylor Obstetrical and Gynaecological Pathology* (Fox H, Wells M, eds). Edinburgh: Churchill Livingstone, 1995: 609–24.

40. Wauters CC, Smedts F, Gerrits LG et al, Keratins 7 and 20 as diagnostic markers of carcinomas metastatic to the ovary. *Hum Pathol* 1995; **26**: 852–5.

41. Loy TS, Calaluce RD, Keeney GL, Cytokeratin immunostaining in differentiating primary ovarian carcinoma from metastatic colonic adenocarcinoma. *Mod Pathol* 1996; **9**: 1040–4.

42. DeCostanzo DC, Elias JM, Chumas JC, Necrosis in 84 ovarian carcinomas: a morphologic study of primary versus metastatic colonic carcinoma with a selective immunohistochemical analysis of cytokeratin subtypes and carcinoembryonic antigen. *Int J Gynecol Pathol* 1997; **16**: 245–9.

43. Berezowski K, Stastny JF, Kornstein MJ, Cytokeratins 7 and 20 and carcinoembryonic antigen in ovarian and colonic carcinoma. *Mod Pathol* 1996; **9**: 426–9.

44. Taal BG, Hageman PC, Delemarre JF et al, Metastatic ovarian or colonic cancer: a clinical challenge. *Eur J Cancer* 1992; **28**: 394–9.

45. Pavelic ZP, Pavelic L, Pavelic K, Peacock JS, Utility of anti-carcinoembryonic antigen monoclonal antibodies for differentiating ovarian

adenocarcinomas from gastrointestinal metastasis to the ovary. *Gynecol Oncol* 1991; **40**: 112–17.

46. Pandha HS, Waxman J, Tumour markers. *QJM* 1995; **88**: 233–41.

47. Markman M, The use of serum tumor markers in the management of patients with malignancy. *J Cancer Res Clin Oncol* 1993; **119**: 635–6.

5

Clinical presentation and management of stage IV disease

Paul A Vasey, Stanley B Kaye

INTRODUCTION

Accounting for 16% of all patients at diagnosis, and defined as 'growth involving one or both ovaries with distant metastases' (FIGO, 1986), stage IV ovarian cancer includes a range of presentations from a unilateral pleural effusion to multiple visceral metastases. Because of the occult nature of the initial spread, true staging is most accurately determined at laparotomy. Nevertheless, stage IV disease may be documented simply by pleural fluid aspiration, or by fine-needle aspiration of distant lymphadenopathy without any major surgical procedure being undertaken. Overall, stage IV disease has a dismal prognosis, with less than 5% of patients surviving five years.[1] Indeed, in the pre-cisplatin era, Wharton and colleagues[2] reported a 9% four-year survival rate among women with stage IV disease participating in randomized trials.

However, randomized studies looking at treatment strategies have combined patients with stage IV disease with those with stage III in their analysis. This may not be appropriate, since a meta-analysis of 58 studies of patients with stages III and IV disease demonstrated that for each 10-point increase in the percentage of stage IV patients in the individual study cohort, there was a significant (2.6%, $p = 0.038$) decrease in median survival.[3] Also, Carmichael and colleagues observed no cured stage IV patients in a series of 342 women with stage III/IV ovarian cancer treated with doxorubicin and cisplatin. One conclusion from these data is that stage IV ovarian cancer has a significantly worse prognosis than stage III disease, and should be considered separately in such studies.

But given the wide variations in presentation and tumour volume, what is the evidence that all stage IV patients do badly? Is it possible to identify subgroups which demonstrate diverse natural histories? If so, should selected stage IV ovarian cancer patients be treated more or less aggressively on the basis that they could be expected to have differing prognoses?

In addition, a feature of Wharton's series was that the few long-term survivors had residual disease with tumour diameter of 2 cm or less prior to the initiation of chemotherapy. It is accepted that maximal tumour debulking is advantageous for stage III patients at their initial laparotomy, but what is the evidence for this practice in patients with stage IV disease?

This chapter will discuss the management of three patients with diverse presentations of stage IV ovarian cancer, and seek to address these important clinical questions.

CASE HISTORY 1

A 74-year-old woman with a history of maturity-onset diabetes presented to her general practitioner with a four-month history of general malaise, weight loss, and altered bowel habit. More recently, she had noticed abdominal swelling, and had lost her appetite. She was referred to a general surgical clinic, where she was found to have abdominal distension due to ascites and 3 cm hepatomegaly.

Abdomino-pelvic ultrasound was performed, which confirmed a significant amount of ascitic fluid, and two echogenic lesions in the right lobe of the liver, 4 cm and 3 cm in diameter respectively. A chest X-ray was normal. Renal function was normal, but hepatic enzymes were deranged: alkaline phosphatase (ALP) and aspartate and alanine aminotransferases (AST and ALT) were 2–5 times normal laboratory values. CA125 was 989 U/ml. Barium studies were performed, which revealed mild diverticulosis, but no intrinsic bowel lesion. A computed tomography (CT) scan confirmed hepatic metastases, but also indicated the presence of a 4 cm diameter splenic metastasis, ascites, diffuse peritoneal metastases, and a 6 cm pelvic mass arising from the right adnexa. Abdominal paracentesis was carried out, and 5 litres of straw-coloured fluid was removed. No malignant cells were evident on cytological examination. A liver biopsy was performed, and histological examination revealed metastatic adenocarcinoma, which was poorly differentiated (grade 3) and thought histologically to be of ovarian origin.

CASE HISTORY 2

A 39-year-old mother of two presented to her gynaecologist with a seven-week history of dysmenorrhoea and menorrhagia, abdominal pain, and weight loss. She had a history of presumed irritable bowel syndrome and had had a normal barium enema 12 months previously. Pelvic examination suggested the presence of a swelling arising from the pouch of Douglas. Abdominal examination was normal, apart from a caesarian section scar. Transabdominal ultrasound demonstrated a 10 cm × 8 cm cystic mass arising from the right ovary. In addition, a moderately severe right hydronephrosis was noted. CA125 was 458 U/ml. A chest X-ray demonstrated a small, left-sided pleural effusion. Following diagnostic aspiration, adenocarcinoma cells were demonstrated in this fluid.*

Given that both of these patients have a presumptive diagnosis of ovarian cancer, what should be the next step in their management?

These patients are likely to represent different prognoses within the stage IV grouping. FIGO stage has been shown to correlate closely with five-year survival, although there are marked differences within stages, depending on patient age. Women aged 65–74 years with stage III/IV can be shown to have a 13% five-year survival rate compared with 45% for the under 45s.[1] Moreover, a strong correlation has been observed between stage and grade of tumour,[5] and also with overall survival. In addition, cell types such as clear cell carcinoma appear to be more aggressive on a stage-for-stage basis.[6] But within stage IV disease, the question is whether there are any other prognostic factors that have been clearly identified.

What is the relevance of extent of residual disease prior to chemotherapy?

Residual disease as a prognostic factor for survival in ovarian cancer has been extensively researched. However, very few studies have reported survival data based on the volume of residual disease for individual FIGO stages. The role of initial cytoreductive surgery in patients with stage III ovarian cancer is now well established, resulting in a higher incidence of pathological complete response to subsequent chemotherapy, and, more importantly, an improved overall survival rate for patients with residual disease less than 1–2 cm compared with patients with bulky residual disease.[7] A consensus statement was produced in 1994 at the National Institutes of Health Consensus Development Conference on Ovarian Cancer, which concluded that 'aggressive attempts at cytoreductive surgery as the primary management of ovarian cancer will improve the patient's opportunity for long-term survival' (Final Statement, NIH Consensus Development Conference on Ovarian Cancer, Bethesda, MD, 1994). There are certainly compelling theoretical and clinical arguments for optimal cytoreduction,[8] and these can be described thus:

1. Removal of large tumour masses may improve patient comfort.
2. Adverse metabolic consequences of large tumour masses (e.g. renal failure, hypercalcaemia) can be alleviated, and nutritional status maintained.
3. Debulking large tumour masses may increase the subsequent exposure to chemotherapy and subsequent response by limiting hypoxic 'sanctuary' sites.
4. Better-perfused, smaller residual tumour nodules have a lower proportion of cells in resting/G_0 phase, so increasing the efficacy of chemotherapy.
5. Cytoreduction may abrogate or slow down the production of chemoresistant clones, which develop as a result of random mutations at a rate proportional to the growth rate and number of tumour cells present.[9]

Nevertheless, there is a lack of specific subgroup analysis of stage IV patients in most studies with respect to any benefit of cytoreductive surgery, and it is appropriate to consider whether these patients, most of whom have a poor prognosis, should undergo such a surgical procedure.

Data supporting an initial aggressive surgical approach were produced in a platinum dose–intensity study by the Gynecologic Oncology Group (GOG) in 1995.[10] Here, McGuire and colleagues reported that patients with stage III disease had a better survival (as expected) compared with patients with stage IV, but that, interestingly, non-bulky stage IV disease had a survival roughly equivalent to that of patients with bulky stage III disease. Nonetheless, patients with bulky stage IV disease as a group had the worst prognosis overall, indirectly implying that stage IV patients could benefit from having cytoreductive surgery. In addition, Allen and colleagues[11] performed a meta-analysis of retrospective studies of women with stage III/IV disease (via literature search and personal communications), and concluded that optimal cytoreduction, through maximal surgical effort, was beneficial for stage IV patients. However, in a review of 192 stage IV patients treated at the Royal Marsden Hospital, London, the size of residual disease was not found to be a prognostic factor on univariate and multivariate analysis.[12]

A prospective, randomized study of this issue would be potentially controversial because of the ethical issues raised by the positive benefits reported for the attainment of minimal residual disease following surgery when stages III and IV are grouped together for analysis. Therefore, to date, most of the analyses looking specifically at these issues are based upon retrospective reviews of individual patient series.

What is the evidence in favour of cytoreduction?

One of the first studies to address this question was the retrospective analysis by Goodman and colleagues[13] of the surgery and subsequent survival of 35 women with stage IV disease. This

nstrate any particular sur-
atients considered optimally
clearly this interpretation
of statistical power due to the
ers.

agues[14] performed a retrospective
review of patients with stage IV disease
treated at the University of Pennsylvania Cancer
Center in 1997. Of 47 patients, 26 (55%) were
stage IV by virtue of positive peritoneal cytology
only, and 21 (45%) had hepatic metastases or
extra-abdominal disease. Defining optimal
surgery as a residuum of less than 2 cm, 14
patients (30%) were optimally cytoreduced, and
had a median survival of 37 months. Of these
patients, 7 (50%) had positive pleural effusion
only. The rest had a median survival of 17
months ($p = 0.0295$). Initial cytoreductive procedures were performed with acceptable perioperative morbidity and mortality, with no major
complications reported for the optimally cytoreduced group. Only 3 patients (6%) had
multiple criteria for allocation to stage IV
disease, and therefore it was not possible to
determine whether these patients were prognos-
tically different.

Curtin and colleagues[15] performed a retrospective review of 97 patients with stage IV disease,
92 of whom underwent initial debulking surgery
at the Memorial Sloan-Kettering Cancer Center.
Optimal surgery was defined as 2 cm or less
residuum, and 40 (43%) of the 92 patients
achieved this. Of the 97 patients, 41 (42%) had
positive pleural cytology only, and 20 (21%) had
hepatic disease. Of the 41 patients with malignant plural effusions, 21 (51%) were optimally
debulked, compared with 20 (39%) of the 51
patients with other stage IV criteria. Hepatic
resections were not performed. The overall
median survival for the optimal group was 40
months, compared with 18 months for those
with disease larger than 2 cm ($p = 0.01$). This

survival advantage was maintained for patients
with and without pleural effusions. An additional
favourable significant prognostic factor from this
report was age less than 65 years.

Finally, Munkarah and colleagues[16] from the
MD Anderson Cancer Center reviewed 100
patients with stage IV disease who underwent
surgical cytoreduction prior to receiving
platinum-based chemotherapy. Of these, optimal
surgery (2 cm) was achieved in 31 patients, suboptimal surgery in 61, and undetermined cytoreduction in 8. As in the other studies, stage IV
status was most frequently diagnosed on pleural
fluid aspiration (54 patients), with liver metastases being present in 16. The overall median
survival for optimally debulked patients was 25
months, compared with 15 months for suboptimally debulked patients ($p < 0.02$). No differences were found with respect to the site of
metastatic disease, but, as with other studies, definite conclusions could not be drawn owing to
the small numbers of patients. In the study by
Bonnefoi et al,[12] visceral disease (either hepatic
or pulmonary) did appear to be associated with a
poorer prognosis. Also, patients undergoing
more aggressive surgical procedures (e.g.
splenectomy or intestinal resection) to achieve
optimal cytoreduction did not appear to have a
better survival than those who underwent standard surgery. Postoperative mortality was only
1%, and morbidity was considered acceptable.

Given the retrospective nature of these
studies, can any conclusions be drawn as to what
should be the appropriate initial surgical management of these patients? All three studies
suggest that aggressive cytoreduction should be
pursued for patients with a preoperative diagnosis of stage IV ovarian cancer.

In addition, postoperative morbidity and mortality appears to be no worse than that reported
for stage III patients undergoing similar cytoreductive surgical procedures.[17] Indeed, the

median overall survival for stage IV patients appears better if the tumour residuum is 2 cm or less, wherever the site of the metastatic disease. However, the major discrepancy between these studies is that the overall survival figures for the optimally debulked groups vary considerably, i.e. 25, 37, and 40 months. The 40-month survival rate for stage IV ovarian cancer exceeds that reported for most studies involving randomized comparisons of patients with optimally debulked stage III disease, and therefore a degree of patient selection bias must be involved. In addition, the majority of patients did not obtain optimal debulking, and the factors preventing this from being achieved are not clear. This is particularly relevant, since it has been shown that patients with large-volume intra-abdominal disease prior to resection have a poorer survival than patients with smaller volumes of disease, indicating that intrinsic tumour biology may have particular prognostic significance.[18,19] However, the proportion of patients with ovarian cancer whose tumours can be successfully cytoreduced remains to be established, since a review of the literature reveals a range of 17–87%, depending on several factors, not least of which is the skill and experience of the surgeon (summarized by Ozols et al[20]).

So what are our treatment recommendations for Cases 1 and 2?

The optimal primary management approach for patients like Case 1 (and other similar patients, e.g. extreme old age, serious co-morbid medical diagnosis, or bilateral pulmonary disease compromising pulmonary function) in whom there is likely to be a significant peri-operative mortality risk is not clear. Many would consider a patient with multiple liver lesions unsuitable for a laparotomy, although unifocal hepatic or pulmonary metastases may actually be technically operable. However, as described above, more

aggressive surgical procedures that include hepatic metastasectomy have not been associated with improved survival (although if abdominal disease is debulked, even these patients appear to do better). Case 2 may be considered to have a better prognosis, given her age, good premorbid performance status, and the presence of a small pleural effusion as the only evidence of stage IV disease. One may intuitively conclude from the above data that she would be optimally treated by maximal debulking of her abdomino-pelvic tumour. Data from retrospective studies strongly make the case that if a patient is fit enough to undergo laparotomy, an attempt at optimal debulking should be made, rather than a 'peek and shriek' procedure, which is generally aimed only at establishing the diagnosis of ovarian cancer. As discussed here, most of the reviewed studies indicate that overall survival appears to be improved if optimal surgical cytoreduction is achieved, with no increase in the frequency or severity of postoperative complications. But many patients with stage IV disease are not optimally debulked initially, despite being young and fit enough for such a procedure.

One proposal could be to give all stage IV patients 'induction' chemotherapy, with a view to interval debulking, provided that all metastatic sites respond to chemotherapy. There are some clinical data supporting this rationale: Chambers and colleagues[21] reported a series of 17 patients with presumed ovarian cancer (cytological or histological findings consistent with ovarian adenocarcinoma) who were treated with upfront platinum-based chemotherapy. Eight patients subsequently had surgery, and nine did not (owing to non-response or only stabilization of disease). The median survival for this group was 15 months, similar to the survival of 21 patients with stage IV disease and 38 suboptimally debulked stage III patients treated during the same period with aggressive surgery followed by chemotherapy. Considering these data, a strategy of initial chemotherapy is not unreasonable, since it can be shown that optimal debulking at second (interval) surgery can be performed in up to 70% of patients who were left with bulky disease after initial surgery.[22]

It could be argued that in stage IV disease, neoadjuvant chemotherapy may be more appropriate not only by making subsequent surgery easier, but also by delineating a group of patients *suitable* for such surgery on the basis of chemoresponsiveness (as well as a group unsuitable for surgery because of a lack of response). Also, patients clearly not fit for surgery can be treated with active therapy from the outset. Responding patients can potentially expect easier surgery, enhanced quality of life during chemotherapy, and the likelihood of at least some survival benefit following interval debulking surgery. However, it is not known how to predict accurately which patients are likely to achieve optimal debulking at interval surgery following such neoadjuvant chemotherapy. A set of criteria have been proposed for patients with a preoperative diagnosis of ovarian cancer using specific 'predictive' features visible on CT scanning.[23] This study (51 patients, with the majority stage III, and only 6 stage IV) demonstrated a sensitivity of 92.3% and a specificity of 79.3% in the ability to predict subsequent surgical outcome.

Randomized data supporting interval debulking surgery come from a European Organization for Research and Treatment of Cancer (EORTC) trial of 278 evaluable patients (FIGO stages IIB–IV) who were treated by suboptimal initial surgery (residuum > 1 cm) followed by either (a) six cycles of chemotherapy (cisplatin–cyclophosphamide) or (b) three cycles of the same chemotherapy, interval debulking surgery, and three more cycles of chemotherapy to finish.[24] Progression-free survival and overall survival were both significantly longer in the group that underwent interval debulking surgery ($p = 0.01$), with a six-month increase in median survival demonstrated for these patients. Interval debulking surgery was not associated with death or severe morbidity, and intraoperative complications were observed in only 5% of patients. In total, 64% of tumours were debulked to less than 1 cm following chemotherapy. Forty-four patients with stage IV disease were identified: 23 had interval surgery and 21 did not. Multivariate analysis of this study was not able to clearly identify a group of patients who did not benefit from interval surgery, although it is of note that the demonstrated survival advantage was more substantial if stage IV patients were excluded from the analysis.

This study is the only published prospective, randomized trial on the impact of interval cytoreductive surgery in ovarian cancer to date, and the data presented strongly argue the case for such surgery in suboptimally debulked patients. However, recruitment to this study proceeded before the ready availability of paclitaxel (Taxol) and therefore the impact of this drug (or other, newer, agents such as docetaxel and topotecan) is unknown. In addition, although it is tempting to extrapolate this recommendation to patients with stage IV disease, most patients (156) were in fact stage IIB/III. A second prospective randomized trial of interval debulking (OVO6), which involves platinum–paclitaxel chemotherapy, has just started in the UK under the auspices of the Medical Research Council (MRC).

In stage IV disease, the most appropriate way forward would be to perform a prospective, randomized clinical trial where the primary objective would be to determine whether those patients presenting with apparent stage IV disease need to undergo aggressive initial surgery, or could benefit equally by 'induction' chemotherapy, followed by surgery. A proposed schema for such a trial is outlined in Figure 5.1,

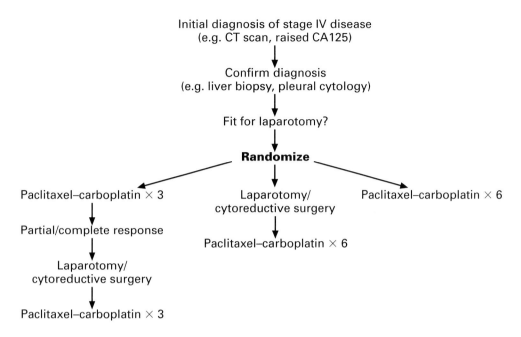

Initial diagnosis of stage IV disease
(e.g. CT scan, raised CA125)

Confirm diagnosis
(e.g. liver biopsy, pleural cytology)

Fit for laparotomy?

Randomize

Paclitaxel–carboplatin × 3

Partial/complete response

Laparotomy/
cytoreductive surgery

Paclitaxel–carboplatin × 3

Laparotomy/
cytoreductive surgery

Paclitaxel–carboplatin × 6

Paclitaxel–carboplatin × 6

Figure 5.1
Proposed 'neoadjuvant' trial in stage IV ovarian cancer. Endpoints are overall survival, quality of life, cost–benefit analysis, optimal cytoreduction achieved, postoperative complications, etc.

and incorporates elements of the recently initiated EORTC trial of neoadjuvant chemotherapy and interval debulking for stage IIIC/IV patients. The main difference proposed here is a no-surgery arm, potentially randomizing a stage IV patient to receive chemotherapy only. Patients with extensive metastatic disease outside the peritoneal cavity would be appropriate candidates for randomization into this trial. Clinicians may feel that patients with only, for example, a pleural effusion as evidence for stage IV disease should not be given a no-surgery option. Any study (or studies) addressing this issue would need to be large enough to make future recommendations with respect to the impact of extent of metastatic disease, and sites of metastatic disease (e.g. hepatic metastases versus pleural effusion) on survival.

For Case 1, we recommended that no attempt

at initial debulking surgery should be made. Instead, we proposed that chemotherapy should be administered, with a view to assessing response and possible interval surgery if appropriate. For Case 2, we did recommend primary debulking surgery; however, there is a case to explore this issue in future trials because of the possible benefits of neoadjuvant chemotherapy. Following surgery, we would then recommend combination chemotherapy (see below).

What actually happened?
Case 1

Following liver biopsy, single-agent carboplatin, dosed to an AUC (area under the concentration-versus-time curve) of 7, was prescribed as primary treatment. After three cycles, CA125 had fallen to 255 U/ml (i.e. >50% fall) and a repeat CT scan demonstrated a partial response in the hepatic disease, and significant improvement at all other disease sites. Liver function tests had normalized. Following a further three cycles of carboplatin, CA125 fell further to 97 U/ml, and a repeat CT scan demonstrated a partial response in the pelvic, hepatic and splenic metastases. A final three cycles of chemotherapy were delivered, and CA125 plateaued at 30–40 U/ml. A follow-up CT scan demonstrated residual disease without further evidence of continuing response. No debulking surgery was attempted. Progression-free survival following completion of chemotherapy was shown to be four months, and the patient subsequently received paclitaxel as salvage therapy.

Case 2

Following percutaneous stenting of the collecting system (urea and electrolytes were normal), the patient was taken to the operating theatre for an exploratory laparotomy. At surgery, no pelvic organs were initially identifiable, owing to the presence of a large tumour mass arising mainly from the right side. Following dissection of both small and large bowel, the ovary was identified, and removed along with the fallopian tube. Subsequently, a total abdominal hysterectomy and removal of the contralateral ovary with tube was performed, along with the omentum. Multiple biopsies were performed. There was no apparent spread of tumour to the retroperitoneal lymph nodes or to the liver. Maximal (<1 cm deposits remaining) debulking was performed. Histopathological examination revealed the presence of a moderately well-differentiated mucinous adenocarcinoma of the ovary, with omental metastases. A postoperative CT scan did not demonstrate any evaluable disease in the abdomen or pelvis, but did confirm the small pleural effusion. Six cycles of chemotherapy with carboplatin and paclitaxel were administered, without any significant complications. CA125 prior to chemotherapy (three weeks post-surgery) was 124 U/ml and fell to 12 U/ml within two treatment cycles. An end-of-treatment CT scan was normal. Current progression-free survival is eight months and ongoing.

What is the most effective chemotherapy regimen for patients with stage IV disease, and should this be different to that administered to patients with disease confined to the peritoneal cavity?

Ovarian carcinoma is classed as a chemosensitive tumour, and activity has been demonstrated following treatment with a wide variety of cytotoxic agents.[25] The platinum agents are among the most active single agents, and meta-analyses have demonstrated that, in terms of survival, platinum-based combinations (cisplatin- or carboplatin-containing) were superior to non-platinum-based combinations and were also superior to single-agent platinum when used at the same dose. In addition, paclitaxel has demonstrated an overall response rate of 24% in platinum-resistant ovarian cancer patients,[27] and 37% in a less heavily pretreated group.[28] A full discussion of the arguments surrounding the use of taxanes in first-line therapy is beyond the scope of this chapter but, following publication of the GOG 111 trial in 1996 (cisplatin–cyclophosphamide versus cisplatin–paclitaxel), most investigators in the USA began to utilize the combination of cisplatin and paclitaxel as the standard treatment for patients with suboptimally debulked stage III/IV ovarian cancer.[29] A European Intergroup trial produced essentially the same survival advantage for its paclitaxel–cisplatin combination, utilizing a patient population that included a significant proportion of optimally debulked stage III patients (and patients with stage II disease).[30]

Despite widespread acceptance of the platinum–paclitaxel combination, patients with stage IV disease still have a poorer prognosis than patients with stage III disease, whether optimally debulked or not. Paclitaxel has been reported to produce an overall response rate of 39% in untreated stage IV patients,[31] and there is no evidence that carboplatin is less active in stage IV than stage III disease. It is therefore unlikely that this poorer survival is due to a difference in the chemosensitivity of stage IV disease. Indeed, Bonnefoi et al[12] reported an overall response rate of 56% (18% complete response) to various chemotherapy regimens in their series of stage IV patients. It appears that patients with stage IV disease who are in good general condition, and without other adverse prognostic factors (e.g. Case 2), should receive the same chemotherapy as stage III patients.

However, given the poor overall survival of these patients, it is reasonable to pilot new treatment approaches, and to test novel, non-cross-resistant chemotherapy agents with the intention of eventual incorporation into front-line therapy. Platinum intensification does not seem to be relevant at clinically achievable doses, although the cumulative dose of platinum may be important.[32] Numerous issues (e.g. dose schedule) still remain regarding the optimal use of paclitaxel. Data suggesting that the addition of doxorubicin to platinum significantly improves survival[33] do not take into account the likely impact of paclitaxel usage, predating as they did the ready availability (economic factors notwithstanding) of this agent. However, some groups are now utilizing three-drug regimens, with platinum–taxane–anthracycline combinations.[34,35] Such regimens produce more myelotoxicity than two-drug platinum–taxane combinations, although they can produce encouragingly high clinical response rates, especially complete responses. Incorporation into first-line regimens of topoisomerase inhibitors such as topotecan (Hycamtin) appears to produce synergistic myelotoxicity, and sequencing issues (e.g. 'doublets' of alternating agents) will need to be addressed if the potential

of cytotoxic compounds like these is to be fully realized. Experience in ovarian cancer with gemcitabine (2',2'-difluorodeoxycytidine), an antimetabolite resembling cytarabine (cytosine arabinoside, Ara-C), is limited, but early phase II reports suggest a degree of non-cross-resistance to platinum.[36] Successful utilization of this agent in front-line combination therapy may depend on the demonstration of a different toxicity profile, although the indications are that haematological toxicity will be an important feature. Similarly, the DACH–platinum compounds typified by oxaliplatin (*trans*-L-(1R)-diaminocyclohexane oxalatoplatinum(II), L-OHP) also exhibit non-cross-resistance with cisplatin and carboplatin. They also have the advantage of being essentially non-myelotoxic at therapeutic doses, thus making combinations with myelosuppressive agents such as topotecan or paclitaxel more feasible.[37] Feasibility studies of each of the above approaches could in the future include patients with stage IV disease in good general condition (ECOG Performance Status 0–1).

For other stage IV patients, single-agent carboplatin is the appropriate treatment. In a large randomized trial, single-agent carboplatin (given every three weeks) was found to be equivalent to a platinum-containing combination (cyclophosphamide–doxorubicin–cisplatin, CAP), and this included patients with stage IV disease.[38] Clearly, single-agent carboplatin has an advantage over any combination regimen in terms of toxicity, and this is particularly relevant for patients with the worst prognosis (e.g. Case 1). For the very frail patient, hormone therapy with antioestrogens or progestational agents may be a reasonable therapeutic option, with a grouped response rate of 10–15% in previously treated patients.[20]

CASE HISTORY 3:
STAGE IV DISEASE PRESENTING WITH LYMPHADENOPATHY

A 48-year-old nulliparous woman presented to her general practitioner with a three-month history of a lump in her groin, with no concomitant systemic symptoms. There was no significant past medical history, and she had been taking no regular medication. On examination, she was found to have right inguinal lymphadenopathy, and was referred to the general surgeons. Rectal and vaginal examinations were unremarkable. Investigations revealed normal haematological indices but a raised erythrocyte sedimentation rate (ESR) of 50 mm/h. Renal and hepatic function were satisfactory. A chest radiograph was normal. Serum CA125 was elevated at 366 U/ml. A double-contrast barium enema was normal, and an abdomino-pelvic CT scan did not demonstrate any abnormality. She was taken to the operating theatre, where an inguinal lymphadenectomy was performed. Histopathological examination revealed that the lymph nodes were replaced by metastatic adenocarcinoma.

Given that the presenting metastatic site and elevated CA125 raised the possibility of a primary site in the ovary, how should this patient now be managed?

The key decision to be made in this relatively young woman with metastatic adenocarcinoma is whether to initiate further invasive investigations in an attempt to find and remove the primary tumour. Finding distant metastatic lymph nodes in the presence of only microscopically involved intraabdominal lymph nodes and an occult primary ovarian cancer is a rare situation, and many of these patients are incorrectly diagnosed as having a tumour of unknown primary site, or perhaps as metastatic breast cancer. In some women with metastatic adenocarcinomas and an unrevealed primary tumour, platinum-based chemotherapy is a reasonable therapeutic option, but in others, a policy of observation ('watchful waiting') is also appropriate. Such management decisions should generally be made on an individual basis, after careful discussion with the patient and family.

The natural ovarian lymphatic drainage occurs along three routes: (a) along the infundibulopelvic ligament to the para-aortic nodes, (b) along the broad ligament and parametrial channels to the pelvic sidewall, external iliac, obturator and hypogastric nodal chains, and (c) along the round ligament to the inguinal lymphatics (see Appendix 1).[39] In order for dissemination of a primary ovarian cancer to occur to lymph nodes outside the peritoneal cavity, and particularly above the diaphragm, involvement of the pelvic and para-aortic lymph nodes is required. Para-aortic lymphadenopathy is more common (67% versus 42%) in stage IV than in stage III disease,[40] which implies that in order to achieve maximal benefit from surgery, these lymph nodes should be resected. In a series of autopsies done on 100 women who died following treatment for ovarian cancer, extra-abdominal lymphadenopathy was uncommon, occurring in the supraclavicular fossa nodes (4%) and inguinal nodes (3%). Metastases to axillary lymph nodes have been reported,[42] but only in one published case as the initial presentation of ovarian carcinoma.[43]

Given the likely coexistence of pelvic and para-aortic lymphadenopathy in patients presenting with distant metastatic lymphadenopathy, it is extremely doubtful that resection (or other local treatment such as radiotherapy) of these distant lymph nodes alone will result in a significant disease-free survival. For this patient, we recommended that an active search for the primary tumour should be performed, and should include either laparoscopy or laparotomy. If an ovarian primary tumour was uncovered, then subsequent surgery should include a pelvic clearance with intent to optimally cytoreduce the disease. Subsequent chemotherapy with six cycles of platinum–paclitaxel would be then recommended.

What actually happened?

Laparoscopy was carried out, which demonstrated a slightly enlarged right ovary, with an irregular capsule. The patient then underwent a laparotomy, and a hysterectomy, bilateral salpingo-oophorectomy, and omentectomy were performed. No peritoneal deposits were noted, and multiple biopsies were performed. Pathological examination of the resected right ovary revealed the presence of a moderately well-differentiated (grade 2) adenocarcinoma with papillary elements and psammoma bodies, with capsular extension and ipsilateral fallopian tube extension. None of the other resected specimens demonstrated tumour. Postoperative chemotherapy was administered with six cycles of carboplatin, AUC 7. She has since been disease-free for four years, although she has now developed a separate primary breast cancer, for which she is now receiving adjuvant chemotherapy.

This case demonstrates the rare but important phenomenon of prolonged survival of some patients presenting with stage IV disease by virtue of extraabdominal lymph node spread. Shetty and colleagues[44] described a similar patient who presented with poorly differentiated carcinoma in left supraclavicular lymphadenopathy (Virchow's node). Despite extensive work-up at the time of this presentation, no primary tumour was uncovered. Four months later, she developed clinically apparent carcinoma of the left ovary, which was surgically treated (by bilateral salpingo-oophorectomy, total abdominal hysterectomy, and omentectomy). Following this she remained progression-free for at least nine years.

A similar clinical scenario was described in 1993 by Kehoe et al.[45] Here, a patient presented with solitary inguinal lymphadenopathy, which was resected and found to represent metastatic poorly differentiated adenocarcinoma. Investigations were unsuccessful in finding a primary tumour, although CT scanning demonstrated a possible abnormality adjacent to the uterus. However, subsequent examination under anaesthesia and laparoscopy did not confirm this finding, and the patient was treated with a policy of 'watchful waiting'. Thirty-three months later, she developed widespread intraabdominal carcinomatosis, and underwent laparotomy. This confirmed the presence of advanced ovarian cancer, and histological review of the previously resected lymph nodes determined the common origin.

The reason for the long progression-free survival seen in cases such as these is not clear, but presumably differences in the biological behaviour of these tumours is a major factor. One could theorize that an immunological mechanism is responsible, in that the host–tumour defences manage to destroy a small, clinically occult primary, without having a significant effect on the metastasis. Another possibility to explain such tumour 'dormancy' is the production of circulating angiogenesis inhibitors such as angiostatin or endostatin from the unresected primary tumour, thus inhibiting the growth of metastases.[46–48]

LEARNING POINTS

- Retrospective data and a meta-analysis strongly suggest that patients with stage IV disease obtain a survival advantage from maximal surgical cytoreduction at initial laparotomy, although randomized trials have not addressed this question.
- Postoperative complications following initial aggressive surgery in stage IV disease do not appear to be more frequent than in stage III patients.

✻ If a laparotomy is planned for patients with stage IV disease, maximal surgical effort is recommended to debulk the intraperitoneal disease.

✻ More extensive surgical procedures, such as hepatic tumour resection, are unlikely to improve the survival of these patients.

✻ It is not known whether a similar survival advantage can be achieved by cytoreductive surgery following 'neoadjuvant' chemotherapy; this could be addressed by a well-designed clinical trial.

✻ There is no evidence that, in general, stage IV patients should receive a different chemotherapeutic regimen, or should be treated differently from patients with bulky stage III disease.

✻ Feasibility studies incorporating new agents may be explored in some patients with extensive disease. These may include more intensive regimens, particularly in younger, fitter patients with stage IV disease.

✻ Patients presenting with seemingly isolated lymph node metastases from ovarian cancer should probably be managed by thorough surgical staging, maximal cytoreduction, and standard chemotherapy, and a proportion of these cases can enjoy a surprisingly long survival.

REFERENCES

1. Yancik R, Ovarian cancer: age contrasts in incidence, histology, disease stage at diagnosis and mortality. *Cancer* 1993; **71**: 517–23.

2. Wharton JT, Edwards CL, Rutledge FN, Long-term survival after chemotherapy for advanced epithelial ovarian carcinoma. *Am J Obstet Gynecol* 1984; **148**: 997–1004.

3. Hunter WR, Alexander NDE, Soutter WP, Meta-analysis of surgery in advanced ovarian carcinoma: Is maximum cytoreductive surgery an independent determinant of prognosis? *Am J Obstet Gynecol* 1992; **166**: 504–11.

4. Carmichael JA, Shelley WE, Brown LB et al, A predictive index of cure versus no cure in advanced ovarian carcinoma patients – replacement of second look laparotomy as a diagnostic test. *Gynecol Oncol* 1987; **27**: 269–78.

5. Russell P, Bannatyne P, *Surgical Pathology of the Ovaries*. New York: Churchill Livingstone, 1989: 539.

6. Vergote IB, Kaern J, Abeler VM et al, Analysis of prognostic factors in stage I epithelial ovarian carcinoma: importance of degree of differentiation and deoxyribonucleic acid ploidy in predicting relapse. *Am J Obstet Gynecol* 1993; **169**: 40.

7. Hoskins WJ, Bundy BN, Thigpen JT et al, The influence of cytoreductive surgery on recurrence-free interval and survival in small-volume stage III epithelial ovarian cancer: a Gynecologic Oncology Group study. *Gynecol Oncol* 1992; **47**: 159–66.

8. Griffiths CT, Surgery at the time of diagnosis in ovarian cancer. In: *Management of Ovarian Cancer* (Blackledge G, Chan KK, eds). London: Butterworths, 1986.

9. Goldie JH, Coldman AJ, A mathematic model for relating the drug sensitivity of tumours to their spontaneous mutation rate. *Cancer Treat Rep* 1979; **63**: 1727–33.

10. McGuire WP, Hoskins WJ, Brady MF et al, Assessment of dose-intensive therapy in suboptimally debulked ovarian cancer: a Gynecologic Oncology Group study. *J Clin Oncol* 1995; **13**: 1589–99.

11. Allen DG, Heintz AP, Touw FW, A meta-analysis of residual disease and survival in stage III and IV carcinoma of the ovary. *Eur J Gynecol Oncol* 1995; **16**: 349–56.

12. Bonnefoi H, A'Hern RP, Fisher C et al, Natural history of stage IV epithelial ovarian cancer. *J Clin Oncol* 1999; **17**: 767–75.

13. Goodman HM, Harlow BL, Sheets EE et al, The role of cytoreductive surgery in the management of stage IV epithelial ovarian cancer. *Gynecol Oncol* 1992; **46**: 367–71.

14. Lui PC, Benjamin I, Morgan MA et al, Effect of surgical debulking on survival in stage IV ovarian cancer. *Gynecol Oncol* 1997; **64**: 4–8.

15. Curtin JP, Malik R, Venkatraman ES et al, Stage IV ovarian cancer: impact of surgical debulking. *Gynecol Oncol* 1997; **64**: 9–12.

16. Munkarah AR, Hallum AV 3rd, Morris M et al, Prognostic significance of residual disease in patients with stage IV epithelial ovarian cancer. *Gynecol Oncol* 1997; **64**: 13–17.

17. Chen SS, Bochner R, Assessment of morbidity and mortality in primary cytoreductive surgery for advanced ovarian carcinoma. *Gynecol Oncol* 1985; **20**: 190–5.

18. Hacker NF, Berek JS, Lagasse LD et al, Primary cytoreductive surgery for epithelial ovarian cancer. *Obstet Gynecol* 1983; **61**: 413–20.

19. Hoskins WJ, Surgical staging and cytoreductive surgery of epithelial ovarian cancer. *Cancer* 1993; **71**: 1534–40.

20. Ozols RF, Rubin SC, Thomas G, Robboy S, Epithelial ovarian cancer. In: *Principles and Practice of Gynecological Oncology*, 2nd edn (Hoskins WJ, Perez CA, Young RC, eds). Philadelphia: Lippincott-Raven, 1997: 919–86.

21. Chambers JT, Chambers SK, Voynick IM, Schwartz PE, Neoadjuvant chemotherapy in stage X ovarian carcinoma. *Gynecol Oncol* 1990; **37**: 327–31.

22. Redman CW, Blackledge G, Lawton FG et al. Early second surgery in ovarian cancer—improving the potential for cure or another unnecessary operation? *Eur J Surg Oncol* 1990; **16**(5): 426–9.

23. Nelson BE, Rosenfield AT, Schwartz PE, Preoperative abdominopelvic computed tomographic prediction of optimal cytoreduction in epithelial ovarian carcinoma. *J Clin Oncol* 1993; **11**: 166–72.

24. van der Burg MEL, van Lent M, Buyse M et al, The effect of debulking surgery after induction chemotherapy on the prognosis in advanced epithelial ovarian cancer. *N Engl J Med* 1995; **332**: 629–34.

25. Ozols RF, Young RC, Chemotherapy of ovarian cancer. *Semin Oncol* 1984; **11**: 251–63.

26. Advanced Ovarian Cancer Trialists Group, Chemotherapy in advanced ovarian cancer: an updated overview of randomised clinical trials. *Br J Cancer* 1998; **78**: 1479–87.

27. McGuire WP, Rowinsky EK, Rosenshein NB et al, Taxol: a unique antineoplastic agent with significant activity in advanced ovarian epithelial neoplasms. *Ann Intern Med* 1989; **111**: 273–9.

28. Thigpen JT, Blessing JA, Ball H et al, Phase II trial of paclitaxel in patients with progressive ovarian carcinoma after platinum-based chemotherapy: a Gynecologic Oncology Group study. *J Clin Oncol* 1994; **12**: 1748–53.

29. McGuire WP, Hoskins WJ, Brady MF et al, Cyclophosphamide and cisplatin compared with paclitaxel and cisplatin in patients with stage III and IV ovarian cancer. *N Engl J Med* 1996; **334**: 1–6.

30. Stuart G, Bertelsen K, Mangioni C et al, Updated analysis shows a highly significant improved overall survival (OS) for cisplatin–paclitaxel as first line treatment of advanced ovarian cancer: mature results of the EORTC–GCCG, NOCOVA, NCNC CTG and Scottish Intergroup trial. *Proc Am Soc Clin Oncol* 1998; **17**: 1394.

31. Gore ME, Rustin G, Slevin M et al, Single agent paclitaxel in patients with previously untreated stage IV epithelial ovarian cancer. *Br J Cancer* 1997; **75**: 710–14.

32. Vasey PA, Kaye SB, Importance of dose intensity in ovarian cancer. In: *Ovarian Cancer: Controversies in Management* (Gershenson DM, McGuire WP, eds). Edinburgh: Churchill Livingstone, 1997: 139–69.

33. A'Hern RP, Gore ME, Impact of doxorubicin on survival in advanced ovarian cancer. *J Clin Oncol* 1995; **13**: 726–32.

34. Hill M, Macfarlane V, Moore J, Gore ME, Taxane/platinum/anthracycline combination therapy in advanced epithelial ovarian cancer. *Semin Oncol* 1997; **24**: S2-34–7.

35. Vasey PA, Reed NS, Davis J et al, Dose-finding

study of carboplatin–epirubicin–docetaxel in advanced epithelial ovarian cancer. *Proc Am Soc Clin Oncol* 1999; **18**: 1490.

36. Lund B, Hansen OP, Hendricks CB et al, Phase II study of gemcitabine (2',2'-difluorodeoxycytidine) in previously treated ovarian cancer patients. *J Natl Cancer Inst* 1994; **86**: 1530–3.

37. Raymond E, Chaney SG, Taamma A, Cvitkovic E, Oxaliplatin: a review of preclinical and clinical studies. *Ann Oncol* 1998; **9**: 1053–71.

38. ICON Collaborators. ICON 2: randomised trial of single-agent carboplatin against three-drug combination of CAP (cyclophosphamide, doxorubicin and cisplatin) in women with ovarian cancer. International Collaborative Ovarian Neoplasm Study. *Lancet* 1998; **352**(9140): 1571–6.

39. Mangan CE, Rubin SC, Rabin DS et al, Lymph node nomenclature in gynaecologic oncology. *Gynecol Oncol* 1986; **23**: 222–6.

40. Chen SS, Lee L, Incidence of para-aortic and pelvic lymph node metastases in epithelial carcinoma of the ovary. *Gynecol Oncol* 1983; **16**: 95–100.

41. Dvoretsky PM, Richard KA, Angel C et al, Distribution of disease at autopsy in 100 women with ovarian cancer. *Hum Pathol* 1988; **19**: 57–63.

42. Duda RB, August CZ, Schink JC, Ovarian carcinoma metastatic to the breast and axillary node. *Surgery* 1991; **110**: 552–6.

43. Hockstein S, Keh P, Lurain JR et al, Ovarian carcinoma initially presenting as metastatic axillary lymphadenopathy. *Gynecol Oncol* 1997; **65**: 543–7.

44. Shetty MR, Virchow's node as a sign of latent tumour of the ovary. *Northwest Common Hosp Med Bull* 1985; **22**: 61–3.

45. Kehoe S, Luesley D, Rollason T, Ovarian carcinoma presenting with inguinal metastatic lymphadenopathy 33 months prior to intraabdominal disease. *Gynecol Oncol* 1993; **50**: 128–30.

46. O'Reilly MS, Holmgren L, Shing Y et al, Angiostatin: a novel angiogenesis inhibitor that mediates the suppression of metastases by a Lewis lung carcinoma. *Cell* 1994; **79**: 315–28.

47. O'Reilly MS, Boehm T, Shing Y et al, Endostatin: an endogenous inhibitor of angiogenesis and tumour growth. *Cell* 1997; **88**: 277–85.

48. Folkman J, Fighting cancer by attacking its blood supply. *Scientific American* 1996; **275**(3 Sept): 116–19.

6

Borderline tumours

Claes Tropé, Janne Kaern

INTRODUCTION

Borderline epithelial tumours of the ovary constitute a special group of tumours with histopathological features and biological behaviour intermediate between those of clearly benign and frankly malignant tumours. They were first described in 1929 by Taylor,[1,2] who referred to them as 'semi-malignant' or 'carcinoma of low malignant potential'. They were further defined in the 1950s by Kottmeier[3] and Woodruff and Novak,[4] but were not formally recognized until 1971.[5] In 1971, this group of tumours was accepted by the International Federation of Gynecology and Obstetrics (FIGO)[6] and in 1973 by the World Health Organization (WHO)[7] as borderline tumours.

These tumours account for approximately 10% of all epithelial ovarian neoplasms, and the peak median age of diagnosis is approximately 10 years earlier than that of invasive epithelial ovarian cancer. This chapter will discuss their surgical and postoperative management, which is particularly important in young women who may wish to have conservative surgery. As patients may survive for many years, it is important to consider the factors that might predict recurrence and prognosis, since a small fraction of these tumours may be truly malignant with the ability to invade and metastasize.

CASE HISTORY

A 35-year-old woman developed abdominal discomfort, and was found to have a pelvic mass with generalized abdominal swelling. On ultrasound, a unilateral multilocular cyst with papillary formations was visualized in the right ovary (Figure 6.1). The serum CA125 and carcinoembryonic antigen (CEA) levels were normal. At laparotomy, there was a cystic right ovarian tumour, which had clearly ruptured prior to removal. In the abdomen, there was no obvious evidence of tumour spread. The patient underwent a hysterectomy, bilateral salpingo-oophorectomy, and infracolic omentectomy. Pathological examination revealed a mucinous 'borderline' ovarian cancer (on the surface of the ovary) of 'low malignant potential' (Figure 6.2). The omentum was negative for malignancy. Cytology of the peritoneal washings contained carcinoma cells.

What is the correct surgical management?
Recommended standard primary surgery for borderline ovarian tumour patients follows the guidelines for invasive ovarian carcinomas: total abdominal hysterectomy, bilateral salpingo-

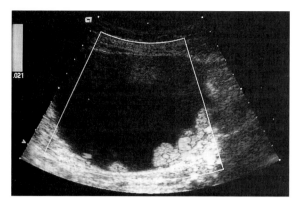

Figure 6.1
Transvaginal sonographic image of a borderline malignant serous cystadenoma of the ovary. This unilocular
cyst had multiple solid papillary projections, which
constitute the most suspicious signs of ovarian malignancy at ultrasonography. (Courtesy of D Timmer-
mann, MD, PhD, Department of Obstetrics and
Gynaecology, University Hospitals, Leuven.)

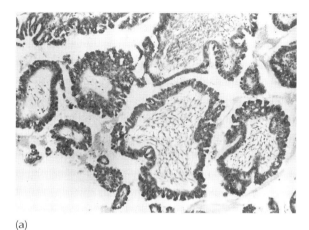

(a)

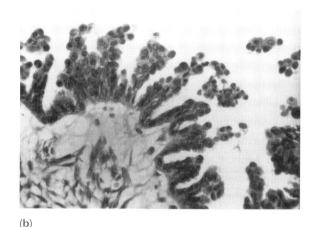

(b)

Figure 6.2
Borderline malignant serous papillary tumour of the
ovary. (a) Broad fibrous papillae, covered by proliferating epithelium (H&E, ×25); (b) characteristic tufting
and budding — note the detached cell clusters at the
end of the papillary formations. Cytologic atypia is
slight to moderate (H&E, ×100). (Courtesy of Ph
Moerman, MD, PhD, Department of Pathology, University Hospitals, Leuven.)

oophorectomy, omentectomy, peritoneal washings, multiple biopsies, and tumour debulking.
For mucinous tumours, appendicectomy is recommended, because these tumours might originate from the appendix. Removal of potential
tumour-infiltrated organs is important. In
advanced stages, tumour debulking surgery has
been performed, but lymph node sampling has
not been part of the standard procedure. Unfortunately, frozen-section diagnosis is not always
accurate. The discrimination of a borderline
ovarian tumour–ovarian carcinoma from a
benign tumour is possible in frozen sections, but
care should be taken in discriminating between a
borderline ovarian tumour and an invasive
ovarian carcinoma. The value of pelvic and para-
aortic lymphadenectomy will be discussed below.

Bilaterality

Mucinous tumours are significantly more likely
to be stage I than serous tumours (84% compared with 67%). The rate of bilateral ovarian
involvement depends on the histological subtype.

For serous tumours, the rate is on average 41%
(range 28–66%), whereas for mucinous tumours,
it is on average 8% (range 0–13%).[8] Although the
standard treatment for all patients is at least
bilateral salpingo-oophorectomy, many young
patients who have not completed childbearing
can be safely treated with unilateral salpingo-

oophorectomy after comprehensive surgical staging, thereby preserving fertility.

Conservative therapy

Recent studies from the Norwegian Radium Hospital (NRH) and the US Gynecologic Oncology Group (GOG) have shown that preservation of reproductive organs[9,10] is feasible. Even ovarian cystectomy has been reported, but the recurrence rate in the ovary is approximately 15%. One of the predictors of relapse is the presence of tumour cells in the resection margins.[11,12] The frequency of persistence or recurrence in 35 patients with serous borderline ovarian tumours treated by unilateral cystectomy, bilateral cystectomy, or unilateral cystectomy with contralateral oophorectomy or salpingo-oophorectomy was retrospectively investigated by Lim-Tan et al.[13] Conservative surgical treatment was performed either because the patients were young and wanted to preserve their fertility or because the nature of the tumour was not determined at the time of surgery. Thirty-three had stage I disease (19 stage IA, 10 stage IB, and 4 stage IC), and two had stage III disease. Four patients with stage I (2 stage IA, 1 stage IB, and 1 stage IC) tumours had persistent or recurrent disease. Although 60% of the patients had additional and, in some cases, definitive operations within relatively short periods after initial cystectomy or cystectomies, 21 had conservation of ovarian tissue and were followed on average for 7.5 years. All stage I patients were alive without evidence of disease after surgical treatment alone. Both stage III patients were treated with 'second-look' laparotomy and cisplatin combination chemotherapy, and were alive four years later. The presence of persistent or recurrent disease correlated with multifocality and involvement of resection margins. Multifocality may be a strong predictor of failure of cystectomy to control the disease. No recurrence of disease was seen in ovaries from which a single cyst had been removed with negative resection margins. Generous sampling of the resection margins of ovarian cysts is very important. To allow conservative surgery, careful evaluation of the extent of disease at the time of operation and meticulous examination of the cystectomy specimen by the gynaecologist and pathologist are desirable to determine the prognosis after cystectomy. Eight of the 19 stage IA patients treated with conservation of ovarian tissue subsequently had normal pregnancies; another three chose not to become pregnant. Conservative surgery is justifiable for some patients with a good prognostic index (see below). Unilateral oophorectomy and omentectomy in stage IA mucinous diploid tumours are indicated in young women who wish to preserve fertility. In stage IA serous tumours, the same procedure is safe if the contralateral ovary is macroscopically normal. Careful inspection of a macroscopic normal contralateral ovary should be sufficient in young women with stage IA disease who wish to remain fertile. As wedge biopsy could lead to reduced fertility, this approach should be avoided. The incidence of infertility after this type of procedure is about 10–20%, and, since the risk of bilaterality is low, this negates its value.[8] In the NRH study,[14] only 4 out of 51 patients with stage IB did not have macroscopic disease in both ovaries, and none of the stage IB patients relapsed. The recurrence rate for conservatively operated stage IA patients was 0–30%.[11,13–16] Survival is not affected if the patients are reoperated upon at recurrence. The corresponding recurrence rate is below 5% for patients with borderline serous tumours who have received relapse treatment.[8,13] Conservatively treated patients need close follow-up. More individualized treatment will probably be possible through the use of modern prognostic parameters such as DNA ploidy.

What is an adequate surgical staging?

Despite the fact that experts have recommended comprehensive surgical staging for many years, most patients referred to university or comprehensive cancer centres after primary surgery have had incomplete surgery. Another common event is that malignancy is not suspected at the initial operation and therefore the abdomen is not properly explored. The question then arises whether the patient should have a further operation. Mucinous tumours confined to one ovary are probably unlikely to be upstaged at a further operation. If evidence of extra-ovarian disease exists, complete surgical staging and appendectomy are indicated. Mucinous tumours with abdominal spread are in 50% of cases claimed to have arisen in the appendix or simultaneously in the appendix and in one or both ovaries.[17–19] For serous tumours, it is reasonable to do a second operation, because they are more likely to be upstaged at a second procedure.

For patients with pseudomyxoma peritonei, recurrence is more common, and these patients often develop bowel obstruction, which eventually is fatal. Repeated surgery with removal of mucinous material is the treatment of choice. The condition is uncommon, and published results of therapy are on retrospective series, often with only a few patients. Limber et al[20] reported that patients with pseudomyxoma peritonei who were not treated had a median recurrence-free survival of 18 months. Chemotherapy administered either intravenously or as an intraperitoneal instillation does not seem to be effective. Subtotal peritonectomies have been performed in a small number of patients, but it is too early to make any statement of the effect on survival of this procedure. Experimental cases have been performed at NRH (data not published), but Sugarbaker and Jablonski[21] have reported that complete stripping of the visceral and parietal peritoneum, followed by intra-peritoneal chemotherapy with 5-fluorouracil (5-FU) and mitomycin C in colorectal and appendiceal cancer resulted in an excellent three-year survival rate of 99%. However, this technique may increase the risk of operative and postoperative complications, with a requirement for total parenteral nutrition.

Leake et al[22] sampled retroperitoneal lymph nodes in 34 women. Out of 12 patients who had pelvic node sampling, 2 had nodal involvement. None of the 7 patients with mucinous tumours had lymph node involvement. However, lymph node involvement does not appear to worsen the prognosis according to our experience and those of others.[14,17] According to Hoskins,[8] the ultimate test of the utility of the more rigorous surgical procedure, which undoubtedly will find unsuspected disease in serous tumours, is its effect on the outcome. At NRH, during the 1960s and 1970s, we did not routinely perform rigorous staging with hysterectomy, bilateral salpingo-oophorectomy, infracolicomentectomy, and diaphragmatic and lymph node resection. Therefore, many of our patients had been understaged according to FIGO – but these procedures do not seem to be necessary in FIGO stage I borderline tumours, since the 15-year survival rate was 95%. Furthermore, none of the patients had recurrent disease in the lymph nodes. We do not consider lymph node sampling to be indicated on a routine basis in borderline ovarian tumours. In the NRH study,[14] none of the 148 patients with serous stage I tumours died of disease. In none of these were lymph node biopsies performed.

Should this patient receive any postoperative therapy?

Adjuvant treatment for borderline ovarian tumours is of questionable value. At the National Institute of Health (NIH) Consensus Conference on Ovarian Cancer in 1994,[23] it was stated that there was no role for postoperative therapy, even in those with advanced disease. Most patients have stage I disease and a very low risk of recurrence. Only a few randomized trials of treatment of early-stage epithelial ovarian carcinoma including borderline tumours have been reported.[24–26] The quoted series consisted of 55, 51, 83, and 67 evaluable patients respectively, and they reached no conclusion regarding optimum treatment for this disease.[26] Between 1970 and 1988, at the NRH, we have studied the efficacy of adjuvant therapy in four prospective randomized trials in 253 patients with epithelial borderline tumours of the ovary (Table 6.1).[26] The overall corrected and crude survival rates for

stage I patients were 99% and 94% respectively. Adjuvant treatment did not seem to improve the overall corrected survival. On the contrary, toxicity was added, with small bowel complications after radiation therapy, neurotoxicity after cisplatin, and bone marrow toxicity after thiotepa. We concluded that patients with stage I borderline tumours should not receive any adjuvant treatment. A meta-analysis conducted by Kurman and Trimble[27] on 953 patients with serous borderline tumours showed that more patients died of treatment-related complications (12 patients) than of progressive disease (8 patients). Reports from Yale University,[11] MD

Table 6.1   Prospective randomized studies in 253 patients with borderline tumours of the ovary, stage I–II, conducted at the Norwegian Radium Hospital between 1970 and 1988[a]

Study	Date	Treatment[b]		No. of patients
1	1970–1974	Radical surgery	Pelvic external irradiation	36
			Pelvic external irradiation + i.p. ^{198}Au	38
2	1975–1977	Radical surgery i.p.^{198}Au or i.p.^{32}P	Control	20
			Thiotepa	22
3	1982–1988	Radical surgery	Control	39
			Thiotepa	29
4	1982–1988	Radical surgery	i.p. ^{32}P	32
			Cisplatin	37

[a] From reference 26, with permission.
[b] i.p., intraperitoneal; ^{198}Au, radioactive gold; ^{32}P, radioactive phosphorus.

Anderson Cancer Center,[28] and Massachusetts General Hospital[29] were also unable to identify any survival benefit associated with adjuvant chemotherapy or radiotherapy. Thirty-two patients with stage III optimal debulked borderline tumours were included in the prospective randomized GOG trial of cisplatin/cyclophosphamide with or without doxorubicin.[29] No significant difference in corrected survival was observed between any of the groups in the above-mentioned randomized studies. This could have been expected, since thousands of patients are required if a difference in corrected survival is to be detected between groups of patients with a survival rate of 90% or higher. Such a trial would be difficult to perform even in a multicentre setting, since borderline tumour are relatively uncommon. The GOG closed their Protocol 72 on ovarian borderline tumours owing to slow recruitment and because too few patients relapsed. Patients were randomized to observation or treatment with six courses of melphalan.[29] Radiotherapy has been suggested by Fernandez and Daly,[30] and Sandenbergh and Woodruff[31] have used intraperitoneal radioactive chromic phosphate,[31] but the results are as uninformative as with chemotherapy. The GOG have proposed studies of hormonal therapy for borderline tumours. These have included evaluation of an antiprogestational or antioestrogenic agent. However, such trials are probably not feasible, since the incidence of recurrent disease is low and we live in an era of limited financial support for clinical research.[17] Prospective phase II studies might be more appropriate for patients with progressive recurrent disease. In conclusion, our patient did not receive any postoperative treatment.

What is the epidemiology of borderline tumours?

Borderline tumours of the ovary have been reported in Caucasian, black African, Chinese, Japanese, and Indian populations.[17] Among the Caucasian population, they are reported to comprise approximately 4–14% of all ovarian malignancies.[8,32,33] Katsube et al[34] reported that in the Denver Metropolitan area, 20% of all epithelial ovarian malignancies were of borderline type. At the NRH and other large institutions, the incidence is lower – usually about 12%, with a range of 9–20%.[8,14,33] This probably reflects the trend not to refer patients with borderline tumours to tertiary centres. The lifetime risk of developing a borderline tumour for women in the USA is between 1 : 200 and 1 : 300.[8]

Few population-based studies on borderline ovarian tumours are available.[35] In total, 2343 borderline tumours were diagnosed in Norway between 1970 and 1993 (Table 6.2).[76] The age-adjusted incidence rate has increased since 1970, reaching 4.8 per 100 000 person-years in 1989–1993 (Figure 6.2). In Finland, there has been a 50% increase in the age-adjusted incidence rate of borderline tumours between the periods 1973–1977 and 1988–1992, whereas the incidence rate of ovarian cancer remained stable during this time period.[37] In Norway, the incidence rate increased with age up to 45–49 years, after which the rate stabilized (Figure 6.3).[36] The median age at diagnosis was 53 years (27% were younger than 40 years of age), compared with about 60 years for women with invasive carcinoma.[17] This latter observation is in agreement with NRH figures[14,36] and with the study published by Rice et al.[38] In the time period 1970–1993, 93% of the borderline tumours were diagnosed as localized tumours (generally reported figures are 80–90%), 0.9% as tumours with regional spread, 4.8% as tumours with distant metastases, and 1.0% as tumours of unknown extent. The proportion of tumours with distant metastases increased from 2.7% in 1970–1973 to 6.6% in 1989–1993. The majority

Table 6.2   Borderline tumours according to histological subtypes in Norway, 1970–1993[a]

Subtype	No. of cases	Percentage
Serous	1010	43
Mucinous	1207	52
Endometrioid	26	1
Clear cell	4	<1
Other	85	4
Unknown	11	<1
Total	2343	100

[a] From reference 36, with permission.

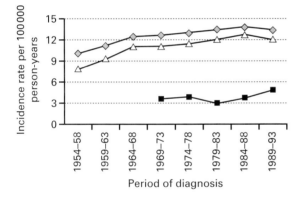

Figure 6.2
Age-adjusted incidence rates for malignant ovarian tumours (◇), epithelial ovarian cancer (△) (1954–1993), and ovarian tumours of borderline malignancy (■) (1970–1993).

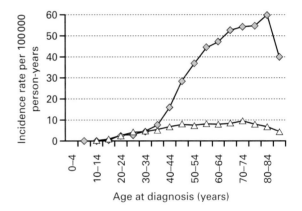

Figure 6.3
Age-specific incidence rates for ovarian cancer (◇) (1970–1993) and tumours of borderline malignancy (△) (1970–1993) in Norway.

of borderline tumours were mucinous (52%), followed by serous tumours (43%).[36] Large differences have, however, been reported in the distribution of the different histological subtypes.[33,39,40] In the nationwide Finnish study mentioned above, 38% of the borderline tumours were classified as mucinous.[37]

In the Norwegian study, the 'borderline' termi-nology was a renaming of ovarian lesions previously diagnosed partly as 'cystadenoma with atypia' and 'partly carcinoma'. It is unknown to us to what extent the two diagnoses have contributed cases to the category of borderline tumours. It is also unknown whether the increase in incidence of borderline tumours is real or merely reflects a shift in classification from carcinomas (and possible benign cystadenomas). Thus, it is possible that the apparent beginning of a decline in the incidence of ovarian cancer since the mid-1980s (and concomitant increase in borderline tumours) is not real.

Are there risk factors associated with the development of borderline tumours?

Limited information exists about risk factors for developing a borderline tumour. Nulliparous women and those with a history of infertility have an increased risk, while pregnancy, breastfeeding, and the use of oral contraceptives have a protective effect. Hypotheses about 'incessant ovulation' and 'ovulatory age' have been proposed for invasive ovarian carcinomas.[41,42] An endocrine disorder may be the basic reason.[43] It is unknown whether some women have a genetic predisposition. Extensive sampling (from both the primary tumour and the implants) and further morphological examination, the identification of new markers for growth-regulatory mechanisms, and genetic studies are needed to improve our knowledge about ovarian neoplasia. These studies may establish whether there is a continuum between benign, borderline, and invasive ovarian tumours (ovarian carcinogenesis).

What are the histopathological features and subtypes of borderline tumours, and how do they relate to outcome?

The histological diagnosis of borderline tumours is based on the following criteria described by Hart and Norris[44] and detailed by Scully:[45] epithelial cellular proliferation (stratification of the epithelial lining of the papillae; and multilayering of the epithelium, mitotic activity, and nuclear atypia) without stromal invasion. To ensure the absence of carcinomatous areas, the tumours must be thoroughly sampled. It is recommended to take one section every 1–2 cm throughout the tumour.[44] Often this important

issue is not described in the published studies. Baak, together with three other distinguished professors in pathology, showed that, despite standardized criteria, there are considerable diagnostic differences when assessing these tumours. They reviewed one representative section of 137 borderline and invasive tumours on two occasions six months apart. Their results were presented by comparing histological diagnosis with survival. The five-year survival rate varied from 80% to 100% and the intra-observer difference in five-year survival rate after their second reading of the slides ranged from 0% to 12%.[46]

Serous borderline tumours

Serous borderline tumours make up between 10% and 15% of all serous ovarian tumours.[47] These tumours have in general a constant and homogeneous histopathological appearance. Bilaterality is reported in from 28% to 66%, with no information about the frequency of micro- or macroscopic bilateral disease. Survival seems to be related predominantly to extra-ovarian spread.[15,48] Extra-ovarian spread and peritoneal implants at the time of diagnosis have been reported in about 35% of patients. There is uncertainty whether these implants are true metastases or manifestations of multifocal in situ lesions of the peritoneum. Both conditions seem to occur, but, according to the literature, the latter occurs most frequently.[15,39,48] Some of these implants will progress to infiltrating cancer, while the majority will either remain stationary or regress after removal of the main ovarian tumour.[49–51] Survival would only be affected by true conversion to invasive disease, corresponding to stage III.[47,48] Foci of endo-salpingiosis and non-invasive implants are often present, suggesting that these implants arise from benign glandular elements of the peritoneal serosa (with potential for Müllerian differentiation). Examination of the nuclear DNA content of the implant and the ovarian tumour might contribute to the differential diagnosis between metastatic lesions and 'in situ' lesions. Recently, in the course of a study of proliferative serous tumours, an aggressive subgroup was identified by Kurman and Trimble,[27] and was called micropapillary serous carcinoma. This tumour has thin micropapillary projections. The mortality rate of the 26 cases that Burks et al[52] published was 15%. Seidman and Kurman[53] found that in 11 patients with micropapillary serous carcinoma, 7 (64%, all of whom had invasive implants) developed recurrences of invasive carcinoma and/or died of tumour. Tumours displaying a micropapillary growth pattern and serous borderline tumours with invasive implants should be classified as carcinomas.[53] In our opinion, and according to Silva et al,[54,55] all serous carcinomas are micropapillary, and if there is no stromal invasion and there are no implants outside the ovary then the tumour will most probably behave like other serous borderline tumours.

Mucinous borderline tumours

Mucinous borderline tumours account for 10–15% of all mucinous ovarian tumours. Grossly, borderline tumours cannot be distinguished from benign cystadenomas or cystadenocarcinomas. These tumours are often large and multilocular, and consist of cysts lined by atypical mucinous cells, which may be stratified (not exceeding three layers in thickness). They can display a different degree of nuclear atypia and mitotic figures. Focal areas of mural thickening, nodularity, or endophytic papillary excrescences are often present. Thus, for proper diagnosis, multiple and extensive sampling for histopathological examination is required. The incidence of bilaterality is low, at about 8%.

Extra-ovarian spread at the time of diagnosis is reported in about 10–15% of cases, nearly always as pseudomyxoma peritonei[39,47] (see below), and not as true peritoneal or omental implants. The mucinous tumours can be separated into endocervical (müllerian type) and intestinal types. Pseudomyxoma is only present in the intestinal type. The prognosis for patients with mucinous borderline tumours is dependent on stage of disease and presence of pseudomyxoma peritonei. The main controversy in mucinous neoplasms is whether a patient with a mucinous tumour in the ovary and in the appendix has two independent primaries, or has a primary appendiceal lesion and a metastatic ovarian lesion (see Chapter 4). We are in agreement with Silva et al,[54] and favour the possibility of multifocality, at least in some cases.

Pseudomyxoma peritonei

Although Rokitansky described this disease in 1842,[56] the term 'pseudomyxoma peritonei' is ascribed to Werth (in 1884).[57] Pseudomyxoma peritonei is characterized by the production of large amounts of cell-poor mucus, which is compartmentalized, in varying degrees, by dense fibrous tissue in the abdominal cavity. The condition may occur in any type of intraabdominal mucinous neoplasm, but originates most often in the appendix or the ovary. The ovarian tumours associated with pseudomyxoma peritonei may range in size from 4 cm to 40 cm. Pseudomyxoma peritonei is a poorly understood condition, and it is unclear whether its continuous production of gelatinous mucus is due to peritoneal implantation of neoplastic mucinous cells or to metaplasia of peritoneal cells into mucinous epithelium, induced by mucin. Beller et al[58] showed that this mucinous substance was 95.9% water, 1.6% lipid, and 2.9% acid sialomucopolysaccharide. In addition to containing CEA, the material is rich in gammaglobulin.[59] Pseudomyxoma peritonei is often associated with pseudomyxoma ovarii, but is not related to pre- or intraoperative rupture of a borderline mucinous tumour.[44] This condition is uncommon,

with a reported frequency of about 15% of mucinous borderline tumours. In the NRH study,[14] 30
of 178 patients (17%) had pseudomyxoma peritonei, and 9 of those 30 were associated with
pseudomyxoma of the appendix (5 with mucinous adenomas with atypia, and 4 with a muco-
coele of the appendix). None of the patients had
pseudomyxoma ovarii. Several reports indicate
that the relapse rate is high and the long-term
survival poor (with a 10-year survival rate of
18%).[8,15,60,61] However, in the NRH study,[14] 80%
of the patients with pseudomyxoma peritonei
survived for 5 years and 60% for 15 years. The
relationship to stage is unclear. Death is usually
due to bowel obstruction.

Non-serous/mucinous borderline tumours

Other types make up about 5% of all borderline
tumours (mixed 2%, endometrioid 2%, clear cell
<1%, and Brenner <1%).[14,35] The endometrioid
type is the most benign type and the clear cell
type has the highest malignant potential. Limited
knowledge exists about the biology and outcome
for patients with these tumours.

How does measurement of cellular DNA content help to define prognosis?

We have searched for new and more objective
prognostic parameters and have analysed the
possible prognostic value of DNA ploidy in a
large number (370) of patients followed over
many years.[9] One-hundred and seventy-four
patients had serous tumour, 178 had mucinous
tumour and 18 had other histological types. The
median follow-up was 149 months (range 15–83
months). A univariate analysis of prognostic variables in women with ovarian borderline tumours
is shown in Table 6.3.

Aneuploid tumours were strongly correlated
with older age, more advanced stage, non-serous
histological type, higher degree of atypia, and the

presence of pseudomyxoma peritonei. The different surgical procedures and the postoperative
treatment modalities, including 'observation',
were equally distributed between the diploid and
aneuploid groups. By univariate analysis, DNA
ploidy, stage, histological type, presence of residual tumour, pseudomyxoma peritonei, tumour
growth on the ovarian surface, tumour size, and
age were of prognostic significance, but degree of
cellular atypia was not.

By Cox multivariate analysis of a subgroup of
315 operated patients without residual disease
and evaluable DNA ploidy, DNA ploidy was the
strongest prognostic factor for long-term survival, followed by stage, histological type (non-
serous/mucinous), and age. The relative risk for
the individual patients could be calculated, and
patients could be divided into risk groups for
treatment decisions. Patients with aneuploid
tumours had a 19-fold increase in the risk of
dying of disease compared with patients with
diploid tumours (Table 6.4). In diploid stage I
tumours, the corrected survival rate observed in
patients who had received adjuvant treatment
was 98.8%, compared with 98.6% in those who
had not. The lowest-risk patients (100% long-
term survival) had diploid stage I serous/muci-
nous tumour, and were less than 40 years old.
The highest-risk patients (<35% long-term survival rate) had aneuploid stage III clear cell
tumours, and were older than 70 years (Table
6.5). DNA aneuploidy has now been reported in
several studies to be an indicator of poor prognosis in borderline tumours.[9,62,63]

DNA content of tumour cells can be measured
by flow cytometry (FCM) and image cytometry
(ICM) analyses. Klemi et al[64] attempted to correlate the distribution of nuclear DNA content,
defined as the ratio of aneuploid to diploid
tumour cells within a single tumour, with prognosis in patients with serous ovarian tumours.
They found aneuploidy in 1% of benign lesions,

Table 6.3 Univariate analysis of prognostic variables in 370 women with ovarian borderline tumours (survival calculated as 15 years' cancer-related survival)[a]

	No. of patients	Survival (%)	Chi-square (p-value)
Ploidy			
Diploid	239	95.9	136.4
Aneuploid	28	36.0	(<0.0001)
Not evaluable	49	97.9	
Stage			
I	311	96.6	74.2
II	20	75.0	(<0.0001)
III	39	57.9	
Age (years)			
>60	232	95.1	9.27
>60	138	84.3	(0. 002)
Histological type			
Serous	174	95.7	
Mucinous	178	88.3	
Other	18	76.2	(0.005)
Grade of atypia			
Mild	127	90.6	NS
Moderate	228	92.3	
Severe	15	80.0	
Size of tumour (cm)			
<10	154	96.7	8.04
>10	216	87.3	(0.005)
Growth on ovarian surface			
Yes	62	79.8	11.70
No	302	94.2	(0.0006)
Peritoneal pseudomyxoma			
Yes	30	60.9	43.15
No	340	94.0	(<0.0001)
Residual tumour			
Yes	6	33.3	43.79
No	364	96.7	(<0.0001)
Surgery[b]			
H + BSO + O	291	92.7	29.39[d]
H + BSO	33	86.3	(<0.0001)
BSO + O[c]	15	55.6	
BSO	17	100.0	
USO	14	100.0	
Postoperative treatment			
Residual postoperative treatment	6	33.3	
Adjuvant	277	91.2	NS
None	87	96.4	
Postoperative adjuvant treatment			
None	87	96.4	NS
Chemotherapy	52	87.6	
Irradiation	185	92.3	
Chemotherapy and irradiation	40	91.5	

[a] From reference 9, with permission.
[b] H, hysterectomy; BSO, bilateral salpingo-oophorectomy; O, omentectomy; USO, unilateral salpingo-oophorectomy.
[c] Including five patients with residual tumour; excluding these five patients, the survival rate was 76.2%.
[d] For patients without residual tumour; chi-square = 3.7, $p > 0.05$.

Table 6.4   Independent prognostic variables identified by Cox multivariate analysis for 15 years' cancer-related survival in 315 ovarian borderline tumours without residual tumour and ploidy estimation[a]

Variable	Coefficient	SD error	*p*-value	Hazard ratio
Ploidy (aneuploidy)	2.975	0.467	<0.001	19.59
Stage: II	2.135	0.633	<0.001	8.46
III	2.296	0.497	<0.001	9.93
Histology (others)	2.145	0.620	<0.001	8.54
Age: 40–70 years	1.263	0.672	0.060	3.54
>70 years	1.680	0.754	0.026	5.37

[a] From reference 9, with permission.

Table 6.5   Risk-group stratification in 315 ovarian borderline tumours without residual tumour according to ploidy, FIGO stage, histological type, and age group (≥40, 40–70, >70 years)[a]

	Low risk (RH 1–10)		Medium risk (RH 11–100)		High risk (RH >100)	
	Stage I	Stage II–III	Stage I	Stage II–III	Stage I	Stage II–III
Diploid						
Serous or mucinous	All ages	≥40 y		>40 y		
Other types	≤40 y		>40 y	≤40 y		>40 y
Aneuploid						
Serous or mucinous			≤70 y		>70 y	All ages
Other types					All ages	All ages

[a] From reference 9, with permission. RH, relative hazard; y, years.

in 17% of borderline tumours, and in 66% of serous invasive carcinomas. They were unable to find any evidence of aggressive behaviour associated with aneuploid tumours in serous borderline tumours.[64] In a Danish retrospective study,[65] DNA ploidy was measured in 121 borderline tumours. These authors found the same frequency of aneuploid tumours as Kaern et al,[9] but DNA ploidy was not associated with prognosis. Another study[66] has also been unsuccessful in showing DNA ploidy as an independent prognostic factor. Harlow et al[67] reported aneuploidy in 5 of 20 (25%) women who died with a diagnosis of a borderline tumour, compared with 9 out of 38 (24%) in surviving patients. However, several studies have confirmed our finding that DNA ploidy is a strong and independent prognostic factor.[62,63] Thus, some disagreement still exists concerning the prognostic value of DNA ploidy. This could partially be explained by the size of the sample analysed and the relatively short follow-up time in most studies. Alternatively, it could be due to a difficulty in the histopathological diagnosis of borderline tumours. Different methods for DNA ploidy analysis may also give contrary results. With FCM, a large number of cells are measured with high resolution, but without morphological control. Small aneuploid stem cell lines, in particular those with high DNA content (DNA index DI >2.5), may be overlooked and the tumour may be falsely classified as diploid. The sensitivity for detection of aneuploid cells is higher by ICM. However, this method is time-consuming, only a few cells are measured, and estimation of S phase has been practically impossible. Fortunately, the technique of ICM is improving, and it will probably replace FCM in the future. In our institution, a tumour is considered diploid only if it is diploid by both methods. Other reasons for differences in results may be associated with the preparation technique, selective cell loss, fixation, staining, measuring device, gating, and subjective assessments of the DNA histograms. Tumour heterogeneity may also contribute to different results. To overcome this problem, two or more different biopsy specimens from each tumour should be analysed. The few FCM studies including estimation of S-phase fraction (SPF) in borderline tumours have demonstrated very low values.[68] The diploid borderline tumours have lower SPF than diploid invasive tumours. This probably

reflects the slow proliferation of the borderline tumours that contain few replicating stem cell lines. It is also very important that the cell suspension used for DNA analysis is examined by the cytologist in order to be sure that the sample is representative.

While DNA ploidy assessments help to define the risk of recurrence, other factors are also involved, since some patients with diploid tumours succumb.

Is measurement of the proliferation marker Ki-67 useful in borderline ovarian tumours?

Henriksen et al[69] examined the expression of Ki-67 antigen in normal ovarian epithelium, benign and borderline ovarian tumours, and ovarian carcinomas. Immunohistochemical staining for Ki-67 was noted in none of the normal ovaries, 2 out of 11 (18%) benign tumours, 7 out of 9 (78%) borderline tumours, and 36 out of 45 (80%) ovarian carcinomas. They found a correlation of Ki-67 expression, flow-cytometric S-phase fraction, and DNA ploidy, but only 9 borderline tumours were analysed. Garzetti et al[70] found a significantly higher expression of the Ki-67 antigen in 28 serous ovarian carcinomas compared with 10 benign serous cystadenomas and 16 serous borderline tumours. Expression of Ki-67 in borderline tumours was intermediate between that of benign lesions and carcinomas.[70,71]

How useful is morphometry in defining risk of recurrence?

In 1981, Baak et al[72] showed that computer-assisted quantitative microscopic analysis was able to distinguish between benign, borderline, and malignant ovarian tumours. They applied this analysis in a blinded fashion to 20 ovarian tumours (19 borderline tumours and 1 invasive carcinoma). Morphometry identified the adenocarcinoma and the two patients with borderline tumours who died (two high-risk patients). They concluded that morphometry may be used to identify those patients who might not need adjuvant chemotherapy. However, their study included too few patients to draw any meaningful conclusions.

Three morphometric parameters seemed important: the mean nuclear area, the mean nuclear perimeter, and the mean of the short axis of the nucleus.[72] The prognostic value of the addition of morphometric parameters and DNA cytometric measurements to well-known prognostic factors in borderline tumours has been studied by Baak et al.[73] Morphometric measurements were performed in 303 tumours (279 diploid and 24 aneuploid tumours) out of the 321 borderline tumours with DNA ploidy assessments in the study by Kaern et al.[9] Multivariate analysis showed that DNA ploidy was the strongest independent prognostic parameter. The mean nuclear area and FIGO stage were also independent factors, whereas the histological subtype was of minor importance. Therefore DNA flow or image cytometry and morphometric analysis should be routinely applied in borderline ovarian tumours.

What can be learned about borderline tumours from study of serum tumour markers, cell surface receptors, growth factors, oncogenes, and tumour suppressor genes?

The prognostic value of CEA, CA19-9, and oestrogen and progesterone receptors does not seem as important in borderline ovarian tumours as in invasive ovarian carcinoma.[8,74–76]

Serum CA125 in borderline ovarian tumours

Although borderline tumours are quite common, the value of CA125 as a tumour marker in this type of tumour has not been investigated in depth.[75] We showed that serum CA125 was elevated preoperatively in 90% of the patients (18 of 20 tumours). The corresponding figures in other reports have varied between 46% and 75%.[38,77,78] In contrast to invasive ovarian carcinoma, we found no significant relationship between the preoperative CA125 level and FIGO stage. This could reflect the benign biological behaviour of this group of tumours, or it could be due to the relatively small number of patients studied. Rice et al[38] reported that all five patients with stage I had normal levels, while six of eight with advanced stages had elevated levels. We did not find any difference in the serum CA125 level between serous and mucinous tumours.[75] It is possible that borderline tumours have different biological behaviour from invasive serous cancer, so that CA125 levels were lower. Alternatively, the finding that mucinous tumours were significantly larger than serous ones may have overshadowed any difference in CA125 levels. We also showed that a greater tumour burden is needed to give an elevated serum CA125 level in borderline tumours than in invasive ovarian cancer. The serum CA125 levels were elevated in 90% of the patients in the preoperative group with a tumour mass of median 10 cm diameter, but in the group with sampling four weeks after surgery, serum CA125 levels were elevated in only 67% of patients with residual tumour of 2 cm or more and in none of patients with residual tumour less than 2 cm. In addition, no difference in the CA125 levels was found between patients with or without residual disease after surgery. Unlike in cases of invasive ovarian cancer, a postoperative serum CA125 level over 35 U/ml in patients with borderline tumours and no residual disease after primary surgery did not imply poorer prognosis. However, the observation time was relatively short, so a definite conclusion cannot be drawn.

Serum CA125 levels in patients with borderline tumours tended to correlate with response to chemotherapy. However, the limited number of patients with residual disease after primary surgery or at disease relapse who had elevated serum CA125 levels will hamper the clinical application of this finding. Only one of six patients with disease relapse in our study[75] had an elevated serum CA125 level. Of the five patients who had CA125 serum level less than 35 U/ml at that time, one had a serum CA125 level of 55 U/ml at the time of primary surgery. Thus, serum CA125 level is of limited value as a tumour marker in patients with borderline tumours. Although elevated serum CA125 levels were observed in 90% of the patients, this did not correlate with FIGO stage. Serum levels were only elevated in 9% of samples obtained postoperatively from patients with residual disease. None of the patients without residual disease after primary surgery with an elevated serum CA125 level relapsed. Serum CA125 levels were elevated in only 17% of patients with disease relapse.

Growth factors

Henriksen et al[76] studied markers of different growth regulatory mechanisms in benign, borderline, and malignant tumours, compared with normal ovaries. The significance of these markers in the malignant group was also evaluated by comparing clinical and pathological variables. Platelet-derived growth factor (PDGF) and its receptors showed no expression in normal ovarian epithelium or benign tumour cells, but PDGF and PDGFα receptors stained positive in tumour cells in a substantial number of borderline and malignant tumours. Furthermore, expression of PDGF receptors in malignant tumours was strongly correlated with decreased survival even in advanced disease.

Expression of oncogenes and tumour suppressor genes

Germline mutations in the BRCA1 and BRCA2 genes are known to be associated with an increased risk of breast and/or ovarian carcinoma. However, there is uncertainty about the heritable basis of borderline ovarian tumours and whether these tumours represent an early form of invasive disease. This has been addressed by Gottlieb et al,[79] who analysed the rates of BRCA1 and BRCA2 mutations in Ashkenazi Jewish patients with borderline ovarian tumours. Forty-six patients with borderline tumours and 54 patients with invasive epithelial ovarian cancers were studied. One (2.2%) of the 46 patients with borderline tumours was identified as a carrier of the BRCA1 mutation, and no patients were found to carry the BRCA2 mutation. They concluded that invasive epithelial and borderline ovarian tumours appear to differ in their genetic predisposition and in the molecular mechanisms underlying their genesis.

Wong et al[80] studied the prevalence and significance of HER2/neu amplification in 34 borderline-type tumours of the ovary. The HER2/neu gene was amplified in 5 out of 34 borderline tumours (15%), but none of the 20 specimens of normal ovaries showed amplification. They did not find any correlation between HER2/neu amplification and cell type or atypia of tumour. Their study suggested that HER2/neu amplification occurs infrequently in early invasive and borderline ovarian tumours, making it unlikely that such an amplification is an early event in ovarian carcinogenesis.

Lu et al[81] have found evidence for multifocal origin of bilateral and advanced human serous borderline ovarian tumours. They studied whether bilateral or extra-ovarian serous borderline lesions were metastases from the original tumour or represented separate primary tumours. DNA specimens from multiple tumour sites and normal tissue controls were obtained in eight women with bilateral or extra-ovarian serous borderline tumours. The pattern of loss of heterozygosity (LOH) at the androgen receptor locus on the X chromosome was evaluated in the multiple tumour sites. Multifocality was defined when alternate patterns of X-chromosome inactivation occurred. In two out of eight patients, the left and right ovarian tumour sites had different androgen receptor alleles inactivated, indicating that the bilateral tumours were derived independently. Their results suggest that bilateral and advanced-stage serous borderline ovarian tumours are multifocal in origin, which is in contrast to invasive epithelial ovarian cancer, which has been shown to be unifocal in origin.

Previous studies have demonstrated a frequent LOH at chromosome 6q, in particular 6q 24–27 locus, in human epithelial ovarian cancer. This suggests that an ovarian-cancer-specific tumour suppressor gene may be located at this chromosomal region. The pattern of LOH at chromosome 6q in borderline ovarian tumours has been analysed by Rodabaugh et al.[82] They have used polymerase chain reaction (PCR) amplification of tandem repeat polymorphism to study the pattern of allelic loss at chromosome 6q in borderline ovarian tumours. DNA extracted from 45 borderline tumours and 25 invasive tumours was used. The invasive tumours demonstrated the highest percentage of LOH (4 out of 15) at the 6q 25–27 locus site. In contrast, the borderline ovarian tumours did not show any LOH at this locus. Furthermore, no other primer pair showed LOH in more than one borderline tumour. Their results display a sharp contrast in the pattern of LOH between invasive and borderline ovarian tumours, and suggest that LOH at chromosome 6q may not be involved in the development and progression of borderline ovarian tumours.

Lee et al[83] investigated a series of 19 human ovarian carcinomas and 17 borderline ovarian tumours to determine the LOH on chromosome 17p and possible concurrent p53 gene mutations. The p53 mutation was observed in 7 of 19 (36.8%) malignant ovarian tumours, and it was predominantly observed in tumours with allelic loss on 17p. Although 9 out of 17 borderline ovarian tumours showed shifted bands on single-strand conformation polymorphism analysis, only one case was proven to have a point mutation in direct sequencing. Lee et al[83] also found positive p53 immunoreactivity in 3 of the 17 borderline ovarian tumours. They concluded that loss or inactivation of tumour suppressor gene function by chromosome 17p allelic deletions or p53 mutations are important genetic changes in ovarian cancer and borderline tumours.

At the NRH, Skomedal et al[84] have studied the frequency of p53 and MDM2 protein overexpression in a series of 27 borderline ovarian tumours and 347 stage I ovarian carcinomas, and investigated these two proteins as prognostic markers. p53 and MDM2 alterations were detected in 15% and 4% of borderline tumours, respectively. The level of p53 alterations in borderline tumours (15%) in the NRH study is in agreement with reported frequencies of 3–14% in some studies,[85–88] but not with others.[89–92] Our results suggest that p53 abnormalities play a crucial role and MDM2 abnormalities a minor role in the development of borderline and early ovarian carcinoma. There was, however, no significant correlation between p53 or MDM2 alterations and survival. We agree with Lipponen et al[88] that p53 oncoprotein overexpression is not a feature of borderline ovarian tumours, and therefore p53 expression analysis has no value in predicting the prognosis of these tumours. If there is an orderly progression from a benign or borderline tumour to early and further to advanced invasive ovarian cancer, then p53 involvement in the carcinogenesis is a late event. This is in contrast to the results of Klemi et al,[85] who investigated the occurrence of p53 expression by immunohistochemistry in benign, borderline, and malignant serous ovarian tumours, and also studied the correlation of p53 with survival. Twenty-four (53%) of the 45 histopathologically malignant tumours were positive for p53, whereas neither the 6 benign nor the 10 borderline tumours showed positive staining. Klemi et al[85] claimed that p53 immunostaining may have diagnostic value in discriminating between borderline and malignant serous ovarian tumours. They also indicated the importance of p53 as a prognostic factor for survival.

Mok et al[93] noted when using RNA fingerprinting (RAP) strategy and Northern blot analysis, a differentially expressed sequence *DOC2*, which is detectable in all normal human ovarian surface epithelial cell cultures, but not in ovarian cancer cell lines and tissue. The *DOC2* gene is located on 5p13. In situ immunohistochemistry performed on normal ovaries and on benign, borderline, and invasive ovarian tumour tissues showed downregulation of DOC2 protein. When *DOC2* was transfected into the ovarian carcinoma cell line SKOV3, the stable transfectants showed significantly reduced growth rate and ability to form tumours in nude mice. The data of Mok et al[93] suggest that downregulation of *DOC2* may play an important role in ovarian borderline carcinogenesis.

What is the long-term outcome of patients with borderline ovarian tumours?

We have recently examined histology-specific prognostic trends in five-year relative survival of 2343 patients with ovarian borderline tumours based on data from the population-based cancer Registry of Norway.[94] The age-adjusted five-year survival rate remained almost constant at about 93% between 1970 and 1993. In general, the survival of patients with serous tumours was lower than that of patients with mucinous tumours. The age-adjusted one-, three-, five-, and 10-year relative survival rates of patients with mucinous tumours were 98%, 97%, 97%, and 95%, respectively, while for patients with serous tumours they were 96%, 93%, 90%, and 90%. The relative risk of dying increased with age at diagnosis (Table 6.6). Much of the large increase by age was explained by the increase in mortality of intercurrent disease. The five-year relative survival rate in patients aged 0–44 was 99%, while it was 85% in patients aged 75–89 years. Before the 1970s, borderline tumours may have been recorded as well-differentiated carcinomas. Consequently, the improvement in prognosis observed from the 1950s onwards may have been underestimated. However, some of these tumours are biologically aggressive, and in the two NRH studies with long follow-up already mentioned, a tendency to late recurrences and death from disease was shown.[14,33] In general, the outcome of borderline tumours is favourable, and has remained unchanged since the 1970s.

The predictors of long-term outcome may be summarized from the results of the retrospective study from the NRH of 370 borderline tumours treated between 1970 and 1982. Kearn et al[14] showed by multivariate analyses only three independent prognostic factors for disease-free and long-term survival; these were FIGO stage ($p < 0.0001$), histological type ($p = 0.014$), and age ($p = 0.012$). A low-risk group (100% disease-free survival) was characterized by stage I disease, serous histology, and age less than 40 years. A high-risk group (75% or higher risk of dying of disease) had serous or mucinous tumours, stage II–III disease, and age greater than 70 years, or had a non-serous–mucinous tumour and stage II–III disease. The inclusion of DNA ploidy in the multivariate analysis showed that it was the strongest prognostic factor for long-term survival, followed by stage, histological type, and age.

Table 6.6   Multivariate survival analysis of patients with borderline tumours diagnosed between 1970 and 1993 with a five-year follow-up: relative risk of dying according to age, stage, period of diagnosis, and histology[a]

	Relative risk[b]	95% confidence interval	No. of patients
Age (years)			
0–44	1.00	Referent	803
45–64	4.70	2.46–8.99	843
65–74	11.09	5.84–21.05	430
75–89	34.16	18.23–64.02	245
Stage			
Localized	1.00	Referent	2165
Regional spread	2.52	0.80–7.96	21
Distant metastases	1.78	1.08–2.94	112
Unknown	1.14	0.36–3.57	23
Period			
1970–1973	1.00	Referent	331
1974–1978	1.52	0.95–2.42	459
1979–1983	1.42	0.88–2.29	372
1984–1988	1.07	0.66–1.72	495
1989–1993	1.24	0.75–2.05	664
Histology			
Serous	1.00	Referent	994
Mucinous	0.72	0.54–0.95	1202
Other	1.30	0.79–2.12	125

[a]From reference 94, with permission.
[b]Adjusted for all other variables in the table.

LEARNING POINTS

✤ DNA ploidy, morphometry, FIGO stage, histological type, and age are independent prognostic factors in patients with epithelial ovarian borderline tumours without residual tumour after primary surgery.

✤ Primary surgery should consist of bilateral oophorectomy, omentectomy, and peritoneal washings. Total abdominal hysterectomy is optional if the curettage specimen is negative. Retroperitoneal lymph node sampling is unnecessary.

✤ Secondary cytoreductive surgery is recommended for patients with recurrent disease, and repeated laparotomies are indicated in patients with pseudomyxoma peritonei. The value of peritonectomy is uncertain.

❖ Conservative surgery (unilateral salpingo-oophorectomy – without the need for random biopsy of a normal-looking contralateral ovary) is indicated for young fertile women with diploid stage IA tumours who have not completed their family. As intraoperative DNA ploidy analysis is not possible, further surgery is necessary if the DNA analysis indicates aneuploidy, or if the histological examination reveals disseminated disease.

❖ Routine use of postoperative adjuvant treatment is not indicated outside protocols in patients with stage I or II or optimally debulked stage III tumours. Borderline tumours respond poorly to chemotherapy.

❖ Oestrogen replacement should be given to patients to prevent cardiovascular disease, osteoporosis, and climacteric disorders.

REFERENCES

1. Taylor HC, Malignant and semi-malignant tumours of the ovary. *Surg Gynecol Obstet* 1929; 48: 204.

2. Taylor HC, Alsop WE, Spontaneous regression of peritoneal implantations from ovarian papillary cystadenoma. *Am J Cancer* 1932; **16**: 1305.

3. Kottmeier HL, The classification and treatment of ovarian tumours. *Acta Obstet Gynecol Scand* 1952; **31**: 313.

4. Woodruff JD, Novak ER, Papillary serous tumors of the ovary. *Am J Obstet Gynecol* 1954; 67: 1112.

5. Ingelman-Sundberg A, Classification and staging of malignant tumors in the female pelvis. *Acta Obstet Gynecol Scand* 1971; **50**: 1.

6. Kottmeier HL, Kolstad P, McGarrity KA et al, *Annual Report on Results of Treatment in Gynecologic Cancer*, Vol 17. Stockholm: Radiumhemmet, 1973.

7. Serov SF, Scully RE, Sobin LH, *International Histological Classification of Tumors*, No. 9. *Histological Typing in Ovarian Tumors*. Geneva: World Health Organization, 1973.

8. Hoskins PJ, Ovarian tumors of low malignant potential: borderline epithelial ovarian carcinoma. In *Epithelial Cancer of the Ovary* (Lawton FG, Neijt JP, Swenerton KD, eds). London: BMJ Publishing, 1995: 112.

9. Kaern J, Tropé CG, Kristensen GB et al, DNA ploidy, the most important prognostic factor in patients with borderline tumors of the ovary. *Int J Gynecol Cancer* 1993; **3**: 349.

10. Barnhill DR, Kurman RJ, Brady MF et al, Preliminary analysis of the behavior of stage I ovarian serous tumors of low malignant potential: a Gynecologic Oncology Group study. *J Clin Oncol* 1995; **13**: 2752–6.

11. Chambers JT, Merino MJ, Kohorn EI et al, Borderline ovarian tumors. *Am J Obstet Gynecol* 1988; **159**: 1088.

12. Leake JF, Currie JL, Rosenschein NB et al, Long term follow-up of ovarian tumors of low malignant potential. *Gynecol Oncol* 1992; **47**: 150–8.

13. Lim-Tan SK, Cajigas HG, Scully RE, Ovarian cystectomy for serous borderline tumors: a follow-up study of 35 cases. *Obstet Gynecol* 1988; **72**: 775–81.

14. Kaern J, Tropé CG, Abeler VA, A retrospective study of 370 borderline tumors of the ovary treated at the Norwegian Radium Hospital from 1970 to 1982. A review of clinicopathologic features and treatment modalities. *Cancer* 1993; **71**: 1810–20.

15. Kliman L, Rome RM, Fortune DW, Low malignant potential tumors of the ovary: a study of 76 cases. *Obstet Gynecol* 1986; **68**: 338–44.

16. Tazelarr HD, Bostwick DG, Ballon SC et al, Conservative treatment of borderline ovarian tumors. *Obstet Gynecol* 1985; **66**: 417.

17. Trimble EL, Trimble LC, Epithelial ovarian tumors of low malignant potential. In: *Cancer of the Ovary* (Markman M, Hoskins WJ, eds). New York: Raven Press, 1993: Chap 31.

18. Ronnett BM, Kurman RJ, Schmookler BM et al, Pseudomyxoma peritonei in women: a clinicopathologic analysis of 30 cases with emphasis

on site of origin, prognosis, and relationship to ovarian mucinous tumors of low malignant potential. *Hum Pathol* 1995; **26**: 509–24.

19. Seidman JD, Elsayed AM, Sobin LH et al, Association of mucinous tumors of the ovary and appendix. A clinicopathologic study of 25 cases. *Am J Surg Pathol* 1993; **17**: 22–34.

20. Limber GK, King RE, Silverberg SG, Pseudomyxoma peritonei: a report of ten cases. *Ann Surg* 1973; **178**: 587–93.

21. Sugarbaker PH, Jablonski KA, Prognostic features of 51 colorectal and 130 appendiceal cancer patients with peritoneal carcinomatosis treated by cytoreductive surgery and intraperitoneal chemotherapy. *Ann Surg* 1995; **221**: 124–32.

22. Leake JF, Rader JS, Woodruff JD et al, Retroperitoneal lymphatic involvement with epithelial ovarian tumors of low malignant potential. *Gynecol Oncol* 1991; **42**: 124–30.

23. NIH Consensus Development Panel on Ovarian Cancer, Ovarian cancer: screening treatment, and follow-up. *JAMA* 1995; **273**: 491.

24. Creaseman WT, Park R, Norris H et al, Stage I borderline ovarian tumors. *Obstet Gynecol* 1982; **59**: 93–6.

25. Young RC, Walton LA, Ellenberg SS et al, Adjuvant therapy in stage I and II epithelial ovarian cancer. Results of two randomized trials. *N Engl J Med* 1990; **322**: 1021–7.

26. Tropé C, Kaern J, Vergote IB et al, Are borderline tumors of the ovary overtreated both surgically and systemically? A review of four prospective randomized trials including 253 patients with borderline tumors. *Gynecol Oncol* 1993; **51**: 236–43.

27. Kurman RJ, Trimble CL, The behaviour of serous tumour of low malignant potential: are they ever malignant? *Int J Gynecol Pathol* 1993; **12**: 120–7.

28. Gershenson DM, Silva EG, Serous ovarian tumors of low malignant potential with peritoneal implants. *Cancer* 1990; **65**: 578–85.

29. Sutton GP, Bundy BN, Omura GA et al, Stage III ovarian tumors of low malignant potential treated with cisplatin combination therapy (a Gynecologic Oncology Group study). *Gynecol Oncol* 1991; **41**: 230–3.

30. Fernandez RN, Daly JM, Pseudomyxoma peritonei. *Arch Surg* 1981; **115**: 409–14.

31. Sandenbergh HA, Woodruff JD, Histogenesis of pseudomyxoma peritonei. *Obstet Gynecol* 1977; **49**: 339–45.

32. Koonings PP, Campbell K, Mishell DR et al, Relative frequency of primary ovarian neoplasms: a 10-year review. *Obstet Gynecol* 1989; **74**: 921–6.

33. Aure JC, Hoeg K, Kolstad P, Clinical and histologic studies of ovarian carcinoma. Long-term follow-up of 990 cases. *Obstet Gynecol* 1971; **37**: 1–9.

34. Katsube Y, Berg JW, Silverberg SG, Epidemiologic pathology of ovarian tumors: histopathologic review of primary ovarian neoplasms diagnosed in the Denver Standard Metropolitan Statistical Area, 1 July–31 December 1969 and 1 July–31 December 1979. *Int J Gynecol Pathol* 1982; **1**: 3–16.

35. Levi F, Franceschi S, La Vecchia C et al, Epidemiologic pathology of ovarian cancer from the Vaud Cancer Registry, Switzerland. *Ann Oncol* 1993; **4**: 289–94.

36. Bjørge T, Engeland A, Hansen S et al, Trends in the incidence of ovarian cancer and borderline tumours in Norway. 1954–1993. *Int J Cancer* 1997; **71**: 780–6.

37. Auranen A, Grenman S, Mäkinen J et al, Borderline ovarian tumors in Finland: epidemiology and familial occurrence. *Am J Epidemiol* 1996; **144**: 548–53.

38. Rice LW, Berkowitz RS, Mark SD et al, Epithelial ovarian tumors of borderline malignancy. *Gynecol Oncol* 1990; **39**: 195–8.

39. Russel P, Borderline epithelial tumours of the ovary: a conceptual dilemma. *Clin Obstet Gynaecol* 1984; **11**: 259.

40. Ewertz M, Kjaer SK, Ovarian cancer incidence and mortality in Denmark, 1943–1982. *Int J Cancer* 1988; **42**: 690–6.

41. Fathalla MF, Incessant ovulation – a factor in ovarian neoplasia? *Lancet* 1971; **ii**: 163.

42. Cassagrande JT, Louie EW, Pike MC et al, Incessant ovulation and ovarian cancer. *Lancet* 1979; **ii**: 170.

43. Whittemore AS, Wu ML, Pfaffenbarger RS et al, Epithelial ovarian cancer and the ability to conceive. *Cancer Res* 1989; **49**: 4047–52.

44. Hart WR, Norris HJ, Borderline and malignant mucinous tumors of the ovary. *Cancer* 1973; **31**: 1031–45.

45. Scully RE, *Tumors of the Ovary and Maldeveloped Gonads. Atlas of Tumor Pathology,* Second Series, Fascicle 16. Washington, DC: Armed Forces Institute of Pathology, 1979.

46. Baak JP, Langley FA, Talerman A et al, The prognostic variability of ovarian tumor grading by different pathologists. *Gynecol Oncol* 1987; **27**: 166–72.

47. Fox H, The concept of borderline malignancy in ovarian tumours: a reappraisal. *Curr Top Pathol* 1989; **78**: 111–34.

48. Tasker M, Langley FA, The outlook for women with borderline epithelial tumours of the ovary. *Br J Obstet Gynaecol* 1985; **92**: 969–73.

49. Bell DA, Weinstock MA, Scully RE, Peritoneal implants of ovarian serous borderline tumors: histologic features and prognosis. *Cancer* 1988; **62**: 2212–22.

50. Bell DA, Scully RE, Serous borderline tumours of the peritoneum. *Am J Surg Pathol* 1990; **14**: 230–9.

51. Bell DA, Ovarian surface epithelial–stromal tumors. *Hum Pathol* 1991; **22**: 750–62.

52. Burks RT, Sherman ME, Kurman RJ, Micropapillary serous carcinoma of the ovary: distinctive low-grade carcinoma related to serous borderline tumors. *Am J Surg Pathol* 1996; **20**: 1319–30.

53. Seidman JD, Kurman R, Subclassification of serous borderline tumours of the ovary into benign and malignant types. A clinicopathologic study of 65 advanced stage cases. *Am J Surg Pathol* 1996; **20**: 1331–45.

54. Silva EG, Kurman RJ, Russel P et al, Symposium: ovarian tumours of borderline malignancy. *Int J Gynecol Pathol* 1996; **15**: 281.

55. Silva EG, Tornos C, Zhuang A et al, Tumor recurrence in stage I ovarian serous low malignant potential neoplasms. *Mod Pathol* 1996; **9**: 987 (abst).

56. Fraenkel E, Uber das sogenannte pseudomyxoma peritonei. *Munch Med Wsch* 1901; **48**: 965.

57. Werth R, Pseudomyxoma peritonei. *Arch Gynecol Obstet* 1884; **24**: 100.

58. Beller FK, Zimmerman RE, Niemhaus H, Biochemical identification of mucus of pseudomyxoma peritonei as the basis for mucolytic treatment. *Am J Obstet Gynecol* 1986; **155**: 970–3.

59. Sutton GP, Ovarian tumors of low malignant potential in ovarian cancer. In: *Ovarian Cancer* (Rubin SC, Sutton GP, eds). New York: McGraw-Hill, 1993: 425.

60. Nakashima N, Nagasaka T, Oiwa N et al, Ovarian epithelial tumors of borderline malignancy in Japan. *Gynecol Oncol* 1990; **38**: 90–8.

61. Rutgers JL, Scully RE, Ovarian müllerian mucinous papillary cystadenomas of borderline malignancy. A clinicopathologic analysis. *Cancer* 1988; **61**: 340–8.

62. Friedlander ML, Russell P, Taylor IW et al, Flow cytometric analysis of cellular DNA content as an adjunct to the diagnosis of ovarian tumours of borderline malignancy. *Pathology* 1984; **16**: 301–6.

63. Drescher CW, Flint A, Hopkins MP et al, Prognostic significance of DNA content and nuclear morphology in borderline ovarian tumors. *Gynecol Oncol* 1993; **48**: 242–6.

64. Klemi PJ, Joensuu H, Kiilholma P et al, Clinical significance of abnormal nuclear DNA content in serous ovarian tumors. *Cancer* 1988; **62**: 2005–10.

65. Andersen ES, Nielsen K, Nielsen RH, Borderline epithelial tumours of the ovary. In: *Proceedings of IGCS (International Gynecologic*

Cancer Society), Third Biennial Meeting, Cairns, Australia, 1991 (abst).

66. Seidman JD, Norris HJ, Griffin JL et al, DNA flow cytometric analysis of serous ovarian tumours of low malignant potential. *Cancer* 1993; **71**: 3947–51.

67. Harlow BL, Fuhr JE, McDonald TW et al, Flow cytometry as a prognostic indicator in women with borderline epithelial ovarian tumors. *Gynecol Oncol* 1993; **50**: 305–9.

68. Kühn W, Kaufmann M, Feichter GE et al, DNA flow cytometry, clinical and morphological parameters as prognostic factors for advanced malignant and borderline ovarian tumors. *Gynecol Oncol* 1989; **33**: 360–7.

69. Henriksen R, Ovarian Carcinogenesis. A Study of Markers for Growth Regulatory Mechanisms in Epithelial Ovarian Cancer. Thesis, Uppsala University, 1994.

70. Garzetti GG, Ciavattini A, Goteri G, Ki-67 antigen immunostaining (MIB monoclonal antibody) in serous ovarian tumors: index of proliferation activity with prognostic significance. *Gynecol Oncol* 1995; **56**: 169.

71. Trimble E, Kaern J, Tropé C, Management of borderline tumors of the ovary. In: *Ovarian Cancer: Controversies in Management* (Gershenson DM, McGuire WP, eds). Churchill Livingstone: New York, 1998: 195.

72. Baak JP, Blanco AA, Kurver PH et al, Quantitation of borderline and malignant mucinous ovarian tumors. *Histopathology* 1981; **5**: 353–60.

73. Baak JP, Abeler VM, Broechaert MAM et al, Morphometry and DNA cytometry have strong and additional prognostic value in borderline ovarian tumours with long term follow up. Poster presentation at the Pathological Society of Great Britain and Ireland, Free University Amsterdam, 171st Meeting, 5–7 July 1995.

74. Trimble CL, Trimble EL, Management of epithelial ovarian tumors of low malignant potential. *Gynecol Oncol* 1994; **55**: 52–67.

75. Makar A Ph, Kaern J, Kristensen GB et al, Elevation of serum CA 125 level as a tumor marker in patients with borderline ovarian tumors. *Int J Gynecol Cancer* 1993; **3**: 299.

76. Henriksen R, Funa K, Wilander E et al, Expression and prognostic significance of platelet-derived growth factor and its receptors in epithelial ovarian neoplasms. *Cancer Res* 1993; **53**: 4550–4.

77. Tholander B, Taube A, Lindgren A et al, Pre-treatment serum levels of CA 125, carcinoembryonic antigen, tissue polypeptide antigen, and placental alkaline phosphatase, in patients with ovarian carcinoma, borderline tumors, or benign adnexal masses: relevance for differential diagnosis. *Gynecol Oncol* 1990; **39**: 16–25.

78. Mogensen O, Mogensen B, Jakobsen A, CA 125 in the diagnosis of pelvic masses. *Eur J Clin Oncol* 1989; **25**: 1187–90.

79. Gotlieb WH, Friedman E, Bar-Sade RB et al, Rates of Jewish ancestral mutation in BRCA1 and BRCA2 in borderline ovarian tumors. *J Natl Cancer Inst* 1998; **90**: 995–1000.

80. Wong YF, Cheung TH, Lam SK et al, Prevalence and significance of HER-2/neu amplification in epithelial ovarian cancer. *Gynecol Obstet Invest* 1995; **40**: 209–12.

81. Lu KH, Bell DA, Welch WR et al, Evidence for the multifocal origin of bilateral and advanced human serous borderline ovarian tumors. *Cancer Res* 1998; **58**: 2328–30.

82. Rodabaugh KJ, Welch WR, Bell DA et al, Detailed deletion mapping of chromosome 6q in borderline ovarian tumors. *Proc Annu Meet Am Assoc Cancer Res* 1995; **36**: A3246.

83. Lee JH, Kang YS, Park SY et al, p53 mutation in epithelial ovarian carcinoma and borderline ovarian tumor. *Cancer Genet Cytogenet* 1995; **85**: 43–50.

84. Skomedal H, Kristensen GB, Abeler VM et al, TP53 protein accumulation and gene mutation in relation to overexpression of mdm2 protein in ovarian borderline tumours and stage I carcinomas. *J Pathol* 1997; **181**: 158–65.

85. Klemi PJ, Takahasi S, Joensuu H et al, Immunohistochemical detection of p53 protein in borderline and malignant serous

ovarian tumors. *Int J Gynecol Pathol* 1994; **13**: 228–33.

86. Kupryjanczyk J, Bell DA, Yandell DW, p53 expression in ovarian borderline tumors and stage I carcinomas. *Am J Clin Pathol* 1994; **102**: 671–6.

87. Berchuck A, Kohler MF, Hopkins MP et al, Overexpression of p53 is not a feature of benign and early-stage borderline epithelial ovarian tumors. *Gynecol Oncol* 1994; **52**: 232–6.

88. Lipponen P, Yliskoski M, Syrjanen K et al, Overexpression of p53 in borderline ovarian tumors. *Anticancer Res* 1995; **15**(5A): 1765.

89. Teneriello MG, Ebina M, Linnoila RI et al, p53 and Ki-ras gene mutations in epithelial ovarian neoplasm. *Cancer Res* 1993; **53**: 3103–8.

90. Zheng J, Benedict WF, Xu HJ et al, Genetic disparity between morphologically benign cysts contiguous to ovarian carcinomas and solitary cystadenomas. *J Natl Cancer Inst* 1995; **87**: 1146–53.

91. Kiyokawa T, Alteration of p53 in ovarian cancer: its occurrence and maintenance in tumor progression. *Int J Gynecol Pathol* 1994; **13**: 311–18.

92. Kappes S, Milde-Langosch K, Kressin P et al, p53 mutations in ovarian tumors, detected by temperature-gradient gel electrophoresis, direct sequencing, and immunohistochemistry. *Int J Cancer* 1995; **64**: 52–9.

93. Mok SC, Chan WY, Wong KK et al, DOC-2, a candidate tumor suppressor gene in human epithelial ovarian cancer. *Oncogene* 1998; **16**: 2381–7.

94. Bjørge T, Engeland A, Hansen S et al, Prognosis of patients with ovarian cancer and borderline tumours diagnosed in Norway between 1954 and 1993. *Int J Cancer* 1998; **75**: 663–70.

7
Laparoscopic surgery for an assumed benign mass

J Baptist Trimbos, Frank-Willem Jansen

INTRODUCTION

It is generally accepted that ovarian cancer should preferably not be treated by laparoscopic surgery. This point of view is based on two assumptions:

1. Rupturing of a malignant ovarian cyst during surgery can cause dissemination of tumour cells. Slow leakage of ovarian cancer cells into the abdominal cavity can adversely effect the prognosis of the patient.[1,2]
2. A further objection to laparoscopic surgery is the increased risk of trocar site metastases.[3,4]

Laparoscopic removal of malignant ovarian cysts should be avoided preoperatively by an optimal clinical diagnosis. By discriminating preoperatively between a benign and possibly malignant cyst, the chances of removing an ovarian cancer by a laparoscope should be reduced. In this respect, the most important preoperative parameters are the patient's age, the ultrasonographic qualities of the cyst and the serum level of tumour markers.

Acute spillage during surgery may not necessarily worsen the prognosis if appropriate action is taken. It would be reasonable to assume that the risk from acute surgical spillage is small

or negligible because the duration of spillage is brief and there is every opportunity to clean the potentially contaminated operating field with saline or sterile water.[2] A number of studies have failed to confirm that acute spillage during surgery is an adverse prognostic factor.[5–7] Furthermore, the risk of leaking cancer cells can be diminished or even minimized by using endoscopic pouch bags during laparoscopic surgery. This will diminish the occurrence of trocar site tumour implants. However, even after taking these precautions, the risk of tumour seeding remains, and the use of laparoscopic surgery for ovarian cancer should therefore be discouraged.

CASE HISTORY

A 53-year-old patient had symptoms of abdominal fullness and mechanical pressure on her urinary bladder. Her history included a hysterectomy for fibroids and a radical vulvectomy with lymph node dissection for a stage I well-differentiated squamous cell carcinoma of the vulva. Pelvic ultrasonography suggested a simple ovarian cyst 7 cm in diameter. A laparoscopic examination was performed, and a mobile right ovarian cyst was seen without additional pelvic abnormalities. The other ovary looked normal, as did the remainder of the peritoneal cavity. One hundred and twenty-five millilitres of yellowish fluid was aspirated and the cyst disappeared completely. The cytological examination showed macrophages and a mixed inflammatory cell population. No atypical cells were found.

She returned six weeks later because of pelvic pain, and pelvic examination showed an additional right-sided cystic pelvic mass and a possible mass on the left side as well. She was referred to a department of gynaecological oncology. A laparotomy was performed eight weeks after the initial laparoscopic examination. The right ovary contained an 8 cm cystic mass with surface excrescences. The left ovary was concealed in a tumour mass involving the sigmoid colon and bladder peritoneum. Numerous metastatic nodules were present on the sigmoid colon and its mesentery, and the omentum contained a 10 cm metastasis. Carcinomatosis peritonei was present. Histopathological examination showed a poorly differentiated serous adenocarcinoma of the right ovary with extensive peritoneal metastases. After cytoreductive surgery, treatment with combination therapy was instituted.[2]

How can we discriminate a benign cyst from a malignant cyst preoperatively?

Age

With increasing age, the relative risk that an ovarian cyst is malignant increases. Koonings et al[8] showed in a retrospective study that the relative frequency of malignant epithelial ovarian tumours increased during every decade up to the age of 60. Before age 50, 13% of ovarian tumours were malignant, whereas this figure rose to 45% in postmenopausal women. Table 7.1 shows the relative risk for the occurrence of malignancy in patients with an ovarian cyst versus the patient's age.[8] The findings show that the risk of ovarian malignancy is particularly relevant in postmenopausal patients.

Table 7.1   Relative risk of malignancy in patients with an ovarian cyst

Age (years)	Relative risk of malignancy
<10	2
20	1
30	3.4
40	8.6
50	11.3
60	12.1
70	7.2

Ultrasonography

Recent developments in ultrasonography have led to this non-invasive technique being regarded as the most accurate method to define the size, shape and internal structure of pelvic cystic tumours. In various studies, the relation between ultrasonographic characteristics and the risk of malignancy has been assessed.[9–11] It could be demonstrated that ultrasound examination could accurately predict the risk of ovarian cancer in the case of an ovarian cyst. The following characteristics are relevant.

Size

Transvaginal ultrasonography can adequately determine the size of a cystic pelvic tumour. This method is more accurate than manual pelvic examination.[12] Also, the interobserver variation between diameters of ovarian cysts measured by ultrasound was shown to be minimal.[13]

The size of an ovarian cyst is important, because the chance of malignancy of an ovarian tumour increases with tumour diameter. Allen and Hertig[14] found cysts greater than 15 cm in

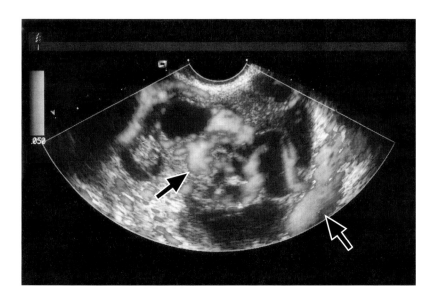

Figure 7.1
Transvaginal sonographic image of an ovarian carcinoma (arrows). The tumour is multilocular, with solid components and areas of very strong neovascularization on colour Doppler imaging. (Courtesy of D Timmerman, MD, PhD, Department of Obstetrics and Gynaecology, University Hospitals, Leuven.)

diameter to be malignant in 56% of cases, compared with 40% in cases with sizes between 5 cm and 15 cm and 4% in cases of cysts smaller than 5 cm. Unilocular cysts smaller than 10 cm were rarely found to be malignant.[15,16] Rulin and Preston[17] demonstrated a significant relation between cyst diameter and ovarian malignancy in postmenopausal patients. In cysts smaller than 5 cm, the occurrence of malignancy was 1 out of 32. Eleven per cent of cysts between 5 cm and 10 cm were malignant, and 64% of cysts greater than 10 cm.

Internal structure

Unilocular, echolucent cystic tumours of the ovary up to 10 cm in diameter are predominantly benign, even in postmenopausal women.[11,18–20] Ovarian cysts larger than 10 cm, however, can be malignant unless they are completely echolucent.[9,21] The presence of thin septa inside the cyst can be seen in a variety of ovarian cysts, such as luteal cysts and dermoid cysts, but also in cases of ovarian malignancy[19] (Figure 7.1). The thick-

ness of an internal septum is relevant in this respect. It has been shown that septae smaller than 2 mm in thickness can be regarded as an indication that the cyst is benign.[19,20,22] In the case of thicker septae, the chances of malignancy are enhanced. This is also true for papillary formations within the cyst.[23] When part of the ovarian tumour is not completely echolucent, the risk of malignancy is also increased,[9] especially if the tumour is larger than 5 cm.[9,11]

Relation to the adjacent structures

Sharp outside edges of an ovarian cyst can be considered as a benign characteristic.[19,20] Blurred edges can be caused by tumour excrescences or adhesions to adjacent structures, and these features may be related to malignancy.

Additional findings

In the case of ascites, there is a strong suspicion of ovarian cancer.[18] This is also true when local thickening of the omentum is seen.[10]

Table 7.2   Predictive value (%) of tumour marker (CA125 ⩾ 35 U/ml) for ovarian cancer with (+) or without (−) ultrasound findings suspicious for malignancy; subdivision has been made according to the menopausal status of the patient.[35]

| | CA125 ⩾ 35 U/ml | | | |
| | Premenopausal | | Postmenopausal | |
	−	+	−	+
Positive predictive value	36	80	94	100
Negative predictive value	87	87	80	91

Ultrasonography appears to be a very valuable diagnostic tool to distinguish between benign and malignant ovarian cysts. However, the predictive value for a benign cyst (91–98%) is more reliable than the predictive value for malignancy (50–74%).[10,18,20]

de Priest et al[24] developed a morphology index based on three criteria: tumour volume, structure of the wall and structure of the septa. Every item could be scored from 0 to 4, giving a total morphology index ranging from 0 to 12. In total, 213 women were studied. In 169 cases, a benign ovarian cyst was found with a mean morphology index of 3.3 (±1.8). Patients with a malignant tumour had a significantly higher index: 7.3 (±1.9).

Colour Doppler flow ultrasonography permits the assessment of vascularization in ovarian tumours. The resistance and pulsatility index of blood vessels within the tumour can be determined. The sensitivity and specificity for detection of ovarian cancer with these methods were 68% and 97.4% respectively.[25,26] Apart from the significance of these indices, the location of the vessels within the tumour might be an important factor. In malignant tumours, these vessels are located in the centre of the tumour in over 65% of cases, compared with 5% in benign tumours.[27] The initial expectations of colour Doppler flow measurements were high, but later studies could not demonstrate superior qualities compared with conventional ultrasonography.[28–32]

Tumour markers

The tumour marker CA125 can be used as a diagnostic method to detect epithelial ovarian cancer.[33] However, the specificity of the marker can be problematic, especially in premenopausal women with various conditions such as endometriosis, trophoblastic disease, pelvic inflammatory disease or fibromyomas.[34] Finkler et al[35] combined CA125 levels with ultrasound findings and the menopausal status of 94 patients. The predictive value of a combination of these three parameters is shown in Table 7.2.

From these findings, it was shown that CA125 levels in premenopausal patients without the additional ultrasound findings are worthless for

Table 7.3   Therapeutic efficacy of aspiration (A) or fenestration (F) by laparoscopy (L) or ultrasonography (US)

Ref	L or US	A or F	No. of cases	Follow-up (months)	Recurrence %
37	US	A	34	—	41
38	L	A	91	9–40	8
39	L	A	45	6–48	11
39	US	A	15	6–18	53
40	L	F	104	20	8
41	US	A	34	—	41
42	US	A	21	6–12	67
43	US	A	34	6–20	53

predicting the presence of ovarian cancer. Vasilev[36] analysed patients younger than 50 years with an ovarian tumour and a raised CA125 level (>35 U/ml). In 85% of cases (34 out of 40), they found benign ovarian tumours. However, the combination of a raised CA125 level and a post-menopausal status can predict ovarian cancer in the context of an ovarian tumour in almost 100% of cases, especially if ultrasonographic findings are included. It can be concluded that CA125 tumour marker analysis in premenopausal patients has a high sensitivity but too low a specificity to predict ovarian malignancy. In postmenopausal patients, it is a useful diagnostic method to distinguish between a benign and a malignant ovarian tumour.

From the data and discussion above, it can be concluded that a prerequisite for the proper surgical management of ovarian cysts is the preoperative discrimination between a benign and a malignant lesion. The combination of patient age (menopausal status) and ultrasonographic findings is an essential diagnostic tool to permit an adequate prediction of a possible malignant con-

dition. In postmenopausal women, the serum level of the tumour marker CA125 is an important value, since a value greater than 35 U/ml is associated with a high specificity for a malignant condition.

What are the different laparoscopic techniques? How can we avoid spillage or trocar site metastases at laparoscopy?
Aspiration and fenestration
Aspiration and fenestration are simple methods, but carry distinct drawbacks and risks. The therapeutic efficacy of these methods is low. In Table 7.3, recurrence rates of ovarian cysts after aspiration or fenestration are summarized. In 8–67% of cases, the cyst recurred.

Although the therapeutic efficacy is rather low, aspiration of ovarian cysts is still widely performed. In a systematic survey in the Netherlands between 1992 and 1994, it was shown that laparoscopic aspiration and fenestration were amongst the 10 most frequently performed laparoscopic operations in the country.[43]

Apart from the poor therapeutic effect of

aspiration and fenestration, the diagnostic accuracy of cytological assessment of the cyst fluid is also problematic. It was shown that cytological examination of cyst fluid resulted in an adequate diagnosis of ovarian cysts in less than 60% of cases.[23] False-negative findings are involved, and this can be hazardous for the patient in the case of an underlying malignant condition. The 95% confidence limits for true-positive and true-negative cytological results of ovarian cyst aspirates have been calculated to be 9–99% (mean 67%) and 80–97% (mean 91%), respectively. Therefore reliance on cytological results is clearly unsatisfactory and dangerous.[2,45] Also, the 65% predictive value of this method in discriminating between functional and neoplastic cysts is low.[46]

Regarding the poor therapeutic results and the unreliable diagnostic accuracy of aspiration and fenestration, this kind of surgery for the treatment of ovarian cysts cannot be recommended as a routine clinical policy. Complete cystectomy with additional histological assessment of the cyst wall or oophorectomy are more reliable methods to deal with these conditions.

Tumour spill

Laparoscopic management of ovarian cysts risks intraoperative cyst rupture. It is not completely clear in what way the patient's prognosis is affected by tumour spill. The literature gives conflicting results, mainly based on retrospective evaluation.[1,5,47] To shed some light on this controversy, Trimbos and Hacker[2] postulated that the time of rupture of a malignant ovarian cyst might be relevant for the patient's prognosis. In this hypothesis, acute rupture during surgery is considered not harmful, but chronic preoperative spill of continuously leaking malignant cells increases the likelihood of peritoneal implantation and worsens the prognosis. This hypothesis of a relationship between the duration of tumour spill and later tumour implantation is supported

by the report of Maiman et al.[48] They described 42 cases of ovarian cancer reported by the Society of Gynecologic Oncologists in the USA, in response to a survey concerning the 'laparoscopic management of ovarian neoplasms subsequently found to be malignant'. When the delay between laparoscopic examination and eventual diagnosis of ovarian cancer was less than four weeks, 32% of patients had stage III or IV disseminated ovarian cancer. When the delay had been more than four weeks, this was the case in 75% of patients.[2] Vergote et al[49] recently performed an extensive meta-analysis of the literature. In their analysis of 1286 patients with early ovarian cancer, they found that preoperative rupture of malignant cysts was a significant factor for an adverse prognosis. Rupture during surgery showed a trend towards poor prognosis, but this was not statistically significant.[49]

The aspiration or fenestration of a potentially malignant ovarian cyst is likely to provoke chronic tumour spill, especially when cytological assessment of the aspirate is inadequate and the eventual diagnosis of ovarian cancer delayed. Therefore this kind of surgery should be avoided.

Laparoscopic cystectomy

Laparoscopic cystectomy has the advantage of preserving ovarian function, but carries the risk of intraoperative cyst rupture, and spill of the cyst fluid cannot be entirely avoided. In the classic technique, the ovarian surface is incised over 3–5 cm using a unipolar electrode. The cyst wall can then be dissected from the normal ovarian tissue by pulling or hydrodissection; often the cyst will rupture during this procedure. The cyst is then further extracted and removed. Thereafter the operating field is thoroughly rinsed.

It is controversial whether the ovarian capsule should be sutured after the procedure. Leaving the ovary open does not seem to provoke more adhesion formation.[50] Animal experiments

Table 7.4 Incidence of malignancy in laparoscopically removed postmenopausal ovarian tumours with normal ultrasound and CA125 findings

Ref	No. of cases	Cyst size (cm)	Carcinoma (%)
52	25	3–9	0
53	44	1–12	0
54	55	6.6	0
Authors' own series	20	2.5–7	0

showed the same results.[51] Because of the inherent risk of spillage of cyst fluid, ovarian cystectomy by the laparoscope cannot be recommended in postmenopausal women.

Laparoscopic oophorectomy

Laparoscopic oophorectomy causes ovarian loss, but the procedure can be performed without appreciable spill by using an endoscopic pouch. A laparoscopic oophorectomy has been reported in a number of papers in postmenopausal patients with ovarian masses that were preoperatively assessed as benign. Table 7.4 shows the results of four studies reporting on such cases (benign ultrasound criteria and a normal CA125).

A 1990 survey by the American Association of Gynecologic Laparoscopists[55] showed only 53 (0.4%) cases of unsuspected ovarian cancer in 13 739 cases of laparoscopic ovarian cyst surgery. So, it can be concluded that the risk of finding an unexpected ovarian cancer in carefully selected patients is very low. Canis and coworkers[56] found that, after careful preoperative and intraoperative evaluation, 7 out of 92 (7.6%) postmenopausal patients managed by laparoscopy had ovarian cancer or a borderline tumour. All of these lesions were considered suspicious at the time of laparoscopy, and were managed by immediate laparotomy.[56]

LEARNING POINTS

- According to the above-mentioned findings and considerations, a number of recommendations can be made for the clinical management of ovarian masses. Figures 7.3 and 7.4 summarize the clinical directives in cases of premenopausal and postmenopausal patients respectively.

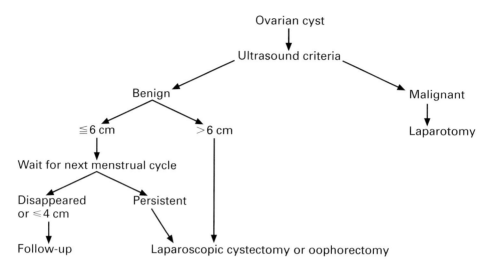

Figure 7.3
Clinical policy in cases of ovarian cysts in premenopausal patients.

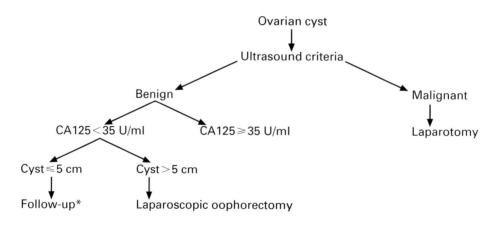

*Ultrasound and CA125 follow-up is indicated

Figure 7.4
Clinical policy in cases of ovarian cysts in postmenopausal patients.

REFERENCES

1. Webb MJ, Decker DG, Mussey E, Williams IJ, Factors influencing survival in state I ovarian cancer. *Am J Obstet Gynecol* 1973; **116**: 222–6.

2. Trimbos JB, Hacker NF, The case against aspirating ovarian cysts. *Cancer* 1993; **72**: 827–35.

3. Gleeson NC, Nicosia SV, Mark JE et al, Abdominal wall metastasis from ovarian carcinoma after laparoscopy. *Am J Obstet Gynecol* 1993; **169**: 522–3.

4. Childers JM, Agua KA, Surwit EA et al, Abdominal wall tumor implantations after laparoscopy for malignant conditions. *Obstet Gynecol* 1994; **84**: 765–9.

5. Dembo AJ, Davy M, Stenwig AG et al, Prognostic factors in patients with stage I epithelial ovarian cancer. *Obstet Gynecol* 1990; **75**: 263–73.

6. Sevelda P, Dittrich C, Salzer H, Prognostic value of the rupture of the capsule in stage I epithelial carcinoma. *Gynecol Oncol* 1989; **35**: 321–2.

7. Sjövall K, Nilsson B, Einhorn N, Different types of rupture of the tumor capsule and the impact on survival in early ovarian carcinoma. *Int J Gynecol Cancer* 1994; **4**: 333–6.

8. Koonings PP, Campbell K, Mishell DR, Grimes DA, Relative frequency of primary ovarian neoplasms: a 10 years review. *Obstet Gynecol* 1989; **74**: 921–5.

9. Moyle JW, Rochester D, Sider L et al, Sonography of ovarian tumors: predictability of tumortype. *Am J Radiol* 1983; **141**: 985–91.

10. Hermann UJ, Locker GW, Goldhirsch A, Sonographic patterns of ovarian tumors: prediction of malignancy. *Obstet Gynecol* 1987; **69**: 777–81.

11. Andolf E, Jörgensen C, Cystic lesions in elderly women diagnosed by ultrasound. *Br J Obstet Gynaecol* 1989; **96**: 1076–9.

12. Grandberg S, Wikland M, A comparison between ultrasound and gynecologic examination for detection of enlarged ovaries in a group of women at risk for ovarian carcinoma. *J Ultrasound Med* 1988; **7**: 59–62.

13. Higgins RV, Nagell JR, Woods CH, Interobserver variation in ovarian measurements using transvaginal sonography. *Gynecol Oncol* 1990; **39**: 69–71.

14. Allen MS, Hertig AI, Carcinoma of the ovary. *Am J Obstet Gynecol* 1949; **58**: 640–3.

15. Grandberg S, Relationship of macroscopic appearance to the histologic diagnosis of ovarian tumors. *Clin Obstet Gynecol* 1993; **36**: 363–75.

16. Maiman M, Laparoscopic removal of the adnexal mass: the case of caution. *Clin Obstet Gynecol* 1995; **38**: 370–9.

17. Rulin MC, Preston AI, Adnexal masses in postmenopausal women. *Obstet Gynecol* 1987; **70**: 578–81.

18. Benecerraf BR, Jinkler NJ, Wojciechowski C, Knapp RC, Sonographic accuracy in the diagnosis of ovarian masses. *J Reprod Med* 1990; **35**: 491–5.

19. Lerner JP, Timor-Tritsch IE, Federman A, Abramovish G, Transvaginal ultrasonographic characterisation of ovarian masses with an improved, waited scoring system. *Am J Obstet Gynecol* 1994; **170**: 81–5.

20. Sassone AM, Trimor-Tritsch IE, Artner A et al, Transvaginal sonographic characterizations of ovarian disease: evaluation of a new scoring system to predict ovarian malignancy. *Obstet Gynecol* 1991; **78**: 70–6.

21. Nagell J, Higgins RV, Donaldson ES et al, Ovarian cancer screening in asymptomatic postmenopausal women by transvaginal sonography. *Cancer* 1991; **68**: 458–62.

22. Kurjak A, Predanic M, New scoring system for prediction of ovarian malignancy based on transvaginal color Doppler sonography. *J Ultrasound Med* 1992; **11**: 631–5.

23. Granberg S, Norström A, Wikland H, Comparison of endovaginal ultrasound and cytological examination of cystic ovarian tumors. *J Ultrasound Med* 1991; **10**: 9–14.

24. de Priest PD, Varner E, Powel J et al, The efficiency of a sonographic morphology index in

identifying ovarian cancer: a multi-institutional investigation. *Gynecol Oncol* 1994; **55**: 174–8.

25. Weiner Z, Thaler I, Beck D et al, Differentiating malignant from benign ovarian tumors with transvaginal color flow imaging. *Obstet Gynecol* 1992; **79**: 159–62.

26. Oram DH, Jeyarajah AR, The role of ultrasound and tumour markers in early detection of ovarian cancer. *Br J Obstet Gynaecol* 1994; **101**: 939–45.

27. Strigini FAL, Gadduci A, Del Bravo B et al, Differential diagnosis of adnexal masses with transvaginal sonography, color flow imaging and serum CA 125 assay in pre- and post-menopausal women. *Gynecol Oncol* 1996; **61**: 68–72.

28. Wu C, Lee CN, Chen TM et al, Factors contributing to the accuracy in diagnosing ovarian malignancy by color Doppler ultrasound. *Obstet Gynecol* 1994; **84**: 605–8.

29. Timor-Tritsch IE, Lerner JP, Monteaguado A, Santos R, Transvaginal ultrasonographic characterization of ovarian masses by means of color flow-directed Doppler measurements and a morphologic scoring system. *Am J Obstet Gynecol* 1993; **168**: 909–13.

30. Bromley B, Goodman H, Benecerraf BR, Comparison between sonographic morphology and Doppler waveform for the diagnosis of ovarian malignancy. *Obstet Gynecol* 1994; **83**: 434–7.

31. Vos MC, Brölman HAM, Bal H, Distinguishing the benign and the malignant adnexal mass: the predictive value of transvaginal ultrasonography, transvaginal color Doppler flow and CA 125 level. *Gynaecol Endosc* 1995; **4**: 183–7.

32. Timmerman D, Bourne TH, Tailor A et al, A comparison of methods for preoperative discrimination between malignant and benign adnexal masses: the development of a new logistic regression model. *Am J Obstet Gynecol* 1999; **181**: 57–65.

33. Bast RC, Feeney M, Lazarus H et al, Reactivity of a monoclonal antibody with human ovarian carcinoma. *J Clin Invest* 1981; **68**: 1331–5.

34. Dixia Ch, Schwartz PE, Kinguo L, Zhan Y, Evaluation of CA 125 levels in differentiating malignant from benign tumors in patients with pelvic masses. *Obstet Gynecol* 1988; **72**: 23–7.

35. Finkler NJ, Benecerraf B, Lavin BI et al, Comparison of serum CA 125, clinical impression and ultrasound in the pre-operative evaluation of ovarian masses. *Obstet Gynecol* 1988; **72**: 659–64.

36. Vasilev S, Serum CA 125 levels in the preoperative evaluation of pelvic masses. *Obstet Gynecol* 1988; **71**: 751–6.

37. Canis M, Mage G, Pouly JL et al, Laparoscopic diagnosis of adnexal cystic masses: a 12-year experience with long-term follow-up. *Obstet Gynecol* 1994; **83**: 707–12.

38. Larsen JF, Pederson OD, Gregersen E, Ovarian cyst fenestration via the laparoscope. *Acta Obstet Gynecol Scand* 1986; **65**: 539–42.

39. Montenari L, Saviotti C, Zara C, Aspiration of ovarian cysts: laparoscopy or echography. *Acta Eur Fertil* 1987; **18**: 45–7.

40. De Wilde RL, Recurrence of functional ovarian cysts after laparoscopic fenestration. *Am J Obstet Gynecol* 1989; **161**: 839.

41. du Crespigny LCh, Robinson HP, Davoren RAM, Fortune DW, The simple ovarian cyst: aspirate or operate? *Br J Obstet Gynaecol* 1989; **96**: 1035–9.

42. Khaw KI, Walker WJ, Ultrasound guided fine-needle aspiration of ovarian cysts: diagnosis and treatment in pregnant and non-pregnant women. *Clin Radiol* 1990; **41**: 105–8.

43. Giorlandino C, Raramanni C, Muzia L et al, Ultrasound guided aspiration of ovarian endometriotic cysts. *Int J Gynaecol Obstet* 1993; **43**: 41–4.

44. Jansen FW, Kapiteyn K, Hermans J, Trimbos-Kemper GCM, A survey on (operative) laparoscopy in the Netherlands in 1992. *Eur J Obstet Gynecol Reprod Biol* 1996; **64**: 105–9.

45. Diermaes E, Rasmussen J, Sorensen I, Hasch E, Ovarian cysts: management by puncture. *Lancet* 1987; **i**: 1084.

46. Jansen FW, Tanahatoe S, Veselic M, Trimbos JB, Laparoscopic aspiration of ovarian cysts: an unreliable technique in primary diagnosis of (sonographically) benign ovarian lesions. *Gynaecol Endosc* 1997; **6**: 363–7.

47. Sainz-del Custa R, Goff B, Fuller A et al, Prognostic importance of intra-operative rupture of malignant ovarian epithelial neoplasms. *Obstet Gynecol* 1994; **84**: 1–7.

48. Maiman M, Seltzer V, Boyce J, Laparoscopic excision of ovarian neoplasms subsequently found to be malignant. *Obstet Gynecol* 1991; **77**: 563–5.

49. Vergote IB, Fyles AW, Bertelsen K et al, Meta-analysis of 1286 patients with FIGO stage 1 invasive ovarian carcinoma: rupture of the cyst is a prognostic variable. *Int J Gynecol Cancer* 1997; **7**(S): 20.

50. Canis M, Mage G, Wattiez A et al, Second-look laparoscopy after laparoscopic cystectomy of large ovarian endometriomas. *Fertil Steril* 1992; **58**: 617–19.

51. Lin P, Pagidas K, Iulandi I, Arseneau J, Ovarian cystectomy with and without suturing in an animal model. *Gynaecol Endosc* 1996; **5**: 165–7.

52. Parker WH, Berek JS, Management of selective cystic adnexal masses in postmenopausal women by operative laparoscopy: a pilot study. *Am J Obstet Gynecol* 1990; **163**: 1574–7.

53. Mann WJ, Reich H, Laparoscopic adnexectomy in postmenopausal women. *J Reprod Med* 192; **37**: 254–6.

54. Shalev E, Eliyaku S, Peleg D, Isabari A, Laparoscopic management of adnexal cystic masses in postmenopausal women. *Obstet Gynecol* 1994; **83**: 594–6.

55. Hulka J, Parker W, Surrey M, Phillips J, Management of ovarian masses – AAGL 1990 survey. *J Reprod Med* 1992; **7**: 599–602.

56. Canis M, Mage G, Pouly J et al, Laparoscopic diagnosis of adnexal cystic masses: a twelve year experience with long-term follow-up. *Obstet Gynecol* 1994; **83**: 707–12.

8
Fallopian tube cancer

Richard R Barakat

INTRODUCTION

Fallopian tube cancer is a rare gynecologic malignancy. The disease is similar to serous papillary ovarian cancer, and is managed in a similar manner. As a rule, the disease is more likely to produce early symptoms and be diagnosed earlier than ovarian cancer. On the other hand, because the fallopian tube is open to the peritoneal cavity, even very early cancers require adjuvant chemotherapy. Fallopian tube cancers also appear to have an increased incidence of metastases to the pelvic and para-aortic lymph nodes. These tumors are treated surgically in a similar fashion to ovarian cancers and respond as well as these (if not slightly better) to platinum-based chemotherapy.

CASE HISTORY

A 63-year-old woman presented with a complaint of colicky left lower quadrant pain, a watery vaginal discharge, and postmenopausal spotting. An endometrial biopsy was benign. The serum CA125 level was elevated at 480 U/l. At laparotomy the patient was found to have a complex mass involving the left fallopian tube. This was removed in its entirety, along with an enlarged left para-aortic node that contained metastatic disease.

What are the clinical and pathologic characteristics of fallopian tube cancer?

Primary cancer of the fallopian tube ranks among the rarest of gynecologic malignancies, composing approximately 0.31–1.11% of the total,[1] with an average annual incidence of 3.6 per million women per year.[2] It tends to metastasize intra-abdominally in a manner similar to ovarian cancer and therefore has been assumed to have the same biological characteristics. However, unlike ovarian cancer patients, who experience delays in diagnosis because of the insidious onset of the disease, patients with fallopian tube cancers frequently display symptoms and present earlier. The majority of cases occur in women in their mid-50s. The most common presenting symptom is abnormal postmenopausal vaginal bleeding. The degree of bleeding depends on the patency of the cornual end of the tube and whether or not the fimbriated end is occluded. Without occlusion of the distal end of the tube, blood would pass mostly into the peritoneal cavity. Other common symptoms include pain and leukorrhea. The term 'hydrops tube profluens' was coined by Latzko to describe the sudden discharge of amber fluid from the vagina in cases of tubal cancer.[1] Distension of the tubal lumen by blood and secretions produces a colicky type of pain, causing the patient to seek medical attention earlier. In published series,[3–10] approximately two-thirds of patients present with disease confined to the tube or pelvis.

In many series, exfoliative cervicovaginal cytology has been reported to be positive in as many as 40–60% of women with tubal cancer.[1,10–12] In some series, however, abnormal Pap smears were distinctly uncommon (<20%).[13–21] When present, the neoplastic cells are often indistinguishable from those shed from endometrial adenocarcinoma. The initial evaluation of a patient presenting with adenocarcinoma on Pap smear requires evaluation of the cervix and endometrium to rule out these more common sources of an abnormal Pap smear. If this workup is negative, the patient may ultimately require a laparoscopy to rule out the fallopian tube or ovary as the site of the abnormal cervical cytology.

Determination of serum CA125 levels does not aid the early detection of fallopian tube cancer, since elevated serum levels are usually associated with advanced primary cancer of the fallopian tube, uterus, or ovary.[22] However, it does help monitor patients in whom the diagnosis has already been established, since serum CA125 is almost always a reliable indicator of recurrent cancer.[23]

Pathology of tubal cancer
Gross appearance
In the majority of cases (95%), the tumor is unilateral.[24] The gross appearance of the fallopian tube is typically enlarged, deformed, or fusiform, with agglutination of the fimbriae and, frequently, distal obstruction (Figure 8.1). When the tumor is confined to the mucosa, the tube is generally soft to palpation, and the initial impression of the surgeon is that a hematosalpinx, pyosalpinx, or hydrosalpinxis is present, which is often associated with pelvic inflammatory

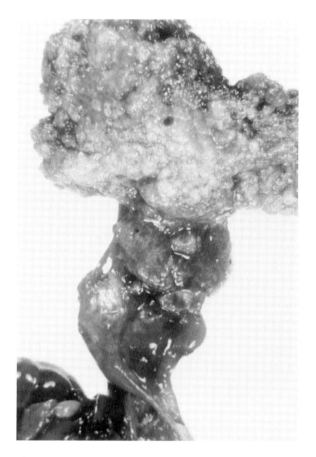

Figure 8.1
The gross appearance of the fallopian tube is typically enlarged, deformed, or fusiform.

disease.[18,25] Turbid fluid frequently fills the lumen, with a friable, exophytic, papillary, or nodular mass affixed to the mucosal surface. The most frequent site of origin is the ampulla, followed by the infundibulum.[19,20,26] Multiple mucosal nodules may be present or the entire lumen may be replaced by a necrotic mass. With more advanced disease, the tumor penetrates the muscular wall and serosa of the tube, and extension to the ovary may result in a conglomerate tubo-ovarian mass. In this situation, the distinction of tubal cancer from that of the ovary may not be possible.

Microscopic appearance

Half of all tubal cancers display a serous histology, with the majority being poorly differentiated. Other common histologic features include tumor giant cells, psammoma bodies, and squamous metaplasia. Endometrioid carcinomas (Figure 8.2) are the next most frequent histologic subtype, followed by clear cell and undifferentiated cancers.

Because the gross and microscopic characteristics, as well as the pattern of spread of fallopian tube cancer closely resemble those of ovarian cancer, it is sometimes difficult to accurately determine the site of origin of a tumor that forms a solid or cystic tubo-ovarian mass. In the past, some investigators have quite reasonably designated such tumors as tubo-ovarian cancers.[27,28] In 1950, Hu et al[28] proposed criteria for differentiating primary from metastatic cancer that involves the fallopian tube. These criteria include the following:

1. Grossly, the main tumor is in the tube.
2. Microscopically, the mucosa chiefly should be involved and should show a papillary pattern.
3. If the tubal wall was found to be involved to a great extent, the transition between benign

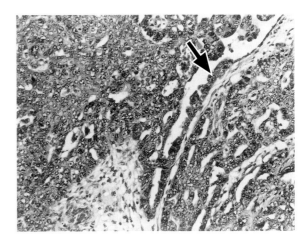

Figure 8.3
Note the in situ carcinoma on the luminal surface and the infiltrating adenocarcinoma beneath it (400×, H&E)..

and malignant epithelium should be demonstrable (Figure 8.3).

Many tumors of probable tubal origin fail to meet these stringent criteria. Since fallopian tube cancers are relatively rare, it would seem logical to be restrictive in their definition. In this way, particular features of their pathogenesis, epidemiology, pathology, and clinical behaviour will not be obscured by the inclusion of cases that might be of ovarian origin. The incidence of fallopian tube cancer, however, is likely to be underestimated, since a conglomerate mass involving the adnexa is more likely to be considered ovarian in origin than a much rarer tubal primary.

Staging of fallopian tube cancer

Staging of fallopian tube cancer is based on a modification of the International Federation of Gynecology and Obstetrics (FIGO) staging of ovarian carcinoma as first proposed by Dodson et al.[29] In 1992, FIGO formally established a staging classification for fallopian tube cancer (see Appendix 2).[30]

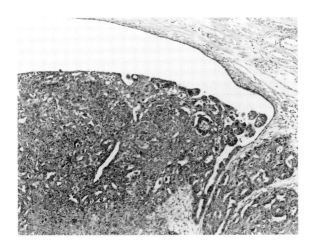

Figure 8.2
Poorly differentiated endometrioid adenocarcinoma of the fallopian tube protruding into the lumen (100×, H&E).

How should fallopian tube cancer be managed?

Surgery

Fallopian tube cancer is rarely diagnosed preoperatively. The surgeon confronted with the diagnosis intraoperatively must therefore be prepared to perform the appropriate staging procedure. Improper staging procedures may erroneously lead to the downstaging of patients with more advanced disease. The importance of proper staging is highlighted by the tendency of fallopian tube cancer to metastasize to lymph nodes. Tamimi and Figge[31] reported a 53% incidence of lymph node metastases in 15 patients with tubal cancer. Five patients had disease in the para-aortic nodes, and, in two of these, this finding was the only evidence of metastases. Similarly, Schray et al[32] noted a 35% incidence of nodal metastases in 34 patients. Five of nine patients with extrapelvic nodal metastases would otherwise have been classified as having stage I disease.

Patients with residual tumor mass of less than 1 cm after surgery are reported to have a higher survival rate than patients with larger residual tumor burdens, a situation identical to that observed in ovarian cancer. Surgical therapy for fallopian tube cancer should therefore follow similar guidelines as employed in ovarian cancer.

The role of second-look surgery in the management of fallopian tube cancer is similar to that for ovarian cancer. The theoretical rationale for this procedure, based on experience with ovarian cancer,[33] would be to determine the effectiveness of front-line therapy and provide information on disease status not reliably obtainable by non-invasive means. A review of approximately 86 cases of second-look procedures for tubal cancer reported in the medical literature[5,9,10,15,34–40] revealed that although 61% of these were negative, information regarding surgical stage prior to administration of chemotherapy or radiation was not always available. Barakat et al[34] reported the largest experience to date regarding second-look laparotomy in tubal cancer. Twenty-one of 35 platinum-treated patients had a negative second-look. With a mean follow-up of 50 months, only four (19%) have had recurrence. This contrasts with advanced-stage ovarian cancer patients treated with platinum-based chemotherapy, among whom approximately 50% will experience recurrence following a negative second-look procedure, with a median interval of 14 months to recurrence.[41] Based on their experience, the authors recommend second-look surgery for patients with stage II–IV tubal cancer to assess tumor status more accurately, allowing for secondary cytoreduction and further treatment if necessary.

Chemotherapy

The prognosis of patients with fallopian tube cancer has generally been regarded as poor, with an overall survival that parallels that of epithelial ovarian cancer.[3–10] Attempts to find a means for improving survival have been hampered by the lack of a uniform staging system[9,31,42] and disagreement as to what constitutes optimal therapy of the disease. Schiller and Silverberg,[42] in a retrospective review of 76 published cases of fallopian tube cancer, documented the important relationship between the depth of invasion by tumor and survival. A crude five-year survival rate of 91% was found for intramucosal lesions, 53% for tumors with mucosal wall invasion, and 25% or less for cases in which the tumors penetrated the tubal serosa. Using these data, they proposed a staging system for fallopian tube cancer based in part on the depth of invasion. A study by Peters et al[3] confirms the importance of depth of invasion in predicting survival. Thus, the pathologist who examines a fallopian tube that contains tumor is recommended to provide information on the depth of invasion, the presence of lymphatic or capillary space involvement, and the degree of histologic differentiation. Since the fallopian tube is a hollow viscus that communicates with the peritoneal cavity, all patients except those with in situ disease should receive adjuvant treatment.

Because of its rarity, most reports concerning adjuvant treatment from any single institution have been small,[34,43–45] while larger studies[3,7] have spanned long time periods during which various modalities were employed. In early-stage disease, pelvic radiation has not been shown to improve survival,[5,34] while whole-abdominal irradiation may be beneficial.[34] In advanced-stage disease, neither whole-abdominal irradiation[9,34–38,45] nor alkylating agents used singly or in combination[22] have significantly impacted upon survival.

Early reports[36,40,43] of the sensitivity of fallopian tube cancer to cisplatin-based combination chemotherapy have been verified by more recent observations of a 75% response rate to this therapy[46,47] in small numbers of patients. Morris et al[48] reported a surgically documented response rate of 53% in 18 patients treated with cisplatin, doxorubicin, and cyclophosphamide. Barakat et al[49] reported on 38 cases of primary fallopian tube cancer treated at Memorial Sloan-Kettering Cancer Center between 1979 and 1989. The overall five-year survival rate for the entire group was 51%, with a median of 61 months, with no difference between the seven patients with early-stage disease compared with the 31 with advanced-stage disease. Excluding patients with stage I disease, those patients who had no residual disease following primary cytoreductive surgery had a significant increase in five-year survival over that of patients with any residual disease. These results with platinum-based combination therapy compare favorably with other regimens used to treat advanced tubal cancer (Table 8.1).

Table 8.1   Summary of series reporting on stage III and IV fallopian tube cancer[a]

Study	No. of patients	No. of platinum-treated patients	Overall 5-year survival rate (%)
Raju et al (1981)[4]	4	2 (50%)	25
Roberts et al (1982)[5]	31	0 (0%)	6
Denham et al (1983)[6]	41	2 (5%)	18
Eddy et al (1984)[7]	33	1 (3%)	5
McMurray et al (1986)[8]	10	2 (20%)	14
Podratz et al (1986)[9]	21	3 (14%)	19
Peters et al (1989)[47]	29	12 (41%)	15
Pfeiffer et al (1989)[10]	17	0 (0%)	6
Barakat et al (1991)[49]	31	31 (100%)	51
Total	217	53 (25%)	17

[a] Adapted from reference 49, with permission.

Fallopian tube cancer appears to respond favorably to platinum-based multiagent chemotherapy. Little information exists regarding the combination of paclitaxel with platinum, which is now the standard regimen for advanced epithelial ovarian cancer; however, one would expect the results to be similar.

SUMMARY

Primary carcinoma of the fallopian tube is a rare disease, which is best treated by total abdominal hysterectomy and bilateral salpingo-oophorectomy. Early-stage disease requires comprehensive staging, while patients with more advanced disease may benefit from tumor debulking. Adjuvant chemotherapy should be used in all cases except for those with in situ disease.

LEARNING POINTS

❋ Abnormal vaginal bleeding, a vaginal discharge, and pelvic pain are the most common presenting symptoms of fallopian tube cancer.

❋ Patients with fallopian tube cancer will have abnormal Pap smears in 20–60% of cases.

❋ The majority of fallopian tube cancers are of the papillary serous type, but endometrioid, clear cell, and undifferentiated cell types are also seen.

❋ The surgical therapy of fallopian tube cancer is similar to that of ovarian cancer, with the most important prognostic factor being the size of residual disease following the initial surgical procedure.

❋ Even very early fallopian tube cancers require adjuvant chemotherapy, since the peritoneal cavity is at risk due to the fact that the fallopian tube is open to the cavity.

❋ Fallopian tube cancers are best treated with platinum-based multiagent chemotherapy.

❋ The role of second-look surgical reassessment is controversial, but most authorities who favor second-look operations for ovarian cancer also utilize the procedure in the management of fallopian tube cancer.

REFERENCES

1. Sedlis A, Primary carcinoma of the fallopian tube. *Obstet Gynecol Surv* 1961; **16**: 209–26.
2. Rosenblatt KA, Weiss WA, Schwartz SM, Incidence of malignant fallopian tube tumors. *Gynecol Oncol* 1989; **25**: 236–9.
3. Peters WA, Anderson WA, Hopkins MP et al, Prognostic features of carcinoma of the fallopian tube. *Obstet Gynecol* 1986; **71**: 757–62.
4. Raju KS, Barker GH, Wiltshaw E, Primary carcinoma of the fallopian tube. *Obstet Gynecol* 1981; **88**: 1124–9.
5. Roberts JA, Lifshitz S, Primary adenocarcinoma of the fallopian tube. *Gynecol Oncol* 1982; **13**: 301–8.
6. Denham JW, MacLennan KA, The management of primary carcinoma of the fallopian tube: experience of 40 cases. *Cancer* 1983; **53**: 166–72.
7. Eddy GL, Copeland LJ, Gershenson DM et al, Fallopian tube carcinoma. *Obstet Gynecol* 1984; **64**: 546–52.
8. McMurray EH, Jacobs AJ, Perez CA et al, Carcinoma of the fallopian tube: management and sites of failure. *Cancer* 1986; **58**: 2070–5.
9. Podratz KC, Podczaski ES, Gaffey TA et al, Primary carcinoma of the fallopian tube. *Am J Obstet Gynecol* 1986; **154**: 1319–26.
10. Pfeiffer P, Morgensen H, Amtrup F, Honroe E, Primary carcinoma of the fallopian tube. *Acta Oncol* 1989; **28**: 7–11.
11. Johnston GA, Primary malignancy of the fallopian tube: a clinical review of 13 cases. *J Surg Oncol* 1983; **24**: 304–9.
12. Muntz HG, Tarraza HM, Granai CO, Fuller AF, Primary adenocarcinoma of the fallopian

tube. *Eur J Gynaecol Oncol* 1989; **4**: 239–49.

13. Amendola BE, LaRouere J, Amendola MA et al, Adenocarcinoma of the fallopian tube. *Surg Gynecol Obstet* 1983; **157**: 223–7.

14. Benedet JL, White GW, Fairey RN et al, Adenocarcinoma of the fallopian tube: experience with 41 patients. *Obstet Gynecol* 1977; **50**: 654–7.

15. Harrison CR, Averette HE, Jarrell MA et al, Carcinoma of the fallopian tube: clinical management. *Gynecol Oncol* 1989; **32**: 357–9.

16. Henderson SR, Harper RC, Salazar OM et al, Primary carcinoma of the fallopian tube: difficulties in diagnosis and treatment. *Gynecol Oncol* 1977; **5**: 168–79.

17. Meng ML, Gan-Gao, Scheng-Sun, Bao AC, Jung ZA, Diagnosis of primary adenocarcinoma of the fallopian tube. *J Cancer Res Clin Oncol* 1985; **110**: 136–40.

18. Momtazee S, Kempson RL, Primary adenocarcinoma of the fallopian tube. *Obstet Gynecol* 1968; **32**: 649–56.

19. Pinto MM, Bernstein LH, Brogan DA et al, Immunoradiometric assay of CA 125 in effusions: comparison with carcinoembryonic antigen. *Cancer* 1987; **59**: 218–22.

20. Semrad N, Watring W, Fu YS et al, Fallopian tube adenocarcinoma: common extraperitoneal recurrence. *Gynecol Oncol* 1986; **24**: 230–5.

21. Yoonessi M, Carcinoma of the fallopian tube. *Obstet Gynecol Surv* 1979; **34**: 257–70.

22. Niloff JM, Klug TL, Schaetzl E, Elevation of serum CA 125 in carcinomas of the fallopian tube, endometrium, and endocervix. *Am J Obstet Gynecol* 1984; **148**: 1057–8.

23. Tokunaga T, Miyazaki K, Matsuyama S, Serial measurement of CA 125 in patients with primary carcinoma of the fallopian tube. *Gynecol Oncol* 1990; **36**: 335–7.

24. Alvarado-Cabrero I, Young RH, Vammakas EC, Carcinoma of the fallopian tube: a clinicopathological study of 105 cases with observations on staging and prognostic factors. *Gynecol Oncol* 1999; **72**: 367–79.

25. Anbrokh YM, Macroscopic characteristics of cancer of the fallopian tube. *Neoplasma* 1970; **17**: 557–64.

26. Kneale BLG, Attwood HD, Primary carcinoma of the fallopian tube: report of 13 cases. *Am J Obstet Gynecol* 1966; **94**: 840–8.

27. Green TH, Scully RE, Tumors of the fallopian tube. *Clin Obstet Gynecol* 1962; **5**: 886–906.

28. Hu CY, Taymor ML, Hertig AT, Primary carcinoma of the fallopian tube. *Am J Obstet Gynecol* 1950; **59**: 58–67.

29. Dodson MG, Ford JH, Averette HE, Clinical aspects of fallopian tube carcinoma. *Obstet Gynecol* 1970; **36**: 935–9.

30. Pettersson F, Staging rules for gestational trophoblastic tumors and fallopian tube cancer. *Acta Obstet Gynecol Scand* 1992; **71**: 224–5.

31. Tamimi HK, Figge DC, Adenocarcinoma of the uterine tube: potential for lymph node metastases. *Am J Obstet Gynecol* 1981; **141**: 132–7.

32. Schray MF, Podratz KC, Malkasian GD, Fallopian tube cancer: the role of radiation therapy. *Radiother Oncol* 1987; **10**: 267–75.

33. Rubin SC, Lewis JL, Second-look surgery in ovarian carcinoma. *Crit Rev Oncol Hematol* 1988; **8**: 75–91.

34. Barakat RR, Rubin SC, Saigo PE et al, Second-look laparotomy in carcinoma of the fallopian tube. *Obstet Gynecol* 1993; **82**: 748–51.

35. Brown MD, Kohorn EI, Kapp DS et al, Fallopian tube carcinoma. *Int J Radiat Oncol Biol Phys* 1985; **11**: 583–90.

36. Deppe G, Bruckner HW, Cohen CJ, Combination chemotherapy for advanced carcinoma of the fallopian tube. *Obstet Gynecol* 1980; **56**: 530–2.

37. Eddy GL, Copeland LJ, Gershenson DM, Second-look laparotomy in fallopian tube carcinoma. *Gynecol Oncol* 1984; **19**: 182–6.

38. Guthrie D, Cohen S, Carcinoma of the fallopian tube treated with a combination of surgery and cytotoxic chemotherapy. *Br J Obstet Gynecol* 1981; **88**: 1051–3.

39. Hirai Y, Chen J-T, Hamada T et al, Clinical and cytologic aspects of primary fallopian tube

carcinoma: a report of 10 cases. *Acta Cytol* 1987; **31**: 834–40.

40. Jacobs AJ, McMurray EH, Parham J et al, Treatment of carcinoma of the fallopian tube using cisplatin, doxorubicin, and cyclophosphamide. *Am J Clin Oncol* 1986; **9**: 436–9.

41. Rubin SC, Hoskins WJ, Saigo PE et al, Prognostic factors for recurrence following negative second-look laparotomy in ovarian cancer patients treated with platinum-based chemotherapy. *Gynecol Oncol* 1991; **42**: 137–41.

42. Schiller HM, Silverberg SG, Staging and prognosis in primary carcinoma of the fallopian tube. *Cancer* 1971; **28**: 389–95.

43. Andriole GL, Garnick MB, Richie JP, Unusual behavior of low-grade, low-stage transitional cell carcinoma of bladder. *Urology* 1985; **25**: 524–6.

44. Cornog JL, Currie JL, Rubin A, Heat artifact simulating adenocarcinoma of fallopian tube. *JAMA* 1970; **214**: 1118–19.

45. Creasman WT, Lukeman J, Role of the fallopian tube in dissemination of malignant cells in corpus cancer. *Cancer* 1972; **29**: 456–7.

46. Maxson WZ, Stehman FB, Elbright TM et al, Primary carcinoma of the fallopian tube: evidence for activity of cisplatin combination therapy. *Gynecol Oncol* 1987; **26**: 305–13.

47. Peters WA, Anderson WA, Hopkins MO, Results of chemotherapy in advanced carcinoma of the fallopian tube. *Cancer* 1989; **63**: 836–38.

48. Morris M, Gerhenson DM, Burke TW et al, Treatment of fallopian tube carcinoma with cisplatin, doxorubicin, and cyclophosphamide. *Obstet Gynecol* 1990; **76**: 1020–4.

49. Barakat RR, Rubin SC, Saigo PE et al, Cisplatin-based combination chemotherapy in carcinoma of the fallopian tube. *Gynecol Oncol* 1991; **42**: 156–60.

9

Ovarian tumour with unexpected pathology: granulosa cell tumour

Nicoletta Colombo

INTRODUCTION

Ovarian cancer is usually of the epithelial type. However, approximately 7% of malignant ovarian tumours are sex cord stromal tumours (Table 9.1). Approximately 70% of malignant sex cord stromal tumours are granulosa cell tumours. Most of these occur in premenopausal women, but they may occur at any age. About 15% are juvenile granulosa cell tumours, found in infancy or before puberty. Granulosa cell tumours usually have a typical clinical appearance. As they are rare, there is still much to be learnt about their biology and management. Most patients present with early (localized) disease, but recurrences may occur. In this chapter, the typical history and management are discussed.

CASE HISTORY

A 56-year-old woman, para 2, had a two-month history of lower abdominal discomfort, and a sense of fullness in the pelvis and rectal pressure. She had reached the menopause at age 50, and a routine physical examination and Pap smear one year previously were normal. She had complained of irregular vaginal bleeding and breast enlargement with tenderness for four months. Her past medical and family history were unremarkable.

On physical examination, she appeared healthy. The blood pressure was 1–30/80 mmHg. There was no cervical, supraclavicular, axillary, or inguinal lymphadenopathy. The breasts were firm and were

Table 9.1   World Health Organization classification of sex cord stromal tumours
Granulosa stromal cell
Granulosa cell
Thecoma–fibroma
Androblastomas (Sertoli–Leydig cell tumours)
Well-differentiated Sertoli cell (Pick's adenoma)
Intermediate differentiated
Poorly differentiated
Heterologous
Lipid cell tumours
Gynandroblastomas
Unclassified

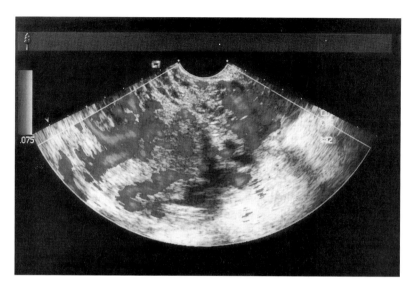

Figure 9.1
Transvaginal sonographic image of a granulosa tumour. The tumour is mainly solid, with multiple cystic areas and foci of very strong neovascularization on colour Doppler imaging. (Courtesy of D Timmerman, MD, PhD, Department of Obstetrics and Gynaecology, University Hospitals Leuven.)

tender on palpation, and no nodules were palpable. Examination of the heart and lungs was normal. The abdomen was soft, and no masses were palpable. There was some tenderness to deep palpation in the left lower quadrant of the abdomen, but there was no rebound tenderness. There was no evidence of intraperitoneal fluid, the liver and spleen were not palpable, and bowel sounds were normal. The external genitalia appeared normal. Bartholin's, urethral, and Skene's glands were unremarkable. The introitus was parous, the vagina was well epithelialized, and the cervix was clean and small. On bimanual and rectovaginal examination, the size of the uterus was normal. On the left side, an approximately 10 cm × 8 cm solid, firm, partially mobile mass was palpable. The cul-de-sac was free of masses or induration. The right ovary was not palpable.

Laboratory data: haematological and biochemical tests and urinalysis were normal. Intravenous urography, cystoscopy, barium enema, and sigmoidoscopy disclosed no abnormalities. A Pap smear showed no atypical cells. Maturation index revealed 80% superficial and 20% intermediate cells. A pelvic ultrasound confirmed a 10 cm × 8 cm solid left

adnexal mass, located posterior and to the left of the uterus (Figure 9.1). The serum CA125 and carcinoembryonic antigen (CEA) levels were in the normal ranges.

What is the management of a solid, mobile ovarian mass in a postmenopausal woman?

An adnexal mass in a postmenopausal woman is highly suspicious for an ovarian neoplasm, and should be explored surgically.

The patient was prepared for surgery, and an exploratory laparotomy was performed through a midline incision. A 10 cm × 8 cm left ovarian tumour was found. The tumour was intact and mobile. There were no excrescences on the surface, and no ascites was present. The contralateral ovary was normal. The cut surface of the ovary contained a firm, yellowish solid tumour (Figure 9.2). Peritoneal washings were obtained, and the material was submitted for cytological examination. Complete examination of the upper abdomen, including the liver, diaphragms, omentum, and para-aortic nodes, failed to reveal any lesions. The left ovary was removed and submitted to pathology for frozen section.

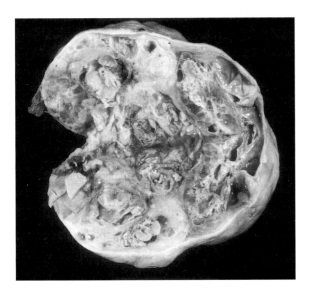

Figure 9.2
Adult granulosa cell tumour with intact lobulated surface without external excrescences. The cut surface shows solid yellow and white zones and areas of cystic degeneration. (Courtesy of Ph Moerman, MD, PhD, Department of Pathology, University Hospitals Leuven.)

What are the differential diagnoses?

A solid yellowish tumour (usually stage Ia) in a postmenopausal tumour is suggestive of a sex cord stromal tumour. The appearance is not typical of an ovarian germ cell tumour, which would be uncommon in this age group. The most frequent malignant sex cord stromal tumour is a granulosa cell tumour. This tumour often produces oestrogens, which may explain the vaginal bleeding, breast tenderness, and high maturation index of the vaginal cells on cytological examination. The serum tumour markers for epithelial tumours such as CA125 and CEA are usually normal.

Histological examination confirmed the diagnosis of a granulosa cell tumour.

What is the appropriate surgical management of granulosa cell tumours?

The appropriate treatment for granulosa cell tumours in this age group is a total abdominal hysterectomy, and bilateral salpingo-oophorectomy, with systematic evaluation of all serosal surfaces to include the parietal and visceral peritoneum, liver, and undersurface of the diaphragms. Omentectomy, appendectomy, and biopsies of any suspicious lymph nodes should be also carried out. In a young patient with stage I granulosa cell tumour, the possibility of a unilateral salpingo-oophorectomy should be considered when there is a strong desire to preserve fertility.

Granulosa cell tumours are unilateral in 95% of cases, and have an average diameter of 12 cm, with a range from microscopic lesions to masses measuring 40 cm in diameter. They can be solid with focal areas of haemorrhage or necrosis, and cystic areas containing watery, serosanguinous or gelatinous fluid. More rarely, the tumours are predominantly cystic and may resemble a cystadenoma.

On microscopic examination, the tumours contain granulosa cells or, more often, theca cells, fibroblasts or both. Several different patterns can be observed: the microfollicular, macrofollicular, insular, or trabecular patterns are characteristic of the more well-differentiated tumours. The microfollicular pattern is characterized by rosette-like structures (Call–Exner bodies), which contain eosinophilic material and nuclear debris (Figure 9.3). The macrofollicles are really areas of liquefaction in islands of granulosa cells. Large follicles lined by circumferentially arranged cells that resemble Graafian follicles of the newborn infant can also be present. The insular parts of granulosa cell tumours are composed of groups or islands of polygonal cells arranged without polarity, while in the trabecular regions, the cells are arranged in ribbons. The diffuse form of these neoplasms,

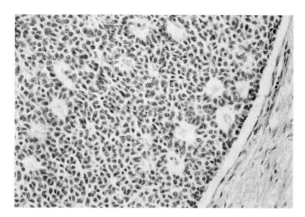

Figure 9.3
Adult granulosa cell tumour showing Call-Exner bodies. (Courtesy of Dr E Benjamin, Department of Histopathology, University College, London.)

often-called 'sacromatoid', may contain polygonal or spindle-shaped cells. Pleomorphism is rarely present, but 2% of these tumours may contain cells with bizarre hyperchromatic nuclei. Mitotic figures are usually scanty.

The definitive pathology report was of an adult-type granulosa cell tumour in the left ovary. The uterus contained glandular endometrial hyperplasia. No malignancy was found in the right ovary, fallopian tubes, omentum, or peritoneal biopsies.

What should the postoperative management of granulosa cell tumours be?

The natural history of these neoplasms includes some peculiar features. In spite of the large size of the lesion at the time of diagnosis, 80–90% of patients will present with stage I disease.[1–3] However, it should be remembered that accurate staging is not available in most reported series. Bilateral ovarian involvement is also unusual, ranging from 0% to 8%. These tumours are considered to be of low-grade malignancy, with a favourable prognosis and a relapse rate of

10–33%. Since these tumours have a propensity for indolent growth, they tend to recur late. The average time to recurrence is between 5 and 10 years,[4] with some recurrences occurring as late as 25 years after the initial diagnosis. The earlier presentation, infrequency of bilaterality, long median time to recurrence (6 years), and long median survival after recurrences (5.6 years) demonstrate a behaviour very different from that of epithelial ovarian cancer.[3] Most authors have reported a 10-year survival rate in excess of 90% for stage I patients.[1–3,5]

The presence of extra-ovarian spread at the time of initial diagnosis carries a much poorer prognosis. Stage III disease, although rare, has a five-year survival rate of 0–22%, similar to that observed for epithelial ovarian cancer.[3] Furthermore, over 70% of patients with recurrent disease will die of granulosa cell tumours, indicating the limitations of non-surgical therapeutic options and possibly a different tumour biology in these cases. The patterns of spread and recurrence indicate that the tumour disseminates by the same routes as epithelial ovarian cancers: exfoliation of clonogenic cells into the peritoneal cavity, direct extension to adjacent organs, and lymphatic and haematogenous metastases.

While stage has been recognized as the most important prognostic factor for granulosa cell tumours, size, rupture, histological subtype, nuclear atypia, and mitotic activity have been correlated with survival. DNA ploidy has recently been correlated with survival. One study demonstrated that DNA ploidy was an independent prognostic factor for survival,[6] while others showed that aneuploidy is significantly associated with other adverse histopathological parameters that may predict outcome (high stage, vascular invasion, nuclear atypia, high mitotic activity), but that it is not by itself a valuable method to predict the biological aggressiveness of granulosa cell tumours.[7,8] Rupture adversely affects survival, but tumour size is not an independent predictor when corrected for stage.[1,4,9,10] Tumours presenting with more advanced stages have a higher grade of atypia and/or more mitotic figures.[1,3,9] Thus histological subtype and DNA ploidy status appear to be of minimal value, since several reports have failed to confirm previous observations of the prognostic value of histological pattern,[1,3,4,9,11] and the reported studies utilizing flow cytometric analysis of DNA content have been inconsistent.[5–7]

The identification of a specific tumour marker would facilitate early detection of recurrent disease. Among proteins derived from granulosa cells, inhibin, follicle-regulating protein, and müllerian-inhibiting substance may be assayed in serum. The granulosa cells of the ovary secrete inhibin, a peptide hormone composed of an α and one or two β subunits.[12] Its major physiological function is to inhibit the secretion of follicle-stimulating hormone (FSH) by the anterior pituitary gland.[13] It functions locally by stimulating progesterone production while inhibiting the production of oestradiol, and serves as a negative regulator of gonadal cell proliferation.[14] Inhibin is expressed in excessive quantities by granulosa cell tumours. In a prospective evaluation of 27 patients with granulosa cell tumours, Jobling et al[15] demonstrated a sevenfold elevation of inhibin levels before surgery, and rising inhibin levels several months before clinical recurrence.

Our understanding of the role of adjuvant therapy in these patients is hampered by the lack of information on the true incidence of recurrence in stage I tumours and on the efficacy of different treatment options. Granulosa cell tumours, which recur, do so in an indolent manner: one-third of recurrences present more than 5 years after diagnosis, one-fifth after 10 years,[16] and some after 25 years.[17] During such a long period of time, a number of patients will die from other causes, making the true estimate of the risk of recurrence more difficult. There have been no reports suggesting a benefit to adjuvant chemotherapy in early-stage granulosa cell tumours. In a retrospective series, Bjorkholm and Petterson[18] reported no benefit to adjuvant irradiation in stage I patients. Currently, there is no basis to recommend adjuvant treatment of any sort following surgery for stage I granulosa cell tumour of the ovary. Appropriate follow-up should include a physical examination with inhibin assay every six months and a computed tomography (CT) scan or abdomino-pelvic ultrasound yearly.

Three years later, the patient developed abdominal discomfort and complained of a sense of fullness in the upper abdomen. An abdominal CT scan revealed a 5 cm × 7 cm mass beneath the right diaphragm. An exploratory laparotomy was performed in this patient, and revealed a 6 cm × 5 cm peritoneal mass arising from the right diaphragm. The mass was surgically excised with apparent free margins. However, widespread tumour nodules were found on the parietal peritoneum, and bowel serosa.

How should a recurrence be managed?

Metastatic lesions and recurrences from granulosa cell tumours have been treated with a variety of different approaches, including surgery, chemotherapy, radiotherapy, and hormonal therapy. The management of patients with recurrent disease should be individualized. Given the characteristic indolent growth pattern of these tumours, surgical resection of disease recurrence is justified in selected patients, depending on the site of relapse. Repeated cytoreduction frequently allows extended palliation. In most cases, the integration of surgery and other treatment modalities such as chemotherapy and/or radiotherapy may allow successful disease control.

What is the role of chemotherapy in recurrent granulosa cell tumours?

Response to chemotherapy has been reported for a number of regimens, but the small number of patients in each series and the admixture of cases with primary advanced and recurrent disease make it difficult to draw definitive conclusions. A response rate of 25% has been reported with single alkylating agents.[19,20] More recently, there have been reports suggesting a possible advantage for multidrug regimens over monotherapy with single alkylating agents. The combination of dactinomycin, 5-fluorouracil (5-FU), and cyclophosphamide has shown activity in 2/2 patients.[20] The Gynecologic Oncology Group (GOG) reported a 20% partial response rate using the combination of vincristine, dactinomycin, and cyclophosphamide in the treatment of advanced or recurrent ovarian granulosa cell tumours.[21] More recently, complete responses have been achieved in patients treated with doxorubicin–cisplatin regimens[22] and with doxorubicin–cisplatin–cyclophosphamide.[23–25] Perhaps the highest activity has been demonstrated with the combination of cisplatin, vinblastine, and bleomycin (PVB). We reported 6 complete and 3 partial responses among 11 previously untreated patients with recurrent and/or metastatic granulosa cell tumours using this regimen.[26] Zambetti et al[27] administered the same regimen to seven patients with granulosa cell tumours, and observed one complete response and three partial responses. In both series, myelosuppression was considerable, with one and two toxic deaths respectively. As in the treatment of germ cell tumours, etoposide has been substituted for vinblastine. Recently, Homesley et al[28] reported the results of a GOG study using bleomycin, etoposide, and cisplatin (BEP) in combination for ovarian granulosa cell tumours and other stromal malignancies. Fourteen out of 38 patients (37%) undergoing second-look laparotomy had a complete remission. With a median follow-up of three years, 11 out of 16 patients in the primary disease category and 21 out of 41 of recurrent patients were progression-free. Although active, this regimen was associated with a considerable toxicity, with two early bleomycin-related deaths. Moreover, severe granulocytopenia was observed in 60% of patients. Thus, while granulosa cell tumours have been shown to respond to platinum-based therapy, toxicity is considerable.

It is clear that the spectrum and severity of toxicity in patients with granulosa cell tumour differ from those observed in younger patients with germ cell tumours. It may be preferable to avoid using bleomycin in the treatment of this disease. Future strategies should include the search for equally or more active, but less toxic, combination regimens. Furthermore, there is a need for alternative treatments after failure of BEP. Paclitaxel should be investigated in patients with refractory granulosa cell tumours; some initial experiences have been encouraging.[29]

Is there a role for radiotherapy in the management of recurrent granulosa cell tumours?

There is little information concerning the use of radiation therapy in advanced or recurrent tumours. Although most reported series include patients treated with radiotherapy, the lack of uniform staging and treatment strategy precludes any definitive conclusions. Neville et al[30] reported on six patients with stage II–III granulosa cell tumours treated with postoperative radiotherapy. All were alive with no evidence of disease, although only one has been followed for longer than 3.5 years. It seems reasonable to conclude that radiotherapy may represent an alternative option to chemotherapy only in patients with small residual disease, and that pelvic radiation can be used to palliate isolated pelvic recurrences.

Other treatments?

Although there is a rationale for the use of hormonal therapy in granulosa cell tumours, clinical experience with this approach is extremely limited. A proportion of tumours express steroid hormone receptors. Responses to medroxyprogesterone acetate and to gonadotropin-releasing hormone (GnRH) antagonists have been reported. Receptors for FSH have been demonstrated in granulosa cell tumours, and FSH has been shown to support the growth of granulosa tumours in nude mice. Fishman et al[31] reported a partial response rate of 50% in a small series, without major side-effects. The clinical evidence of activity for hormonal manipulation in the treatment of granulosa cell tumours remains scanty and anecdotal.

The evidence above suggests that the most appropriate treatment for this patient would be a combination regimen including bleomycin, etoposide, and platinum (BEP). However, this regimen requires monitoring in postmenopausal women.

DISCUSSION

What is the aetiology of sex cord tumours?

Sex cord stromal tumours of the ovary are formed of cells that derive from the sex cords or mesenchyme of the embryonic gonad, and may contain granulosa cells, Sertoli cells, Leydig cells, theca cells, or fibroblasts, singly or in various combinations. These neoplasms represent a minority of ovarian malignancies (7%), and their scarcity limits our understanding of the natural history, management, and prognosis.

While it is generally accepted that both granulosa and Sertoli cells derive from the sex cords of the developing gonad, which originate from the celomic epithelium, disagreement exists about the ultimate fate of the sex cord cells. Some authors believe that granulosa cells are derived from the cortical sex cords while the Sertoli cells originate from medullary cords of mesonephric origin; others believe that sex cord cells differentiate into granulosa or Sertoli cells depending on whether gonadal development is towards an ovarian or testicular pathway. The stromal elements of sex cord tumours can exist in a pure form, or may be admixed with epithelial elements of putative sex cord origin.

Very little is known about the aetiology of these tumours in the human. However, sex cord tumours can be easily induced in animals provided that oocyte depletion has occurred and the pituitary gland is functioning normally. The most accepted hypothesis is that the degeneration of follicular granulosa cells after oocyte loss and the consequent compensatory rise in pituitary gonadotropins induces irregular proliferation and eventually neoplasia of the granulosa cells. This hypothesis is consistent with the observation that most granulosa cell tumours occur soon after the menopause, when oocyte depletion and high levels of gonadotropin are observed. However, this explanation does not account for tumours developing during the reproductive years or even before menarche.

Granulosa cell tumours

Granulosa cell tumours comprise only 5% of all ovarian malignancies, and account for approximately 70% of malignant sex cord stromal tumours.[3,10,32–34] The incidence in developed countries varies from 0.4 to 1.7 cases per 100 000 women per year.[1,32] The average age at the time of diagnosis is 52 years, but granulosa cell tumours have been diagnosed from infancy through to the tenth decade of life. Since the clinical and pathological characteristics of the tumours occurring after the menopause are different from those occurring in children and younger patients, the adult and juvenile granulosa cell types will be considered separately.

Granulosa cell tumours: adult type

The adult type accounts for 95% of all granulosa cell tumours. The main symptoms at presentation include abnormal vaginal bleeding, abdominal distension, and pain.[1,2,32,33] While the latter two symptoms are related to the dimension of the tumour and to possible adnexal torsion-haemorrage and tumour rupture, bleeding anomalies are consistent with the presence of an oestrogen-secreting tumour. Hormone production is frequent, and, as a result, endometrial hyperplasia and even in situ or invasive adenocarcinoma can be found in a substantial proportion of patients with granulosa cell tumours. The reported incidence of hyperplasia ranges from 24% to above 80%. Gusberg and Kardon[35] reported, in a retrospective series of 69 patients, 13% with cystic glandular hyperplasia, 42% with atypical hyperplasia, 5% with adenocarcinoma in situ, and 22% with invasive adenocarcinoma.

Rarely, virilizing changes such as oligomenorrhoea, hirsutism, and other masculinizing signs may be present.

Granulosa cell tumours: juvenile type

About 90% of granulosa tumours occurring in prepubertal girls and many of those seen before the age of 30 years are of this juvenile type. In a clinico-pathological review of 125 cases, Scully's group[36] described 44% of these tumours prior to age 10, and only 3% after the third decade of life. The tumour usually arises in otherwise normal children, although there is a suggestion of a specific association with Ollier's disease (enchondromatosis) and Maffucci's syndrome (enchondromatosis and haemangiosis).[37–40] The majority of prepubertal patients present with clinical evidence of isosexual precocious pseudopuberty. The most consistent clinical sign at presentation is an increasing abdominal girth; infrequently, a surgical emergency is encountered following spontaneous rupture or torsion of the adnexal mass. The frequency of bilaterality is 5%, similar to the adult type, and most tumours present at an early stage.[36]

Pathology

The tumours are largely solid, although cystic forms are occasionally encountered. Microscopic examination reveals a predominantly solid cellular tumour with focal follicle formation and an oedematous, loose stroma. The two characteristic cytological features of the neoplastic juvenile granulosa cells are their rounded, hyperchromatic nuclei and their moderate to abundant eosinophilic or vacuolated cytoplasm. A severe degree of nuclear atypia is seen in 13% of cases, while the mitotic activity is generally higher than that seen in adult granulosa cell tumours.

Clinical behaviour and prognosis

While the propensity for presentation with localized disease is similar to the adult type, there are several different behavioural characteristics. The juvenile form is characteristically aggressive in advanced stages, and the time to relapse and death is short. Only 3 out of 13 cases with advanced disease extracted from two analyses[41,42] were alive, with most recurrences and deaths occurring within three years. As for adult granulosa cell tumours, extra-ovarian spread is the most important prognostic factor. Tumour size, mitotic activity, and nuclear atypia lose their significance when applied to only stage I disease. Furthermore, no impact on recurrence or survival was associated with tumour rupture. In a limited number of patients with advanced disease, aneuploidy was associated with a worse prognosis.[43]

Management

Our understanding of the optimal management of granulosa cell tumours is limited by their scarcity. The diagnosis of a granulosa tumour is often not made until surgery, and a correct frozen section diagnosis can be a challenge even for experienced gynaecological pathologists. If future reproductive potential is not an issue, total hysterectomy and bilateral salpingo-oophorectomy should be performed. In addition, careful surgical staging should be undertaken. This includes a thorough exploration of the abdominal cavity, washings for cytological analysis, multiple biopsies, omentectomy, and pelvic and para-aortic lymph node sampling/dissection. Although no scientific evidence exists about the efficacy of cytoreduction, every effort should be made to remove metastatic disease. Following careful staging and in the absence of extra-ovarian spread, preservation of the uterus and controlateral ovary is reasonable in patients wishing to preserve their fertility. In such cases, endometrial curettage must be performed to rule out concomitant endometrial pathology. There are no data to support any kind of postoperative adjuvant treatment for patients with stage I disease, given the indolent nature of this neoplasm and the overall good prognosis for these cases. Evans et al[5] reported a 9% risk of recurrence in stage IA disease. It would appear that patients with stage I disease based on optimal surgery have a very low risk of recurrence. In Bjorkholm's and Pettersson's retrospective series,[18] there was no observed benefit to adjuvant irradiation in stage I patients.

LEARNING POINTS

❇ Sex cord stromal tumours represent 5% of all ovarian neoplasms, and their rarity constitutes a limitation on our understanding of their natural history and management. Granulosa cell tumours represent the most common histotype (70%).

❇ 95% of cases are at stage I at diagnosis, and are unilateral.

❇ Typically, they have an indolent growth and propensity for late recurrences.

❇ The 10-year survival rate is in excess of 90% for stage I patients.

❇ Surgery is the mainstay of treatment, and can be fertility-sparing in younger patients who desire to preserve their reproductive function.

❇ There are no data to support the use of adjuvant treatment in stage I disease.

❇ Treatment of advanced or recurrent disease should integrate surgery and chemotherapy: repeated cytoreduction frequently affords these patients extended palliation. The most effective chemotherapy regimen is a combination of bleomycin, etoposide, and cisplatin (BEP).

❇ Experience with radiotherapy and hormonal manipulation is limited and mostly anecdotal.

REFERENCES

1. Malmstrom H, Hogberg T, Risberg B et al, Granulosa cell tumours of the ovary: prognostic factors and outcome. *Gynecol Oncol* 1994; **52**: 50.

2. Piura B, Nemet D, Yanai-Inbar I et al, Granulosa cell tumour of the ovary: a study of 18 cases. *J Surg Oncol* 1994; **55**: 71.

3. Bjorkholm E, Silfversward C, Prognostic factors in granulosa cell tumours. *Gynecol Oncol* 1981; **11**: 261.

4. Stenwig JT, Hazekamp JT, Beecham JB, Granulosa cell tumours of the ovary. A clinicopathological study of 118 cases with long-term follow-up. *Gynecol Oncol* 1979; 7: 136.

5. Evans AT, Gaffey TA, Malkasian GD et al, Clinicopathologic review of 118 granulosa and 82 theca cell tumors. *Obstet Gynecol* 1980; **55**: 231.

6. Klemi PJ, Joensuu H, Salmi T, Prognostic value of flow cytometric DNA content analysis in granulosa cell tumour of the ovary. *Cancer* 1990; **65**: 1189.

7. Chadha S, Cornelisse CJ, Schaberg A, Flow cytometric DNA ploidy analysis of ovarian granulosa cell tumours. *Gynecol Oncol* 1990; **36**: 240.

8. Roush GR, El Naggar AK, Abdul-Karim FW, Granulosa cell tumour of ovary: a clinico-pathologic and flow cytometric DNA analysis. *Gynecol Oncol* 1995; **56**: 430.

9. Fox H, Agrawal K, Langley FA, A clinico-pathologic study of 92 cases of granulosa cell tumour of the ovary with special reference to the factors influencing prognosis. *Cancer* 1975; **35**: 231.

10. Bjorkholm E, Silfversward C, Granulosa and theca cell tumours. Incidence and occurrence of second primary tumours. *Acta Radiol Oncol* 1980; **19**: 161.

11. Bjorkholm E, Granulosa cell tumours: a comparison of survival in patients and matched controls. *Am J Obstet Gynecol* 1980; **138**: 329.

12. Burger HG, Inhibin. *Reprod Med Rev* 1992; **1**: 1.

13. Ying S, Inhibins, activins, and follistatins: gonadal proteins modulating the secretion of follicle-stimulating hormone. *Endocrinol Rev* 1988; **9**: 267.

14. Matzuk MM, Finegold MJ, Su JJ et al, Alpha inhibin is a tumour suppressor gene with gonadal specificity in mice. *Nature* 1992; **360**: 313.

15. Jobling T, Mamers P, Healy DL et al, A prospective study of inhibin in granulosa cell tumours of the ovary. *Gynecol Oncol* 1994; **55**: 285.

16. Diddle AW, Granulosa–theca-cell ovarian tumours: prognosis. *Cancer* 1952; **5**: 215.

17. Kolstad P, *Clinical Gynecologic Oncology. The Norwegian Experience.* Oslo: Norwegian University Press, 1986.

18. Bjorkholm E, Pettersson F, Granulosa cell and theca cell tumours: the clinical picture and long term outcome for the Radiumhemmet series. *Acta Obstet Gynecol Scand* 1980; **59**: 361.

19. Malkasian GD, Webb MJ, Jorgensen EO, Observations on chemotherapy of granulosa cell carcinomas and malignant ovarian teratomas. *Obstet Gynecol* 1974; **44**: 885.

20. Schwartz PE, Smith JP, Treatment of ovarian stromal tumours. *Am J Obstet Gynecol* 1976; **125**: 402.

21. Slayton RE, Management of germ cell and stromal tumours of the ovary. *Semin Oncol* 1984; **11**: 299.

22. Jacobs HJ, Deppe G, Cohen CJ, Combination chemotherapy of ovarian granulosa cell tumour with cisplatinum and doxorubicin. *Gynecol Oncol* 1982; **14**: 294.

23. Gershenson DM, Copeland LJ, Kavanagh JJ et al, Treatment of metastatic stromal tumours of the ovary with cisplatin, doxorubicin and cyclophosphamide. *Obstet Gynecol* 1987; **70**: 765.

24. Canlibel F, Caputo TA, Chemotherapy of granulosa cell tumours. *Am J Obstet Gynecol* 1983; **145**: 763.

25. Pectasides D, Alevizakos N, Athanassiou AE, Cisplatin-containing regimen in advanced or recurrent granulosa cell tumours of the ovary. *Ann Oncol* 1984; **3**: 316.

26. Colombo N, Sessa C, Landoni F et al, Cisplatin, vinblastine, and bleomycin combination chemotherapy in metastatic granulosa cell tumour of the ovary. *Obstet Gynecol* 1986; **67**: 265.

27. Zambetti M, Escobedo A, Pilotti S et al, Cisplatinum/vinblastine/bleomycin combination chemotherapy in advanced or recurrent granulosa cell tumours of the ovary. *Gynecol Oncol* 1990; **36**: 317.

28. Homesley HD, Bundy BN, Hurteau JA et al, Bleomycin, etoposide, and cisplatin combination therapy of ovarian granulosa cell tumours and other stromal malignancies: a Gynecologic Oncology Group study. *Gynecol Oncol* 1999; **72**: 131.

29. Tresukosol D, Kudelka AP, Edwards CL et al, Recurrent ovarian granulosa cell tumour: a case report of a dramatic response to Taxol. *Int J Gynecol Cancer* 1995; **5**: 156–9.

30. Neville AJ, Gilchrist KW, Davis T, The chemotherapy of granulosa cell tumours of the ovary: experience of the Wisconsin Clinical Cancer Center. *Med Ped Oncol* 1984; **12**: 397.

31. Fishman A, Kudelka A, Edwards C et al, GnRH agonist (Depot-Lupron) in the treatment of refractory or persistent ovarian granulosa cell tumour (GCT). *Proc Am Soc Clin Oncol* 1994; **13**: 236.

32. Ohel G, Kaneti H, Schenker JG, Granulosa cell tumours in Israel: study of 172 cases. *Gynecol Oncol* 1983; **15**: 278.

33. Pankratz E, Boyes DA, White GW et al, Granulosa cell tumours: a clinical review of 61 cases. *Obstet Gynecol* 1978; **52**: 718.

34. Schweppe KW, Beller FK, Clinical data of granulosa cell tumours. *J Cancer Res Clin Oncol* 1982; **104**: 161.

35. Gusberg SB, Kardon P, Proliferative endometrial response to theca–granulosa-cell tumours. *Am J Obstet Gynecol* 1971; **111**: 633.

36. Young RH, Dickersin GR, Scully RE, Juvenile granulosa cell tumour of the ovary: a clinico-pathological analysis of 125 cases. *Am J Surg Pathol* 1984; **8**: 575.

37. Takeuchi H, Hamada H, Sodemoto Y et al, Juvenile granulosa cell tumour with rapid distant metastases. *Acta Pathol Jpn* 1983; **33**: 357.

38. Tamini HK, Bolen J, Enchrondomatosis (Ollier's disease) and ovarian juvenile granulosa cell tumour. *Cancer* 1984; **53**: 1605.

39. Vaz RM, Turner CH, Ollier's disease (enchrondomatosis) associated with ovarian juvenile granulosa cell tumour and precocious pseudopuberty. *J Paediat* 1986; **108**: 945.

40. Velasco-Oses A, Alonso-Alvaro A, Blanco-Pozo A et al, Ollier's disease associated with ovarian juvenile granulosa cell tumour. *Cancer* 1988; **62**: 222.

41. Plantaz D, Flamant F, Vassal G et al, Tumeurs de la granulosa de l'ovaire chez l'enfant et l'adolescente. *Arch Fr Pediatr* 1992; **49**: 793.

42. Vassal G, Flamant F, Caillaud JM et al, Juvenile granulosa cell tumour of the ovary in children: a clinical study of 15 cases. *J Clin Oncol* 1988; **6**: 990.

43. Jacoby AF, Young RH, Colvin RB et al, DNA content in juvenile granulosa cell tumours of the ovary: a study of early and advanced stage disease. *Gynecol Oncol* 1992; **46**: 97.

44. Young RH, Scully RE, Ovarian sex cord–stromal tumours: recent advances and current status. *Clin Obstet Gynecol* 1984; **11**: 93.

10
Germ cell tumours

Edward S Newlands

INTRODUCTION

Germ cell tumours of the ovary are a rare but an important group of tumours. Overall, they comprise less than 5% of ovarian malignancies, but they account for a significant percentage of malignant ovarian tumours in young women. Since they affect predominantly young women of childbearing age and are usually curable, it is important that they are properly diagnosed and treated.

The average age at diagnosis is 20 years, and an ovarian germ cell tumour should be at the top of the list of differential diagnoses when an ovarian mass is discovered in a girl or young woman. Dysgerminomas account for about 45% of malignant germ cell tumours. The remainder are chiefly endodermal sinus tumours or immature teratomas. Mature teratomas are more commonly found in older women, and about 2–3% will undergo malignant transformation.

Patients may present with localized (stage 1) or advanced disease. Conservative surgery is now commonly performed, since chemotherapy has become so effective in this disease. The case discussed below demonstrates the importance of correct staging and surveillance of these patients. Relapse following early-stage disease is not unusual, and the appropriate use of chemotherapy is usually curative.

CASE HISTORY

A 24-year-old teacher presented in April 1987 with a distended abdomen and heavy vaginal bleeding. Clinical and ultrasound examination confirmed a large pelvic mass. A laparotomy was performed in May 1987, which confirmed a large pelvic mass arising from the right ovary, and a right salpingo-oophorectomy was performed. Staging at the time of laparotomy showed no evidence of disease outside the ovary, but no biopsies were taken and, in particular, the contralateral ovary was not biopsied. Peritoneal washings were taken, but no definite malignant cells were seen. Pathologically, the ovarian mass measured 17 cm × 15 cm × 7 cm, and, histologically, appeared to be a pure dysgerminoma, with the tumour reaching near the surface of the ovary. Postoperatively, her β human chorionic gonadotropin (βhCG: normal range <5 IU/l) and α-fetoprotein (AFP: normal range <10 kU/l) were normal. Following recovery from her laparotomy, regular follow-up was started, and the plan was to repeat the laparoscopy in November 1987.

What should her initial management have been?

Clearly, in a 24-year-old woman presenting with a large lower abdominal mass, it is imperative to get histological confirmation of the nature of the mass. In her case, she had a laparotomy with conservative surgery. Only the tumour involving the right ovary was removed, and surgery was limited to a right salpingo-oophorectomy. Histology confirmed apparently pure dysgerminoma, and her postoperative tumour markers for βhCG and AFP were normal. It is recognized that up to 15% of dysgerminomas can be bilateral. During her laparotomy, she should have had the contralateral ovary biopsied. Therefore, at this stage, she apparently had stage I disease, and a further laparoscopy was planned for some months later.

Discussion

Ovarian germ cell tumours are rare, but account for over half of the malignant ovarian tumours in women under the age of 20.[1] This patient was 24, still young for ovarian adenocarcinoma, and the conservative surgery to preserve her fertility was entirely correct. Postoperatively, she did not have a body computed tomography (CT) scan, nor did she have regular serum tumour markers taken, and nor did she have regular clinical check-ups. In 1987, the options for her further treatment would have included pelvic radiation. Since dysgerminomas are radiosensitive, this can be effective treatment – but it would probably have sterilized her. Cisplatin-containing chemotherapy was already established as being effective in this disease, but its use as an adjuvant in a patient with stage I disease was, and is, a questionable policy owing to the short- and long-term toxicities associated with chemotherapy.

Surveillance for stage I testicular germ cell tumours was established as a safe and reliable policy by the Charing Cross Hospital group in London in 1978. Since it has proved a safe and reliable policy in male patients who could be regularly followed up, we have been using the same policy in patients with stage I ovarian germ cell tumours since the 1970s. The follow-up is quite intensive, involving regular clinical review, serological tumour markers and a laparoscopy three months after the initial laparotomy. We also repeat the CT scan of thorax, abdomen and pelvis three and six months after the initial one, looking for early recurrence, particularly peritoneal disease. The schedule of follow-up used at the Charing Cross Hospital is shown in Table 10.1. Using this policy, we have followed up 24 patients with stage I disease. Two patients with dysgerminoma developed disease in the contralateral ovary at 4.5 and 5.2 years after their first tumour. These are considered to be second primaries rather than recurrence of the original tumour. All patients on the stage I follow-up are alive, apart from one patient who became pregnant during the initial year of follow-up, against medical advice, and on delivery of her child was found to have metastatic disease and died of pulmonary embolism as she was starting chemotherapy. This policy gives a five-year overall survival rate of 95%, with a five-year disease-free survival rate of 68%.[2] The other patients who have relapsed have been salvaged with POMB/ACE chemotherapy (see below). Although the number of ovarian germ cell tumours is small, we have followed over 300 male patients with stage I disease since 1979, and the overall survival rate in these patients at five years is 100%, and at 10 years it is 98%. This policy means that the majority of patients are spared the short- and long-term side-effects of cytotoxic chemotherapy.

Relapse during follow-up

Shortly before the planned second laparoscopy, the patient represented with irregular and heavy periods, loss of appetite, low back pain and abdominal swelling. At the second laparotomy in November 1987, she was found to have a frozen pelvis and

Table 10.1 Follow-up of germ cell tumours (GCT)

GCT stage I follow-up (females)

1st year

Initial surgery	Unilateral salpingo-oopherectomy with biopsies of omentum, contralateral ovary and locoregional lymph nodes, and peritoneal washings for cytology
3–6 weeks after initial surgery	CT chest, abdomen and pelvis
Then monthly	Clinical examination and chest X-ray, alternate visits
3 months after initial surgery	Repeat CT chest, abdomen and pelvis and if normal then second-look laparoscopy
6 months after initial surgery	CT chest, abdomen and pelvis

Clinical examination

1st year	Monthly
2nd year	2-monthly
3rd year	3-monthly
4th year	4-monthly
Years 5–10	6-monthly

Tumour marker follow-up

Samples: serum AFP and βhCG and LDH (regardless of initial value)

0–6 months	2-weekly
7–24 months	4-weekly
25–36 months	8-weekly
37–60 months	12-weekly
After 5 years	6-monthly

CT, computed tomography; AFP, α-fetoprotein; βhCG, β human chronic gonadotropin; LDH, lactate dehydrogenase.

tumour involving the whole of the lower abdomen. No attempt at radical surgery was made. Preoperative tumour markers showed that her βhCG was 4 IU/l and that AFP was 2137 kU/l.

She was referred to the Charing Cross Hospital, and was first seen in November 1987. Clinical examination identified the large abdominal mass, which was confirmed on CT scan of the thorax, abdomen and pelvis. There was no spread of tumour to the chest, but CT scan showed bilateral hydronephrosis from pressure on the ureters in the pelvis.

In November 1987, the patient had unresectable tumour involving the pelvis and lower abdomen, and at this stage her tumour markers were elevated, with a small amount of βhCG production but a significant amount of AFP production. The presence of AFP in the serum at relapse confirmed that there had been a sampling problem in the original tumour, which had appeared histologically as a pure dysgerminoma. AFP is produced by the yolk sac elements in a teratoma – and therefore she must have had a mixed germ cell tumour of the ovary, and the yolk sac component had not been sampled histologically. Dysgerminomas can produce a small amount of βhCG but large amounts of βhCG are typically produced by trophoblasts from a teratoma. The values found in this patient are still compatible with a diagnosis of dysgerminoma, and do not automatically confirm that she had a major trophoblastic element in the tumour. Her CA125 was raised (at 100 U/ml) at the initiation of chemotherapy, reflecting either tumour production of CA125 or peritoneal irritation from the tumour. Clearly, at this stage, she required chemotherapy, and it is now established that cisplatin-containing chemotherapy can cure the majority of patients with spread of their ovarian germ cell tumours.

What is the management of a relapsed ovarian germ cell tumour?

The plasma urea and electrolytes were normal but, in view of the hydronephrosis, the patient was started with reduced-dose chemotherapy with etoposide and cisplatin to shrink the abdominal tumour with the aim of relieving the pressure on the ureters. Once renal function had recovered, she was treated with the POMB/ACE schedule of chemotherapy (Table 10.2). POMB (cisplatin, vincristine (Oncovin), methotrexate, bleomycin by infusion) is essentially alternated with ACE (dactinomycin (actinomycin D), cyclophosphamide, etoposide) at two-weekly intervals unless there is a treatment delay from myelosuppression. Initially, her tumour markers showed a surge on starting chemotherapy, reaching a peak on βhCG of 36 IU/l before returning to normal, and her AFP rose to a peak of 7361 kU/l before reaching the normal range in February 1988 (Figure 10.1). At the end of chemotherapy, there was a residual mass in the pelvis. She had a further laparotomy, and histology showed only necrotic tissue and differentiated teratoma, which was excised (Figure 10.2).

POMB/ACE chemotherapy has long been established as effective treatment for this disease. It was first introduced in 1977, and therefore there is over 20 years' experience in using this schedule of chemotherapy. Because this patient had impairment of renal function at the initiation of chemotherapy, she was given etoposide (100 mg/m² i.v.) and cisplatin (20 mg/m² i.v.) on two consecutive days to shrink the pelvic tumour sufficiently to relieve the hydronephrosis. After the hydronephrosis was relieved, she had POMB/ACE chemotherapy; the details of this treatment have been published on several occasions.[3–6] Her tumour markers returned to normal by early 1988, and she was left with a residual mass in the pelvis, which needed to be resected to confirm whether or not it contained active tumour; in her case, it contained only differenti-

Table 10.2   POMB/ACE schedule

POMB

Day 1	Vincristine	1 mg/m^2 (max. 2 mg) i.v. bolus
	Methotrexate	300 mg/m^2 i.v. infusion
Day 2	Bleomycin	30 mg i.v. infusion over 24 hours
	Folinic acid	15 mg at 24, 36, 48 and 60 hours after start of
	(leucovorin)	methotrexate infusion
Day 3	Cisplatin	120 mg/m^2 i.v. infusion over 12 hours

ACE

Day 1	Etoposide	100 mg/m^2 i.v. infusion
	Dactinomycin	0.5 mg i.v. bolus
Day 2	Etoposide	100 mg/m^2 i.v. infusion
	Dactinomycin	0.5 mg i.v. bolus
Day 3	Etoposide	100 mg/m^2 i.v. infusion
	Dactinomycin	0.5 mg i.v. bolus
	Cyclophosphamide 500 mg/m^2 in 250 ml normal saline over 30 minutes	

The POMB/ACE schedule is administered fortnightly, and alternates between the POMB and ACE regimens after the first two cycles, which are both POMBs.

ated teratoma and necrotic tissue. She therefore went onto regular follow-up, which is a combination of clinical check-ups and regular tumour markers (βhCG, AFP, CA125 and LDH).

What are the acute side-effects of platinum- and etoposide-based chemotherapy of germ cell tumours?

During her chemotherapy, the patient experienced severe nausea and vomiting with each course of cisplatin chemotherapy, and lost a considerable amount of weight. On completion of her chemotherapy and recovery from her laparotomy, she put on weight rapidly, and briefly had painful engorgement of both breasts as her weight increased by approxi-mately 10 kg over two to three months. On completion of treatment, she went onto regular tumour marker and clinical follow-up, and there has been no evidence of recurrence of her disease.

When this patient was treated in 1987, modern antiemetic treatment using 5-HT$_3$ antagonists was not available, and she had significant problems with vomiting from the cisplatin chemotherapy and lost a considerable amount of weight. Fortunately, over the last decade, the introduction of 5-HT$_3$ antagonists, such as granisetron, ondansetron and tropisetron, has transformed the ability to control nausea and vomiting caused by cytotoxic chemotherapy. We

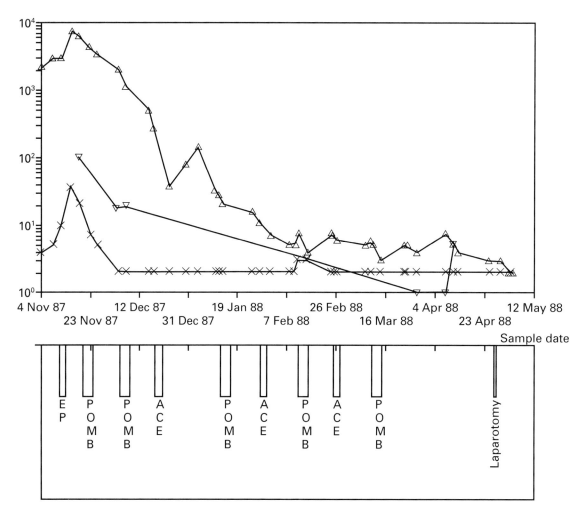

Figure 10.1
Case history patient tumour marker results: X, serum βhCG (IU/l); Δ, AFP (U/ml); ▽, CA125 (U/ml); EP, etoposide, cisplatin; POMB, cisplatin, vincristine, methotrexate, bleomycin; ACE, dactinomycin, cyclophosphamide, etoposide. Chemotherapy was continued until the patient was clearly in tumour marker remission, and then the residual pelvic mass was excised.

introduced the combination of a 5-HT$_3$ antagonist with dexamethasone, and confirmed that with the POMB/ACE schedule of chemotherapy, the addition of dexamethasone doubled the incidence of control of nausea and vomiting to approximately 80%.[7] While the combination of 5-HT$_3$ antagonist and dexamethasone is very effective, and should certainly be used with cisplatin in the POMB/ACE schedule of chemotherapy, there are potentially two complications of dexamethasone that need to be borne in mind: (i) the frequent use of dexamethasone (i.e. weekly) increases the incidence of pneumocystis in patients receiving chemotherapy, and (ii)

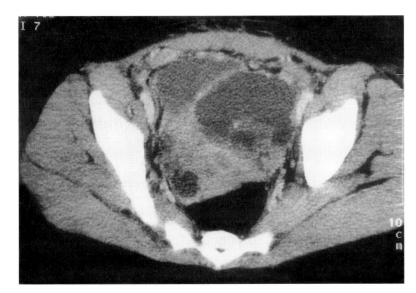

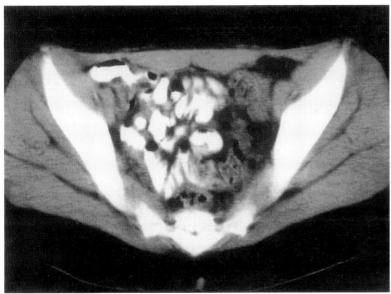

Figure 10.2
Computed tomography (CT) scans of the upper pelvis of a patient with an advanced ovarian germ cell tumour mainly producing AFP (see Figure 10.1). Within the pelvis, there is a mixture of low-density (darker areas) of cystic tumour interspersed with solid tumour, which shows up as white, owing to the uptake of intravenous contrast. The upper image is at the start of chemotherapy and the lower image after completing chemotherapy and a laparotomy to remove mature differentiated teratoma. The patient remains in remission 11 years after completing treatment, and has had two normal pregnancies.

aseptic necrosis of the femoral and humeral heads is a well-recognized complication of dexamethasone treatment, and certainly does occur in patients receiving only brief courses of dexamethasone with their cytotoxic chemotherapy.

Neurotoxicity is a recognized complication of therapy with high doses of cisplatin. When it occurs, there is most commonly a loss of high-tone hearing, and patients should be monitored with audiograms. Peripheral neuritis may occur, but is less common. The symptoms usually improve, but recovery may be incomplete. Careful monitoring of fluid balance before, during and after each course is important to help prevent nephrotoxicity. Improvements in the control of emesis in the last 10 years have reduced the frequency of renal impairment. Neutropenic sepsis is not unusual with intensive therapy with etoposide. However, it is rarely long-lasting.

On completing chemotherapy, the patient rapidly put on weight (around 10 kg) and this increase in body mass can induce a poorly under-stood (presumably endocrine) syndrome of refeeding gynaecomastia. This is much more commonly seen in male patients, but was presum-ably the cause of her temporary breast engorge-ment. Fortunately, with modern antiemetics, this is seen much less commonly now.

What are the effects of chemotherapy on fertility and long-term health?

The patient's periods returned approximately four months after completing chemotherapy, and she was advised not to start a pregnancy until 12 months after her chemotherapy. Her first pregnancy was in 1989 and was entirely normal; this was fol-lowed by a second normal pregnancy in 1993. She continues on annual check-ups and six-monthly serum samples for tumour markers βhCG, AFP, CA125 and lactate dehydrogenase (LDH).

Cytotoxic chemotherapy certainly impairs fertility in both sexes, and it is now routine to perform sperm storage in male patients prior to cytotoxic chemotherapy. Fortunately, in female patients, ovarian function usually recovers between two and six months after completing POMB/ACE chemo-therapy. We have recommended that patients do not try to start a further pregnancy for 12 months after completing cytotoxic chemotherapy to allow adequate follow-up and also to minimize the potential teratogenicity from the chemotherapy. At the last analysis, on patients who had tried to become pregnant and who had not had radical surgery for their germ cell tumour, 42% of these patients had successful pregnancies and there had

been no fetal abnormalities. This patient completed two normal pregnancies successfully.

It is likely that this type of cytotoxic chemotherapy will have an effect on the age of menopause. In an analysis of a large number of patients treated with intensive chemotherapy for gestational trophoblastic tumours, the average age of menopause was brought forward from 52–53 years of age in patients not receiving any chemotherapy to around 47 years of age in those receiving intensive chemotherapy.[8] It is likely that patients receiving either BEP-type chemotherapy (see below) or POMB/ACE chemotherapy will also have the menopause early, and should have hormone replacement therapy at least until they reach their early 50s.

Excellent results can be obtained with chemotherapy in patients with metastatic ovarian germ cell tumours, provided that the combina-tion includes cisplatin and etoposide. One of the considerations in devising POMB/ACE chemo-therapy, which is essentially an alternating regi-men, was that the cumulative dose of each drug would be less than when repeating the same combination with each course of chemotherapy. It has become apparent that one of the complica-tions of this type of combination chemotherapy is the small incidence of induction of second tumours – the main one induced by the combi-nations used in treating germ cell tumours is acute myeloid leukaemia (AML). In a report in over 600 male patients, a similar incidence of induced AML was found in patients given BEP-type chemotherapy as in those receiving POMB/ACE chemotherapy.[9] The majority of patients developing therapy-induced AML die from their second tumour, although occasional patients have been salvaged with marrow trans-plantation. Although uncommon, this real com-plication of cytotoxic chemotherapy confirms that the management of stage I disease should not include chemotherapy as an adjuvant, since it is inevitable that occasional second tumours will be induced. At present, it is not clear that there is a threshold below which it is safe to subject young patients to cytotoxic chemotherapy. The sole patient with an ovarian germ cell tumour who developed AML had a total dose of etoposide of 1200 mg/m^2.

Discussion

Chemotherapy for ovarian germ cell tumours prior to the introduction of cisplastin was unsatisfactory, although some patients were salvaged with a combination of vincristine, dactinomycin and cyclophosphamide. One report showed a remission rate of 28%.[10] More intensive chemotherapy with the same drugs salvages a higher proportion of patients, and this can reach 78% according to one report.[11] Since the introduction in the 1970s of etoposide and cisplatin, these two agents have become the cornerstone of chemotherapy combinations for germ cell tumours of all sites in both males and females. The results of POMB/ACE chemotherapy have been published on a number of occasions,[3–6] and in our most recent report, the three-year survival rate of patients with metastatic disease was 88%, and no relapses have occurred beyond three years after completing treatment. Other combinations containing cisplatin and etoposide have also been used in treating ovarian germ cell tumours; these include BEP chemotherapy (bleomycin, etoposide, cisplatin) (Table 10.3), and in a report by Segelov et al,[12] the five-year survival rate in these patients was 88%.

LEARNING POINTS

❖ It is necessary to be aware of the possibility of an ovarian germ cell tumour.
❖ The age distribution of these tumours is younger than in patients presenting with ovarian adenocarcinoma.

Table 10.3	BEP schedule
Etoposide	100 mg/m^2 i.v. days 1–5
Cisplatin	20 mg/m^2 i.v. days 1–5
Bleomycin	30 mg i.v. infusion[a] weekly
Courses repeated on a three-weekly cycle	

[a] Bleomycin by infusion or intramuscular injection probably reduces the incidence of significant pneumonitis.

❖ Conservative surgery should be performed.
❖ There are problems with histopathological sampling: serum tumour markers can detect yolk sac (AFP) and trophoblast (βhCG).
❖ Careful surveillance is acceptable management for stage I disease.
❖ There is an excellent long-term outlook following cisplatin-containing chemotherapy.
❖ Residual masses at the end of chemotherapy must be removed surgically.
❖ Fertility is usually preserved in female patients receiving cisplatin-containing chemotherapy.
❖ It is necessary to be aware of the long-term complications of cytotoxic chemotherapy.

REFERENCES

1. Altaras MM, Goldberg GL, Levin W et al, The value of cancer antigen-125 as a tumor marker in malignant germ cell tumors of the ovary. *Gynecol Oncol* 1986; **25**: 150–9.
2. Dark CG, Bower M, Newlands ES et al, Surveillance policy for stage I ovarian germ cell tumours. *J Clin Oncol* 1997; **15**: 620–4.
3. Newlands ES, Southall PJ, Paradinas FJ, Holden L, Management of ovarian germ cell tumours. In: *Textbook of Uncommon Cancer* (Williams CJ, Krikorian JC, Green MR, Raghavan D, eds). Chichester: Wiley, 1988: 37–53.

4. Bower M, Fife K, Holden L et al, Chemotherapy for ovarian germ cell tumours. *Eur J Cancer* 1996; **32**: 593–7.

5. Newlands ES, Begent RHJ, Rustin GJS, Bagshawe KD, Potential for cure in metastatic ovarian teratomas and dysgerminomas. *Br J Obstet Gynaecol* 1982; **89**: 555–60.

6. Newlands ES, Holden L, Bagshawe KD, Tumour markers and POMB/ACE chemotherapy in the management of ovarian germ cell tumours (GCTs). *Int J Biol Markers* 1988; **3**: 185–92.

7. Smith DB, Newlands ES, Rustin GJS et al, Comparison of ondansetron and ondansetron plus dexamethasone as antiemetic prophylaxis during cisplatin-containing chemotherapy. *Lancet* 1991; **338**: 487–90.

8. Bower M, Rustin GJS, Newlands ES et al, Chemotherapy for gestational trophoblastic tumours hastens menopause by 3 years. *Eur J Cancer* 1998; **34**: 1204–7.

9. Boshoff C, Begent RHJ, Oliver RTD et al, Secondary tumours following etoposide-containing therapy for germ cell cancer. *Ann Oncol* 1995; **6**: 35–40.

10. Slayton RE, Park RC, Silverberg SG et al, Vincristine, dactinomycin and cyclophosphamide in the treatment of malignant germ cell tumors of the ovary. A Gynecologic Oncology Group study (a final report). *Cancer* 1985; **56**: 243–8.

11. Mann JR, Pearson D, Barrett A et al, Results of the United Kingdom Children's Cancer Study Group's malignant germ cell tumor studies. *Cancer* 1989; **63**: 1657–67.

12. Segelov E, Campbell J, Ng M et al, Cisplatin-based chemotherapy for ovarian germ cell malignancies: the Australian experience. *J Clin Oncol* 1994; **12**: 378–84.

SECTION 3: Relapsed Ovarian Cancer

11
Relapse with ascites within 12 months of diagnosis

Jonathan A Ledermann

INTRODUCTION

A high proportion of patients with advanced ovarian cancer attain a complete clinical remission following surgery and chemotherapy. Most of these patients will relapse and require further treatment. Such treatment is not curative, and careful consideration needs to be given to the choice of treatment – its likely results and the impact of such treatment on the quality of life of the patient. In patients with a symptomatic relapse, there is usually a clear indication for further treatment. Decisions about which of the 'second-line' therapies to use are often based on the type of first-line treatment and the length of time the patient has been free from treatment.

The time to first relapse depends upon the initial stage, degree of surgical debulking and type of first-line chemotherapy. Patients relapsing during treatment or within six months of chemotherapy are defined as being resistant to primary chemotherapeutic drugs, most commonly cisplatin or carboplatin. Later relapse confers a decreasing probability of resistance to re-challenge with the same group of drugs. Markman et al[1] have defined degrees of platinum resistance, and response to several other drugs also appears to depend upon the platinum-free

period.[2] However, newer drugs such as paclitaxel and topotecan that may be active in patients with resistance to platinum-based therapy have increased the choice of therapies available at relapse.

In this chapter, we are faced with the clinical problem of symptomatic relapse occurring within 12 months of diagnosis. Should such patients be given new agents, not previously used in first-line therapy, or re-challenged with the same drugs, allowing alternative drugs to be used for any subsequent relapse? Such decisions need to be based on the evidence of benefit of these two approaches and the side-effects of such treatments.

CASE HISTORY

A 58-year-old woman noticed gradual onset of abdominal swelling over three months and an increase in urinary frequency, particularly at night. There had been some irregularity of her bowel function, with diarrhoea two or three times per day. Her previous health had been good, apart from a benign breast lump discovered 15 months previously. She had had three children, and had reached the menopause 10 years previously. Her mother died, possibly of carcinoma of the ovaries, aged 55. She was found to have ascites, and aspiration revealed adenocarcinoma cells. The serum CA125 was 5422 U/ml. The ultrasound and computed tomography (CT) scan did not show any definite ovarian enlargement, but there was a small right-sided pleural effusion.

After drainage of the ascites, she underwent a laparotomy and was found to have a widespread intraabdominal tumour with nodules throughout the peritoneum, on the bowel and in the subdiaphragmatic region. The omentum was completely replaced by tumour. The ovary was covered by superficial tumour nodules. There was no para-aortic lymphadenopathy. The uterus appeared normal. She underwent a subtotal hysterectomy, bilateral salpingo-oophorectomy and omentectomy. A plaque of tumour measuring approximately 2 cm in diameter was left next to the uterus behind the bladder. The pathology was reported as a poorly differentiated serous carcinoma that partially replaced the ovaries and left fallopian tube. Similar deposits of tumour were seen in the omentum. A right pleural aspirate was performed before treatment, which confirmed the presence of adenocarcinoma. She had FIGO stage IV disease.

Following surgery, she started chemotherapy with carboplatin AUC 5 (area under the concentration and time curve) and paclitaxel 175 mg/m² as a three-hour infusion every three weeks. Six cycles were given between May and August 1997. She tolerated the treatment well, although she developed asymptomatic grade 4 neutropenia on two occasions and required a blood transfusion during treatment. The serum CA125 fell rapidly during treatment, and became normal at the time of the fourth cycle of treatment. An implantation nodule in the right flank from the site of the previous drainage of ascites was no longer palpable after the third cycle of treatment, and a chest radiograph taken at the time of cycle 3 showed the lung fields were clear. At the end of treatment, the serum CA125 was 6 U/ml, and a follow-up CT scan was clear apart from possibly some thickening behind the bladder in the region where the plaque of tumour had remained after surgery. A magnetic resonance image (MRI) of the pelvis showed no mass but a trace of fluid in the pelvis.

She remained well until April 1998, when serum CA125 had risen to 836 U/ml. Over the previous month, she had noticed some lower abdominal discomfort and again an increase in frequency of bowel evacuation and urination. There was no clinical evidence of ascites and the chest was clear. Pelvic examination was normal. A further CT scan was performed and compared with the CT and MRI scans of October. There was now a moderate amount of ascites, and some early thickening of the remaining omentum along the anterior abdominal wall. There was some thickening of the fat in the pelvis but no distinct mass.

Could an early relapse within 12 months have been prevented?

The patient developed clinical, radiological and serological relapse 11 months after the diagnosis of ovarian cancer. This is a typical finding in patients with advanced disease in a 'poor-prognosis' group. Although surgical debulking of the tumour had been performed, the patient had stage IV disease because of the presence of a pleural effusion. In a long-term survival analysis from two trials from the Netherlands Joint Study Group for Ovarian Cancer in which patients received platinum-based chemotherapy, 12% and 14% of patients with stage IV disease were alive at five years.[3] In an analysis of prognostic factors by Redman and colleagues,[4] the median progression-free period for patients with stage IV ovarian cancer treated with combination chemotherapy was 13 months. It is difficult to know what impact platinum–paclitaxel combinations have on these figures. In the Gynecologic Oncology Group (GOG) 111 study in patients with 'poor-prognosis' stage III (>1 cm residual mass after surgery) and stage IV disease, the median progression-free period was 18 months. About one-third of these patients had stage IV disease.[5]

Extension of chemotherapy has been considered as a means of improving the outlook of patients with 'poor-prognosis' disease who attain a clinical remission with first-line therapy. However, there is no evidence that a prolonged course of chemotherapy (8–10 cycles compared with the standard 5 or 6) confers a survival advantage.[6,7] However, Howell et al[8] have used intraperitoneal cisplatin as consolidation, and reported a median survival of more than 49 months in patients who had disease with a maximum diameter of less than 2 cm after initial therapy. High-dose consolidation therapy with bone marrow or peripheral blood stem cell support has also been used. In the largest series from a single centre, 59.9% of 53 patients were alive five years after consolidation therapy with high-dose melphalan or carboplatin and cyclophosphamide. In 19 patients who had a negative second-look operation, 74.2% were alive at five years, but the disease-free survival rate was only 32.8%.[9] Randomized trials in Europe and the USA are in progress, but at the moment there is no indication to recommend either of these approaches in routine clinical practice.

Relapse is often detected either by the presence of rising CA125 levels or by clinical criteria, typically ascites or gastrointestinal symptoms. The approach to asymptomatic relapse is dealt with elsewhere in this book (see Chapter 15). In this patient, there were clinical indications to restart treatment, and in addition the CT scan demonstrated signs of recurrence in the abdomen and pelvis. There was no indication for surgery, since no mass was identified.

What type of chemotherapy should be considered in patients relapsing within 12 months of diagnosis?

Until five years ago, the main choice of treatment was to re-treat with either cisplatin or carboplatin (the first-line agents), alone or in combination with other drugs. In most cases, clinicians used platinum-based therapy in patients relapsing more than six months after completing first-line therapy. The likelihood of a second response to platinum-containing drugs depends on the 'platinum-free interval'. Patients whose tumours progress during initial therapy, have residual stable disease, or relapse within six months after the completion of first-line therapy are classified as 'platinum-resistant'. The tumour response rate to rechallenge with cisplatin or carboplatin is less than 10%. Similar findings have been reported for other classes of drugs given to this group of patients.[2] However, Markman et al[1] reported responses in 27% (6/26) of patients re-treated with cisplatin after a cisplatin-free period of 5–12 months. In the series reported by Gershenson et al,[10] all 19 patients relapsing after a treatment-free interval of 5–81 months (median 26.3 months) responded to re-challenge with cisplatin. The probability of response increases as the platinum-free period lengthens. Thirty-three per cent responded when re-treated between 13 and 24 months, rising to 59% when the interval was greater than 24 months (Table 11.1). Clinical and pathological response rates to carboplatin and cisplatin are similar.[11] Cisplatin is more nephrotoxic and neurotoxic, but carboplatin is more myelosuppressive. Patients treated with cisplatin are often treated with carboplatin at relapse because of the risk of inducing neurotoxicity with cisplatin. However, little is gained by crossing over from cisplatin to carboplatin, or vice versa, because of a lack of tumour response to or progressive disease with that compound. Taylor et al[12] showed that only 5 out of 35 patients

Table 11.1 Tumour sensitivity to cisplatin following relapse.		
Cisplatin-free interval (months)	No. of patients assessable	Total response
5–12	22	6 (27%)
13–24	18	6 (33%)
>24	32	19 (59%)
Adapted from reference 1.		

(14%) responded to the other agent in this situation. Before the introduction of taxanes, some patients were treated with combination schedules such as cisplatin and cyclophosphamide or cisplatin, cyclophosphamide and doxorubicin (Adriamycin). Patients initially given single-agent therapy were often offered combination therapy at relapse. Combination therapy increases toxicity, and some regimens require hospitalization. There is no clear evidence that treatment with combination therapies is superior.

The introduction of two new drugs, paclitaxel and topotecan, with novel modes of action has extended the choices of therapy available at relapse. The antineoplastic drug paclitaxel (Taxol) extracted from the bark of the Pacific yew tree, *Taxus breviofolia*, stabilizes and promotes microtubule assembly. Initial reports of its activity in ovarian cancer demonstrated that some patients whose tumours were platinum-resistant responded.[13] A response rate of 22% (approximate 95% confidence interval 19–25%) was reported in 652 evaluable patients given paclitaxel in a large registration study of cases referred to the National Cancer Institute. Patients had received three or more prior chemotherapy regimens.[14] In a phase II study performed by the GOG, 33% of 27 patients with platinum-resistant disease and 44% of 16 patients with platinum-sensitive disease (defined as progression more than six months after platinum-based therapy) responded. However, the median progression-free interval in the two groups after paclitaxel was only 4 and 4.9 months respectively.[15] The principal toxicity was neutropenia. In the USA, paclitaxel is given as a 24-hour infusion using 135 mg/m^2. In Europe, 175 mg/m^2 is given as a 3-hour infusion. A large European–Canadian study compared these two doses of paclitaxel given either as a 24- or a 3-hour infusion. Response rates and progression-free survival were slightly greater using the higher dose, but the differences were not significant. The infusion time did not affect the response rate, but significantly more neutropenia was seen when the drug was given as a 24-hour infusion.[16]

Following the encouraging results with paclitaxel in relapsed ovarian cancer, the drug was incorporated into first-line therapy. Two large and very similar studies have shown that the combination of cisplatin and paclitaxel (given either by a 24- or a 3-hour infusion) is superior to cisplatin and cyclophosphamide.[5,17] There has now been a shift in practice, and paclitaxel is usually used as first-line therapy. Before this occurred, patients relapsing after platinum were offered paclitaxel. However, most of the data on the use of this drug were in the platinum-refractory group, and the benefit of paclitaxel, alone or in combination with platinum in patients who were potentially platinum-sensitive, is less clear.

An Italian phase II randomized study was performed comparing paclitaxel with CAP (cyclophosphamide, doxorubicin and cisplatin) in patients with a disease-free interval of more than 12 months, but was stopped early. Patients receiving CAP had a significantly longer progression-free survival (18.9 months versus 7.9 months) compared with the group receiving paclitaxel alone.[18] The ICON group (International Collaborative Group for Ovarian Neoplasia) launched a randomized phase III trial in 1996 to compare the addition of paclitaxel to platinum-based chemotherapy in relapsed ovarian cancer. In the ICON 4 study, patients progressing more than six months after the completion of first-line platinum therapy are randomized to a platinum–paclitaxel (cis- or carboplatin) combination or the same dose of platinum alone or in combination without paclitaxel according to the clinician's choice. Initially, most of the patients entering the study had not received paclitaxel as 'first-line' therapy, but the majority of patients entering the study now have received paclitaxel. The trial continues to recruit patients, and will be able to evaluate the use of paclitaxel in relapse in both groups of patients. Some information on the response following re-challenge with paclitaxel at relapse is now available. Rose et al[19] treated 25 patients with recurrent ovarian or peritoneal carcinoma who relapsed a median of 10 months (range 6–30 months) after cisplatin and paclitaxel with a combination of carboplatin and paclitaxel. Eighty-nine per cent of patients with assessable disease responded, and the median duration of response was more than nine months. Furthermore, a loss of platinum resistance has been seen

in some patients who were treated with carboplatin following an earlier failure of platinum-based therapy, provided they had responded to paclitaxel therapy and subsequently had a platinum-free interval greater than 12 months. It is not clear whether paclitaxel was responsible for the renewed sensitivity to carboplatin, or whether the prolonged period from platinum treatment led to loss of platinum resistance.[20]

Topotecan is a semisynthetic water-soluble analogue of camptothecin. It is a specific inhibitor of the enzyme topoisomerase I, which is involved in maintaining the topological structure of DNA. In an early phase II study, antitumour activity was seen in ovarian cancer cases, 80% of whom were considered to have platinum-refractory disease. Patients received 1.5 mg/m^2 intravenously daily for five days every three weeks. Twenty-eight patients were assessable for response, and four of them had partial responses (14%), with a median duration of response of 8.9 months. However, one or more dose reductions were required in 61% of patients, and four patients were hospitalized with febrile neutropenia.[21] Neutropenia and thrombocytopenia are the dose-limiting side-effects of this drug and these toxicities need to be carefully considered in the context of palliative chemotherapy. Gastrointestinal side-effects were mild and alopecia was not severe. In a further study conducted by Creemers et al,[22] 27% of patients defined as 'platinum-sensitive' (progression more than six months after initial treatment) responded. However, myelotoxicity was again quite severe, with 69.1% developing grade 3 or 4 neutropenia. The incidence of febrile neutropenia was only 4.3%, perhaps partly owing to the use of granulocyte colony-stimulating factor (G-CSF), which was given to 20.5% of patients to maintain the dose intensity.[22] The activity of topotecan has been compared with that of paclitaxel, 175 mg/m^2 as a 3-hour infusion, in a randomized study in patients with refractory or relapsing ovarian cancer. Two hundred and twenty-six patients were evaluable for response. Of patients relapsing within six months, 13.3% responded to topotecan and 6.8% to paclitaxel. In the 'late-relapse' group, progressing more than six months after primary therapy, the overall response rates were 28.8% to topotecan and 20% to paclitaxel.[23] All patients were in first relapse, and none had previously received paclitaxel therapy. In the first interim analysis, the median time to progression was longer in the topotecan group: 23.1 weeks compared with 14.0 weeks ($p = 0.002$). However, in the final analysis, the differences were no longer statistically significant (18.9 weeks versus 14.7 weeks; $p = 0.72$). The benefit of second-line chemotherapy with either of these agents was relatively small. Patients were on treatment for a median of about three months and had evidence of progressive disease within a few weeks of the cessation of therapy. However, in patients who had a measurable response to therapy, the median duration of response from the start of treatment was between 21.6 and 25.9 weeks. Thus, it is important to distinguish responders from non-responders early, since the latter benefit little from continuing with these expensive agents.

The indication to use topotecan may increase, since most patients now receive platinum and paclitaxel as first-line therapy. Furthermore, there is now an orally available preparation, which would be particularly attractive for the palliative treatment of relapsed disease. There is less haematological toxicity with oral topotecan,[24] but it is too early to know whether its activity is equivalent to that of the intravenous preparation. Studies are also being performed combining cisplatin or carboplatin with paclitaxel and topotecan. These are myelotoxic regimens, and more work is needed to establish the best schedule and dose.

In the case discussed here, there would have been a reasonable indication to rechallenge with carboplatin alone, since the probability of response would have been about 30%. However, patients who have had carboplatin and paclitaxel as 'first-line' therapy may feel this is inferior to their initial regimen. A further course of both drugs would also have been appropriate. When the results of the ICON 4 trial are available, there may be better guidance about these choices. An alternative would be to offer topotecan, which would be a new drug for this patient and would be less likely to lead to hair loss. Following discussion, the patient decided to be treated with topotecan.

The first dose was started at the end of April 1998 at a dose of 1.0 mg/m² per day for five days every 21 days. A reduced dose was chosen because of the neutropenia experienced with carboplatin and paclitaxel. A total of five cycles of treatment was given, which she tolerated well, although there was again asymptomatic grade 4 neutropenia. There was very little hair loss with this treatment, and the serum CA125 fell from 1150 to 261 U/ml after three cycles. However, after cycle 5 was given, it was clear that the CA125 was rising again. Treatment was stopped in mid-August 1998, by which time the CA125 was 546 U/ml. There had been resolution of the ascites but a CT scan demonstrated a significant pelvic mass lying between the bladder and rectum.

How should one monitor the response to therapy at relapse?

The difficulty in measuring the response of ovarian cancer to chemotherapy using World Health Organization (WHO) criteria is often underestimated, since many patients do not have easily measurable disease. As the serum CA125 is raised in most patients, it is useful to monitor the response to therapy by regular measurements of this tumour marker. A serial fall in the serum CA125 indicates tumour response, and this has been shown to correlate well with response measured by WHO criteria.[25] It is particularly useful to use CA125 response in the palliative setting and when toxic and expensive drugs are used. As there can be a discrepancy between the serum CA125 result and CT response, some clinicians repeat CT imaging half-way through a course of palliative treatment if the serum CA125 is falling. A rising serum CA125 on treatment is a clear sign of tumour progression, which would be an indication to change or stop treatment. It is unclear for how long patients should be treated. Most clinicians would plan to give about six cycles if it appeared that the patient was entering a remission. Consolidation of remission with high-dose therapy has been investigated, but the results do not suggest that sustained remissions are produced. The largest experience in a single centre is from Stiff et al,[26] who reported the results of high-dose chemotherapy in 100 patients. Platinum sensitivity and low tumour bulk were the most important prognostic determinants for a favourable outcome. For 20 patients in this group, the median progression-free survival and overall survival from the date of transplantation were 19 and 30 months respectively. Randomized trials are needed to determine if this approach provides a significant benefit to patients.

The patient had a good symptomatic response to topotecan, and the serum CA125 levels fell but did not reach normal values. The elevation of CA125 on chemotherapy suggested that residual resistant disease was present. A CT scan at the end of therapy confirmed this, showing a persistent pelvic mass.

At the completion of chemotherapy, the patient described a disturbance of bowel function, with discomfort in the pelvis. Because of the symptomatic and enlarging pelvic mass, she was offered palliative radiotherapy to the pelvis, and received 30 Gy in 10 fractions over two weeks. This was completed by early October 1998. However, the serum CA125 continued to rise, and by November it was

3540 U/ml and she had developed generalized ascites again. A further CT scan (Figure 11.1a) showed an ascites with peritoneal infiltration and a reduction in the size of the pelvic mass.

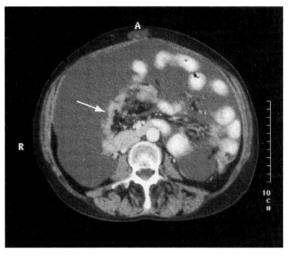

(a)

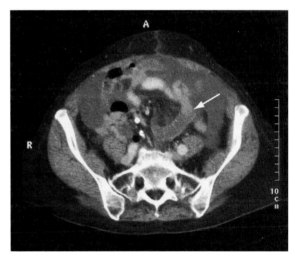

(b)

Figure 11.1
(a) Computed tomography (CT) scan demonstrating widespread ascites with peritoneal infiltration (arrow). (b) CT scan taken at the same time, showing early signs of bowel obstruction, which occurred within two weeks. Oral contrast does not flow freely throughout the small bowel, which shows early dilatation (arrow).

How should one manage progression on 'second-line' therapy?

Relapse on 'second-line' chemotherapy is usually associated with a very poor outcome. In many cases, further chemotherapy may not be appropriate. The decision often rests on trying to obtain a balance between control of symptoms and the side-effects associated with further treatment. In this patient, the choices for chemotherapy included re-treatment with platinum-based drugs, either alone or in combination with paclitaxel, oral chemotherapy with drugs such as etoposide or altretamine, or entry into an experimental therapy programme. Oral etoposide is well-tolerated by patients, and causes little nausea – an important consideration in patients who have a tendency to gastrointestinal disturbances, particularly in the later stages of their disease. However, alopecia is universal, and it is unlikely that survival will be prolonged sufficiently for hair to re-grow. Myelotoxicity is unpredictable; it can be severe, and careful monitoring of the drug is required, particularly in patients with renal dysfunction. In phase II studies, the use of 50 mg twice daily for 14 out of 21 days has produced a response rate of 24%.[27] Progression-free survival following etoposide was longer in patients with platinum-sensitive disease compared with those who were defined as resistant.[28] In practice, in heavily pretreated patients, 7–10 days may be the maximum length of treatment because of myelosuppression.

Altretamine may be useful in patients who are sensitive to platinum-based chemotherapy.[29] In one phase II study, 18 out of 45 (40%) assessable patients responded to 260 mg/m² daily for 14 days every 28 days. Patients had relapsed following platinum-based treatment more than six months previously. A higher response rate was seen in patients with longer treatment-free periods.[30] The main side-effects are nausea and vomiting (which are variable), fatigue, haemato-

Table 11.2   Second-line agents for recurrent ovarian cancer

Paclitaxel
Topotecan
Altretamine[29,30]
Etoposide[27,28]
Docetaxel[31,32]
Liposomal doxorubicin[33]
Gemcitabine[34,35]
Ifosfamide[36,37]
Vinorelbine[38]

logical toxicity and neurotoxicity, particularly with prolonged therapy. Other drugs have been used in the treatment of ovarian cancer; these are summarized in Table 11.2. (See also Chapter 12.)

Caution has to be exercised in interpreting the results of phase II studies for all these agents; there is often considerable variation in the response rate, since some of the patients have received multiple prior therapies, which reduces the chance of further response.[2] In a recent analysis of 704 patients, Eisenhauer et al[39] reported that serous tumour histology and small tumour burden are the most important prognostic determinants of response to a variety of second- or third-line agents. The treatment-free interval correlated with the tumour burden.

This patient had only received one course of carboplatin, which had finished 15 months earlier. She also wished to have a further course of paclitaxel, since these drugs had been so helpful initially. It was not clear at this point whether the probability of response to carboplatin and paclitaxel would be compromised by the recent therapy with topotecan. Her wish was to pursue an active treatment programme, and she was offered cisplatin and paclitaxel.

The first cycle of cisplatin and paclitaxel was given in November 1998, after drainage of ascites. Within a few days of this treatment, the patient developed severe nausea and vomiting and subacute intestinal obstruction (Figure 11.1b). The symptoms settled with conservative management, and she was discharged home in mid-December. When she was reviewed in early January 1999, there had been a significant improvement in all her abdominal symptoms. It had been six weeks since a single injection of chemotherapy, but there was now no evidence of ascites and the serum CA125 had fallen from 5050 to 683 U/ml. Her disease was still sensitive to platinum and paclitaxel, and she decided to embark on a further course of chemotherapy with carboplatin and paclitaxel given three-weekly. She completed this in July 1999, and the CA125 returned to normal. A CT scan was reported showing resolution of the ascites and a residual small abnormality in the pelvis, but no other disease.

In which ways can platinum-based drugs and paclitaxel therapy be given as third-line treatment?

There has been a growing interest in weekly administration of paclitaxel. In a phase I study, doses of 40–100 mg/m^2 per week for 12 weeks were given.[40] The response rate in heavily pre-treated women who had all previously received paclitaxel was 30%. Side-effects were generally mild; hair loss was uncommon, and neutropenia was the dose-limiting toxicity. Furthermore, a response was seen in two women after switching from three-weekly to weekly paclitaxel. In a phase II study giving paclitaxel 80 mg/m^2 as a 1-hour infusion, responses were seen in 13 out of 45 patients (28.9%). Patients received paclitaxel a median of eight months after previous paclitaxel therapy, and responses were evident after a median of seven weeks of treatment.[41] In the Netherlands, schedules of weekly paclitaxel 90 mg/m^2, or four-weekly 200 mg/m^2, combined

with weekly cisplatin 70 mg/m^2 have been studied as first- or second-line therapy. Following six cycles over an eight-week period, patients were continued on carboplatin and paclitaxel on a maintenance schedule. The overall response rate in recurrent disease with a platinum-free interval of more than three months was 94% (17/18).[42] Whether given weekly or in a more conventional schedule, paclitaxel and platinum remains an active second-line regimen in relapsed ovarian cancer.

In this patient, it was not possible to continue with the planned weekly cisplatin and paclitaxel regimen because of gastrointestinal side-effects. However, a single injection of cisplatin and paclitaxel produced a dramatic clinical response, indicating that in this patient the tumour was sensitive to these agents. Continuing therapy with standard doses of carboplatin and paclitaxel resulted in a further complete remission.

Relapsed ovarian cancer remains difficult to treat. However, there is a reasonably wide range of second-line drugs that have comparable activity. For most patients relapsing 6–12 months after completion of initial chemotherapy, there can be a reasonable expectation of response either to the re-introduction of first-line agents or to second-line drugs. The pattern of toxicity varies, and this may influence the choice of therapy.

SUMMARY

The treatment of relapsed ovarian cancer is palliative, and the choice of drugs needs to be considered carefully. A treatment should have a reasonable chance of palliating symptoms and delaying the progression of the disease without producing unacceptable toxicity. The probability of response to any therapy is likely to depend on the treatment-free period although paclitaxel is active in some patients who are clearly resistant to platinum therapy. For platinum-based agents, resistance has been defined as relapse on treatment or within six months of therapy. It must be remembered that this is only a probability of resistance and that it may be a continuous variable within that period. Nevertheless, many clinicians would not use platinum-based chemotherapy in patients whose disease returns within six months.

For this patient and others relapsing over six months, the use of platinum-based drugs, most commonly carboplatin (because of its lower toxicity than cisplatin), is appropriate. Most patients now receive paclitaxel as first-line therapy. The results of ongoing trials should indicate whether these patients should in addition be re-treated with paclitaxel. Like much of clinical medicine, the choices for therapy are often empirical. It may be possible in the future to make predictions based on analysis of tumour samples or tumour DNA as to whether a particular drug or drug combination is likely to be successful. Decisions about therapy based on molecular analysis are likely to save patients from unnecessary side-effects and reduce the costs of therapy to health purchasers.

Careful clinical decisions are needed, and the patient and her family should be involved with the discussion about further therapy. One needs to consider very carefully whether further treatment is appropriate. If so, it is important to ensure that the patient (and physician) maintains the balance between hope and realism. Palliation of symptoms and maintenance of the quality of life are the most important considerations, since treatment is not curative.

LEARNING POINTS

❉ The probability of response to second-line platinum-based drugs, usually carboplatin, depends on the platinum-free interval.

❉ Paclitaxel and topotecan are active agents in patients who are 'platinum-resistant', but it is still unclear whether it is better to use these drugs as 'second-line' agents in patients who might still be platinum-sensitive or wait until further relapse occurs, when platinum resistance is clearly demonstrable.

❉ Patients receiving paclitaxel or topotecan at relapse do not necessarily become platinum-resistant when carboplatin is used at a subsequent relapse.

❉ Treatment of relapsed ovarian cancer is not curative. It is important that patients and their family understand the aims of chemotherapy for relapsed disease. Treatment must be directed at control of symptoms and preservation of the quality of life.

REFERENCES

1. Markman M, Rothman R, Hakes T et al, Second-line platinum therapy in patients with ovarian cancer previously treated with cisplatin. *J Clin Oncol* 1991; **9**: 389–93.
2. Blackledge G, Lawton F, Redman C, Kelly K, Response of patients in phase II studies of chemotherapy in ovarian cancer: implications for patient treatment and the design of phase II trials. *Br J Cancer* 1989; **59**: 650–3.
3. Neijt JP, ten Bokkel Huinink WW, van der Burg MEL et al, Long term survival in ovarian cancer: mature data from the Netherlands Joint Study Group for Ovarian Cancer. *Eur J Cancer* 1991; **27**: 1367–72.
4. Redman JR, Petroni GR, Saigo PE et al, Prognostic factors in advanced ovarian cancer. *J Clin Oncol* 1986; **4**: 515–23.
5. McGuire WP, Hoskins WJ, Brady MF et al, Cyclophosphamide and cisplatin compared with paclitaxel and cisplatin in patients with stage III and stage IV ovarian cancer. *N Engl J Med* 1996; **334**: 1–6.
6. Hakes TB, Chalas E, Hoskins WJ et al, Randomised prospective trial of 5 versus 10 cycles

of cyclophosphamide, doxorubicin and cis-platin in advanced ovarian carcinoma. *Gynecol Oncol* 1992; **45**: 284–9.

7. Lambert HE, Rustin GJ, Gregory WM, Nel-strop AE, A randomized trial of five versus eight courses of cisplatin or carboplatin in advanced epithelial ovarian carcinoma. A North Thames Ovary Group study. *Ann Oncol* 1997; **8**: 327–33.

8. Howell SB, Zimm S, Markman M et al, Long-term survival of advanced refractory ovarian carcinoma patients with small-volume disease treated with intraperitoneal chemotherapy. *J Clin Oncol* 1987; **5**: 1607–12.

9. Legros M, Dauplat J, Fleury J et al, High-dose chemotherapy with hematopoietic rescue in patients with stage III to IV ovarian cancer: long-term results. *J Clin Oncol* 1997; **15**: 1302–8.

10. Gershenson DM, Kavanagh JJ, Copeland LJ et al, Re-treatment of patients with recurrent epithelial ovarian cancer with cisplatin-based chemotherapy. *Obstet Gynecol* 1989; **73**: 798–802.

11. Mangioni C, Bolis G, Pecorelli S et al, Ran-domized trial in advanced ovarian cancer com-paring cisplatin and carboplatin. *J Natl Cancer Inst* 1989; **81**: 1464–71.

12. Taylor AE, Wiltshaw E, Gore ME et al, Long-term follow up of the first randomised study of cisplatin versus carboplatin for advanced epithelial ovarian cancer. *J Clin Oncol* 1994; **10**: 2066–70.

13. McGuire WP, Rowinsky EK, Rosenshein NB et al, Taxol: a unique antineoplastic agent with significant activity in advanced ovarian epithe-lial neoplasms. *Ann Intern Med* 1989; **111**: 273–9.

14. Trimble EL, Adams JD, Vena D et al, Paclitaxel for platinum-refractory ovarian cancer: results from the first 1,000 patients registered to National Cancer Institute Treatment Referral Center 9103. *J Clin Oncol* 1993; **11**: 2405–10.

15. Thigpen JT, Blessing JA, Ball H et al, Phase II trial of paclitaxel in patients with progressive

ovarian cancer after platinum-based chemotherapy: a Gynecologic Oncology Group study. *J Clin Oncol* 1994; **12**: 1748–53.

16. Eisenhauer EA, ten Bokkel Huinink WW, Swenerton KD et al, European–Canadian ran-domised trial of paclitaxel in relapsed ovarian cancer: high-dose versus low-dose and long versus short infusion. *J Clin Oncol* 1994; **12**: 2654–66.

17. Stuart G, Bertelsen C, Mangioni C et al, Updated analysis shows a highly significant improved overall survival (OS) for cisplatin–paclitaxel as first line treatment of advanced ovarian cancer: mature results of the EORTC–GCCG, NOCOVA, NCIC CTG and Scottish Intergroup trial. *Proc Am Soc Clin Oncol* 1998; **17**: 1394.

18. Colombo N, Marzola M, Parma G et al, Pacli-taxel vs CAP (cyclophosphamide, Adriamycin, cisplatin) in recurrent platinum sensitive ovarian cancer: a randomised phase II study. *Proc Am Soc Clin Oncol* 1996; **15**: 279.

19. Rose PG, Fusco N, Fluellen L, Rodriguez M, Second-line therapy with paclitaxel and carbo-platin for recurrent disease following first-line therapy with paclitaxel and platinum in ovarian or peritoneal carcinoma. *J Clin Oncol* 1998; **16**: 1494–7.

20. Kavanagh J, Tresukosol D, Edwards C et al, Carboplatin reinduction after taxane in patients with platinum-refractory epithelial ovarian cancer. *J Clin Oncol* 1995; **13**: 1584–8.

21. Kudelka AP, Tresukosol D, Edwards CL et al, Phase II study of intravenous topotecan as a 5-day infusion for refractory epithelial ovarian carcinoma. *J Clin Oncol* 1996; **14**: 1552–7.

22. Creemers GJ, Bolis G, Gore M et al, Topote-can, an active drug in the second-line treat-ment of epithelial ovarian cancer: results of a large European phase II study. *J Clin Oncol* 1996; **14**: 3056–61.

23. ten Bokkel Huinink W, Gore M, Carmichael J et al, Topotecan versus paclitaxel for the treat-ment of recurrent epithelial ovarian cancer. *J Clin Oncol* 1997; **15**: 2183–93.

24. Gore M, Rustin G, Calvert H et al, A multicentre, randomised, phase III study of topotecan (T) administered intravenously or orally for advanced epithelial ovarian carcinoma. *Proc Am Soc Clin Oncol* 1998; **17**: 349a.

25. Bridgewater J, Nelstrop A, Rustin G et al, Comparison of clinical and CA 125 responses in patients treated with platinum or paclitaxel. *Proc Am Soc Clin Oncol* 1998; **17**: 358a.

26. Stiff PJ, Bayer R, Kerger C et al, High-dose chemotherapy with autologous transplantation for persistent/relapsed ovarian cancer: a multivariate analysis of survival for 100 consecutively treated patients. *J Clin Oncol* 1997; **15**: 1309–17.

27. Seymour MT, Mansi JL, Gallagher CJ et al, Protracted oral etoposide in epithelial ovarian cancer: a phase II study in patients with relapsed or platinum-resistant disease. *Br J Cancer* 1994; **69**: 191–5.

28. Rose PG, Blessing JA, Mayer AR, Homesley HD, Prolonged oral etoposide as second-line therapy for platinum-resistant and platinum-sensitive ovarian carcinoma: a Gynecologic Oncology Group study. *J Clin Oncol* 1998; **16**: 405–10.

29. Lee CR, Faulds D, Altretamine. A review of its pharmacodynamic and pharmacokinetic properties, and therapeutic potential in cancer chemotherapy. *Drugs* 1995; **49**: 932–53.

30. Rustin GJ, Nelstrop AE, Crawford M et al, Phase II trial of oral altretamine for relapsed ovarian carcinoma: evaluation of defining response by serum CA125. *J Clin Oncol* 1997; **15**: 172–6.

31. Piccart MJ, Gore M, Ten Bokkel Huinink W et al, Docetaxel: an active new drug for treatment of advanced epithelial ovarian cancer. *J Natl Cancer Inst* 1995; **87**: 676–81.

32. Kaye SB, Piccart M, Aapro M et al, Phase II trials of docetaxel (Taxotere) in advanced ovarian cancer – an updated overview. *Eur J Cancer* 1997; **33**: 2167–70.

33. Muggia FM, Hainsworth JD, Jeffers S et al, Phase II study of liposomal doxorubicin in refractory ovarian cancer: antitumor activity and toxicity modification by liposomal encapsulation. *J Clin Oncol* 1997; **15**: 987–93.

34. Friedlander M, Millward MJ, Bell D et al, A phase II study of gemcitabine in platinum pretreated patients with advanced epithelial ovarian cancer. *Ann Oncol* 1998; **9**: 1343–5.

35. Lund B, Hansen OP, Theilade K et al, Phase II study of gemcitabine (2',2'-difluorodeoxycytidine) in previously treated ovarian cancer patients. *J Natl Cancer Inst* 1994; **86**: 1530–3.

36. Willemse PH, van der Burg ME, van der Gaast A et al, Ifosfamide given as a 24-h infusion with mesna in patients with recurrent ovarian cancer: preliminary results. *Cancer Chemother Pharmacol* 1990; **26**(Suppl): S51–4.

37. Markman M, Hakes T, Reichman B et al, Ifosfamide and mesna in previously treated advanced epithelial ovarian cancer: activity in platinum-resistant disease. *J Clin Oncol* 1992; **10**: 243–8.

38. Burger RA, DiSaia PJ, Roberts JA et al, Phase II trial of vinorelbine in recurrent and progressive epithelial ovarian cancer. *Gynecol Oncol* 1999; **72**: 148–53.

39. Eisenhauer EA, Vermorken JB, van Glabbeke M, Predictors of response to subsequent chemotherapy in platinum pretreated ovarian cancer: a multivariate analysis of 704 patients. *Ann Oncol* 1997; **8**: 963–8.

40. Fennelly D, Aghajanian C, Shapiro F et al, Phase I and pharmacologic study of paclitaxel administered weekly in patients with relapsed ovarian cancer. *J Clin Oncol* 1997; **15**: 187–92.

41. Abu-Rustum NR, Aghajanian C, Barakat RR et al, Salvage weekly paclitaxel in recurrent ovarian cancer. *Semin Oncol* 1997; **24**(5 Suppl 15): S15-62–7.

42. van der Burg MEL, de Wit R, Stoter G, Verweij J, Phase I study of weekly cisplatin (P) and weekly or 4-weekly Taxol (T): A highly active regimen in advanced epithelial ovarian cancer. *Proc Am Soc Clin Oncol* 1998; **17**: 355a (Abstr 137006).

12

Early relapse (within six months): drug resistance

Willem ten Bokkel Huinink, Stanley B Kaye

INTRODUCTION

Despite the introduction of paclitaxel into the treatment strategy for advanced ovarian cancer, along with cytoreductive surgery, published results still demonstrate relapse-free survival curves that point to a significant number of patients facing early relapse. This chapter will try to deal with factors related to early relapse and measures to salvage these patients.

The majority of patients suffering from ovarian cancer will respond to primary treatment. Only a small percentage of patients, 10% or less, may have progressive disease while on primary treatment with cisplatin/carboplatin and paclitaxel. This is defined as refractory disease. Generally speaking, these patients are considered to have a dismal prognosis, and their poor performance status sometimes precludes additional treatment. A slightly larger number of patients respond initially to the treatment with platinum- and paclitaxel-based chemotherapy, but, not withstanding more or less successful interval debulking surgery, they will have a persistent elevation of the tumour marker CA125 after six courses. Another subset of patients demonstrate normalization of all tumour signs, and, following chemotherapy, a complete remis-

sion at restaging procedures, even at second-look laparotomy. Unfortunately, there are signs of relapsing disease, for example palpable tumour mass and/or a rise of CA125, within six months.

Together, these patients constitute those with early relapse, and they pose difficult problems for the treating physician.

The first issue is whether another attempt to perform surgery on these patients in order to remove the tumour at sites of relapse should be considered. In their review, Berek et al[1] pointed to the limitations of such a procedure. Surgery should essentially only be attempted for palliative measures, for example to alleviate bowel obstruction,[2] since the prognosis of these patients with rapidly progressive recurrent disease is generally very dismal. Palliative measures could include radiotherapy to larger masses, in order to prevent bowel obstruction, vaginal bleeding and other discomfort. In many patients with refractory disease or early relapse, further chemotherapy is considered. The chances of benefit from this treatment requires careful discussion, and the following case illustrates these issues.

CASE HISTORY

A 52-year-old woman was found to have stage III ovarian cancer with bulky residual masses. These could not be adequately removed despite an initial attempt at cytoreductive surgery. She was treated with three courses of carboplatin and paclitaxel, and showed an impressive response in the palpable tumour masses at pelvic examination. Another attempt at cytoreduction[3] was made after three courses, and proved to be successful: only minimal tumour remnants had not been resected at the end of the procedure. Three further courses of the combination of carboplatin and paclitaxel followed, and since CA125 levels had already normalized during the second of these courses, she was considered to be in clinically complete remission and followed thereafter. Unfortunately, at a first examination only two months after completion of the first six courses of chemotherapy, she was found to have a steep rise in her CA125 level. On pelvic examination, an early relapse was found, and this was confirmed on computed tomography (CT) scan. In addition, examination had revealed enlarged left-sided supraclavicular lymph nodes, and signs of lung metastases were also documented on the chest X-ray.

What is the chance of response to further therapy?

The therapeutic measures undertaken to salvage these patients have been very disappointing. In their analyses of prognostic factors predicting response to salvage programmes in patients relapsing from primary treatment for ovarian cancer, several authors have indicated that the time between the last platinum-containing regimen and the documentation of relapse plays a major role.[4] Other important factors include histology, the number of relapsing sites and the size of the tumour mass at relapse.[5] In clinical practice, the time to relapse is most often taken into account as the key factor when considering further treatment options for these patients.[6]

The chance of a response to re-treatment with the same agents (paclitaxel and carboplatin) in the situation of early relapse (within six months) is less than 20%. In the patient with refractory disease (progression while on initial chemotherapy), the chance of a response is minimal. When chemotherapy is contemplated, this should thus involve different drugs. The agent that represents the first clinically available example of a large class of new drugs, topoisomerase I inhibiting agents, is topotecan.[6] This has demonstrable activity in patients who have failed prior therapy with paclitaxel and platinum compounds (with a response rate of 10–20%). It has the advantage of causing relatively little vomiting, but the disadvantage of a cumbersome regimen requiring intravenous administration over five successive days. At the dose of 1.5 mg/m^2 per day, it causes significant myelosuppression. An alternative to consider in this situation is treatment with a new agent, preferably in the context of a controlled clinical trial.

The patient was informed about the treatment options. She consented to treatment within a phase II protocol of a novel platinum analogue that had experimental activity in resistant tumour models. After two courses, however, there was further evidence of disease progression. Despite this, her clinical condition remained satisfactory. There was evidence of increase in the size of lung metastases and in the pelvic mass, leading to further abdominal symptoms, and occasional vomiting. Following further discussion, she was treated with topotecan. After three courses, a clear partial response was noted, with symptomatic benefit. The dose was reduced from 1.5 mg/m^2 per day to 1.0 mg/m^2 per day after three courses, but was generally well tolerated. After six months, however, her condition *deteriorated and she developed acute intestinal obstruction.*

Which drugs could be used in platinum- and taxane-resistant cancer?

Although a series of agents have demonstrated activity in patients with early relapse from standard chemotherapy in ovarian cancer, the response rates remain generally less than 20%. A reasonable option is treatment with topotecan, which is registered for this indication; other agents undergoing evaluation in this context include liposomally formulated doxorubicin (Caeylx),[7] the platinum analogue oxaliplatin[8] and gemcitabine.[9] Another agent, which offers the additional advantage of oral administration, is etoposide, which in this context is generally given at a low dose (50–100 mg/day) for two weeks out of a three-week cycle.[10] It does cause alopecia and myelosuppression, and care is needed in patients with renal impairment. Longer-term treatment is associated with an increased risk of leukaemia. Other oral agents, particularly hexamethylmelamine,[11] are available, but tend to cause more nausea and vomiting. Whichever treatment is chosen, it is important if possible to include the patient in a clinical trial, either randomized or phase II in design.

An important issue in the clinical management of patients with clinically drug-resistant ovarian cancer is the optimal timing of experimental therapy if, following discussion with the patient, this is considered to be justified. In the patient described here, it was considered appropriate to initiate treatment with a novel agent prior to treatment with topotecan. The rationale is that the novel agent is tested in the most optimal situation; however, these treatment choices must be individualized and follow careful discussions in each case.

The patient was readmitted to hospital with acute intestinal obstruction. The family raised the issue of further treatment, but it was clear that her condition was deteriorating rapidly. She died three weeks after being admitted to hospital.

Experimental chemotherapy of ovarian cancer

An important part of the treatment of patients with ovarian cancer is to understand the point at which further experimental chemotherapy is not appropriate. This needs full discussion with the patient and her family. In some situations, patients may be treated within the context of phase I clinical trials even after the failure of phase II agents. However, this will only apply to a selected number of patients. In the context of drug resistance, phase I trials may address the issue of molecular mechanisms. Since mutant *p53* tumour cells are clearly an important element in clinical drug resistance, one novel approach has been the administration of the Onyx-015 adenovirus, which bears an E1B deletion and therefore replicates selectively in drug-resistant tumour cells.[12] A phase I trial using the Onyx-015 adenovirus via an intraperitoneal approach is nearing completion. Similarly, intraperitoneal administration of wild-type p53 protein using an adenoviral vector has been assessed as a way of selectively attempting reversal of ovarian cancer cell resistance, and randomized trials of this approach are underway.

The major problem illustrated by this case is indeed the development of tumour cell resistance to both platinum and taxanes. Resistance to platinum compounds is related in experimental models to four factors:[13,14]

1. Reduction of intracellular drug accumulation
2. Increased DNA repair
3. Cytoplasmic detoxification by mechanisms such as glutathione
4. Mismatch repair deficiency

The key factor is the ability of resistant tumour cells to avoid the process of apoptosis, and a range of signalling factors, including the *p53* gene, are involved in this function. Mutations of the *p53* gene have been noted in clinical series, and correlations with response to chemotherapy have been documented.[15] More recently, mismatch repair deficiency (MMR) has been examined in the laboratory, and evidence has been obtained to indicate that this may be an important feature underlying resistance to agents, including platinum.[16] MMR leads to lack of recognition of platinum–DNA adducts, and it may be detected by assessing the presence of microsatellite instability in tumour samples or even in free tumour DNA in blood samples taken from patients with ovarian cancer. Further studies to examine the clinical relevance of these observations are proceeding.

A number of manoeuvres are being assessed in the clinical situation with the aim of circumventing drug resistance. These include the assessment of buthionine sulphoximine (BSO), which can be demonstrated to reduce cellular levels of glutathione, and experimentally will reverse platinum resistance in ovarian tumour models.[17] There are some data to suggest that tumour glutathione concentrations can predict for response to platinum-based chemotherapy.[18] Drug resistance may be overcome experimentally by increasing the doses used, and clinical trials are proceeding involving high-dose regimens including carboplatin. One of the most interesting trials in this respect is the assessment of weekly administration of cisplatin, which is designed to increase the platinum dose intensity. In studies at the Rotterdam Cancer Centre, a high response rate has been noted in patients with early relapse, and, following earlier combination trials with etoposide, studies are now proceeding combining weekly cisplatin with paclitaxel in a randomized framework.[19]

Novel platinum analogues also merit exploration. Oxaliplatin has demonstrated activity in colorectal cancer, and experimental data indicate its potential in ovarian cancer because of activity in those platinum-resistant tumour models where MMR deficiency has been demonstrated to be a major mechanism.[20] Activity has been noted in patients with refractory ovarian cancer, and randomized trials are proceeding. Another platinum analogue with activity in tumour models resistant to platinum through impaired uptake, increased inactivation and enhanced DNA repair is ZD473,[21] and this is currently undergoing phase II exploration.

Resistance to paclitaxel is also multifactorial. As with platinum compounds, experimental data for several mechanisms have been published, but their clinical relevance remains uncertain. Probably the best-defined mechanism is the P-glycoprotein-mediated process of enhanced drug efflux known as multidrug resistance (MDR). The significance of the MDR phenotype in resistant ovarian cancer is unclear in the clinical situation,[22] although trials of novel MDR-based drug-resistant reversing agents are underway. Significant activity has recently been reported in patients with refractory disease, re-treated with paclitaxel and VX-710, which is a potent inhibitor of both P-glycoprotein-based and multidrug resistance-associated protein (MRP)-based MDR.[23] Mutations in tubulin have also been noted in paclitaxel-resistant tumour models, and novel analogues of this agent are currently being assessed in this context. Interestingly, other tubulin binders, such as the novel agent epothilone, may have particular potential in the context of paclitaxel resistance.

The relationship between p53 function and paclitaxel activity is intriguing. There are clear data indicating that mutant-p53 tumour cells are indeed hypersensitive to paclitaxel, although the reverse is the case for platinum compounds.[24] However, other cell signalling molecules are clearly relevant to the initiation of apoptosis following paclitaxel therapy. These include members of the BAX/BCL2 family, and modulation of the function of these proteins may be relevant to paclitaxel sensitivity.

LEARNING POINTS

✤ Patients whose tumour relapses within six months of completing chemotherapy for ovarian cancer have a poor prognosis. When further chemotherapy has been agreed, this should generally comprise different therapy.

✤ Chemotherapy in this context could include topotecan; oral etoposide is also an option in certain patients. Whenever possible, treatment should be within clinical trials.

✤ Treatment with an experimental agent within phase II trials is also appropriate; this requires careful discussion with each individual patient.

✤ The molecular mechanisms underlying drug resistance, to both platinum compounds and taxanes, require urgent clinical validation, preferably in the context of large clinical trials.

REFERENCES

1. Berek JS, Trompé C, Surgery during chemotherapy and at relapse of ovarian cancer. *Ann Oncol* 1999; **10**(Suppl 1): 3–7.

2. Fernandes JR, Seymour RJ, Suissa S, Bowel obstruction in patients with ovarian cancer: a search for prognostic factors. *Am J Obstet Gynecol* 1988; **158**: 244–9.

3. Van der Burg ME, van Lert M, Buyse M et al, The effect of debulking surgery after induction chemotherapy on the prognosis in advanced epithelial ovarian cancer. Gynaecological Cancer Cooperative Group of the European Organization of Research and Treatment of Cancer. *N Engl J Med* 1995; **332**: 629–34.

4. Markman M, Rothman R, Hakes T et al, Second line platinum therapy in patients with ovarian cancer previously treated with cisplatin. *J Clin Oncol* 1991; **9**: 389–93.

5. Eisenhauer EA, Vermorken JB, Van Glabbeke M et al, Predictors of response to subsequent chemotherapy in platinum pre-treated ovarian cancer: a multivariate analysis of 704 patients. *Ann Oncol* 1997; **8**: 963–8.

6. Ten Bokkel Huinink WW, Gore M, Carmichael JEA, Topotecan versus paclitaxel for the treatment of recurrent epithelial ovarian cancer. *J Clin Oncol* 1997; **15**: 2183–93.

7. Muggia FM, Hainsworth JD, Jeffers SEA, Phase II study of liposomal doxorubicin in refractory ovarian cancer: antitumour activity and toxicity modification by liposomal encapsulation. *J Clin Oncol* 1997; **15**: 987–93.

8. Sessa C, ten Bokkel Huinink W, du Bris A, Oxaliplatin in ovarian cancer. *Ann Oncol* 1999; **10**(Suppl 1): S55–8.

9. Hansen SW, Tuxen MK, Sessa C et al, Gemcitabine in the treatment of ovarian cancer. *Ann Oncol* 1999; **10**(Suppl 1): S51–3.

10. Rose PG, Blessing JA, Mayer AR, Homesley AD, Prolonged oral etoposide as second line therapy for ovarian cancer. A GOG study. *J Clin Oncol* 1998; **16**: 405–10.

11. Markman M, Blessing J, Moore D et al, Hexamethylmelamine in platinum resistant ovarian cancer. A GOG Phase II trial. *Gynecol Oncol* 1998; **69**: 226–9.

12. Heise C, Sampson Johannes A, Williams A et al, Onyx-015 and E1B gene-attenuated adenovirus causes tumor-specific cytolysis and antitumoral efficacy that can be augmented by standard chemotherapeutic agents. *Nature Med* 1997; **3**: 639–45.

13. Johnson S, Laub P, Beesley S et al, Increased platinum-DNA damage tolerance is associated with cisplatin resistance and cross-resistance to various chemotherapeutic agents in unrelated human ovarian cancer cell lines. *Cancer Res* 1997; **57**: 850–6.

14. Fink D, Aebi S, Howell S, The role of DNA mismatch repair in drug resistance. *Clin Cancer Res* 1998; **4**: 1–6.

15. Righetti SC, Dellatorre G, Pilotti S et al, A comparative study of p53 gene mutations, protein accumulation, and response to cisplatin-based chemotherapy in advanced ovarian cancer. *Cancer Res* 1996; **56**: 689–93.

16. Strathdee G, MacKean M, Illand M, Brown R, A role for methylation of the hMLH1 promoter in loss of hMLH1 expression and drug resistance in ovarian cancer. *Oncogene* 1999; **18**: 2335–41.

17. O'Dwyer PJ, Hamilton TC, Young RC et al, Depletion of glutathione in normal and malignant human cells in vivo by buthionine sulfoximine. *J Natl Cancer Inst* 1992; **84**: 264–7.

18. Kikawa J, Minnakawa Y, Canamori Y et al, Glutathione concentration may be a useful predictor of response to second line chemotherapy in patients with ovarian cancer. *Cancer* 1998; **82**: 697–702.

19. Van der Burg MEL, de Wit R, Stoter G et al, Weekly cisplatin in combination with taxol or etoposide is highly active in recurrent and platinum resistant ovarian cancer. *Int J Gynecol Cancer* 1999; **9**(Suppl 1): 28 (Abst A85).

20. Fink D, Zheng H, Nebel S et al, In vitro and in vivo resistance to cisplatin in cells that have lost DNA mismatch repair. *Cancer Res* 1997; **57**: 1841–5.

21. Holford J, Sharp SY, Murrer BA et al, In vitro circumvention of cisplatin resistance by the novel sterically hindered platinum complex AMD473. *Br J Cancer* 1998; **77**: 366–73.

22. Van der Zee A, DeVries EG, Drug resistance factors. In: *Ovarian Cancer 4* (Sharp F, Blackett T, Leake R, Berek J, eds). London: Chapman & Hall, 1996: 221–33.

23. Seiden M, Swenerton K, Matulomis U et al, Phase II study of VX-710 and paclitaxel in women with paclitaxel refractory ovarian cancer. In: *Proceedings of AACR/NCI/EORTC Conference on Molecular Targets and Cancer Therapeutics*, 1999: 108.

24. Wahl AF, Donaldson KL, Fairchild C et al, Loss of normal p53 function confers sensitization to Taxol by increasing G2/M arrest and apoptosis. *Nature Med* 1996; **2**: 72–9.

13

Intestinal obstruction in advanced ovarian cancer

Joke JM Bais, Anca C Ansink, Marten S Schilthuis

INTRODUCTION

Intestinal obstruction in patients with advanced ovarian cancer is a serious complication affecting survival and quality of life. In the presence of intestinal obstruction and progressive disease, palliation is a highly complex issue.

Although surgery is the primary treatment of choice for malignant obstruction, it is now recognized that many patients with advanced ovarian cancer are generally in a poor condition and might not benefit from surgery. These patients require alternative management to relieve distressing symptoms. In this chapter, the indications for surgery and other management strategies such as medical treatment and percutaneous endoscopic gastrostomy are discussed.

CASE HISTORY

A 56-year-old woman was admitted with symptoms of intestinal obstruction (nausea, vomiting and abdominal distension). Three years earlier, a poorly differentiated mucinous cystadenocarcinoma, stage III, of the ovaries was diagnosed. After primary surgery, only minimal residual disease remained. She was treated with six cycles of cyclophosphamide and cisplatin chemotherapy.

Normalization of CA125 was achieved after the third cycle. Twelve months later, recurrent abdominal disease was detected (two lesions, with the largest mass about 5 cm in size), and was successfully treated with six cycles of a combination of cisplatin and paclitaxel. The last course had been administered nine months previously. A recent computed tomography (CT) scan showed peritoneal carcinomatosis and a dilated bowel (Figure 13.1). The serum CA125 was 330 kU/l.

What investigations should be performed in a patient in second relapse with intestinal obstruction demonstrated clinically and on a CT scan of the abdomen?

Initial management of intestinal obstruction

In patients with intestinal obstruction secondary to ovarian cancer, strangulation or perforation is rare. Therefore immediate laparotomy is seldomly required.[1–3] The diagnosis of intestinal obstruction should be confirmed by erect and supine radiographs of the abdomen, showing dilated loops of the intestine and/or air–fluid levels. Initial management in all patients should be conservative. This comprises nasogastric intubation, rectal enemas, and the administration of intravenous fluids. Obstruction due to opiates or

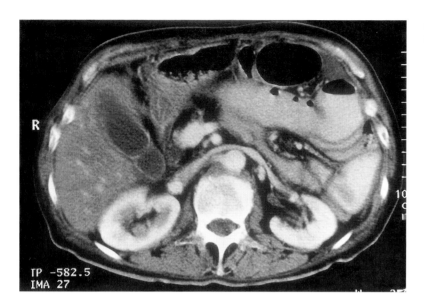

Figure 13.1
CT scan showing dilated bowel.

chemotherapeutic agents, biochemical disorders such as hypercalcaemia or hypokalaemia, or faecal impaction should be excluded.

If faecal impaction is present, physical examination reveals a loaded rectum and palpable faecal masses in the abdomen. When the rectum is empty and impaction is located in the sigmoid or more proximally, the diagnosis is made by abdominal radiographs. Sometimes overflow diarrhoea results from bacterial liquefaction of faecal material blocked in the sigmoid or rectum.[4] If the symptoms do not settle with initial management, investigation is required to determine whether the patient might benefit from surgery.

Successful palliation is usually defined as producing at least two months' survival, but restoration of intestinal function is also an important component. In the studies by Rubin et al[5] and Lund et al[6] intestinal obstruction was resolved in 65% and 32% of patients respectively.

In the studies by Bais et al[7] and Jong et al[8] 68% (13/19) and 53% (28/53) respectively of the patients survived for two months, and in addition gastrointestinal function was partial or completely restored. Thus a considerable number of patients were not successfully treated, often because of inoperability or persistent obstruction caused by a paralytic ileus. Inoperability may be due to multiple sites of obstruction and/or proximal small bowel obstruction. Relief of the latter by surgery would result in a short bowel syndrome. The absence of any clinical improvement and recovery of intestinal function may be due to a motility disorder resulting from the presence of carcinomatosis.

It is essential to rule out multiple obstruction sites and a paralytic ileus before any surgical intervention.

Bowel contrast studies can distinguish between mechanical obstruction and a paralytic bowel. Such studies demonstrate the site of obstruction and the presence of multiple sites of obstruction. In a paralytic bowel, the transit time of radiographic contrast is prolonged.

Suspected small intestinal obstruction

Small bowel obstruction may be detected as follows:

1. A small bowel follow-through with barium or water-soluble medium (e.g. Gastrografin) contrast studies can be used.
2. A small bowel double-contrast enema or enteroclysis can be performed.

A small bowel follow-through contrast study with barium may convert a tight partial obstruction into complete obstruction by becoming inspissated above the level of the blockage. This can result in serious problems in inoperable patients.[1] Barium should also be withheld in patients when intestinal perforation is suspected. Contrast studies with water-soluble medium (e.g. Gastrografin) would be preferable in such cases.[9] A disadvantage of water-soluble contrast material is that it is too dilute to give precise information about pathological changes in the distal small bowel. Moreover, its hyperosmolarity may aggravate prestenotic fluid overload.[9] Follow-through contrast studies are also informative regarding intestinal transit time.

In a small bowel double-contrast enema, methylcellulose distends the small bowel with radiolucent liquid, leaving a thin coating of barium on the mucosal surface.[10] With enteroclysis, barium and air are infused through a tube inserted into the duodenum. This is more accurate in localizing lesions resulting from adhesions, acute or chronic radiation enteritis, or partial obstruction by tumour.[9–11] Lack of distensibility of the small bowel when enteroclysis is used usually reflects encasement of the intestines by tumour, and should be regarded as a sign of poor prognosis.

In the series of Clarke-Pearson et al[12] (with 49 patients), evaluation by barium contrast studies showed evidence of tumour involvement of the intestinal wall that was confirmed at surgery in 75% of cases. Conversely 56% (5 of 9 patients) with no radiographic evidence of intestinal involvement by tumour were found at surgery to have tumour as the primary cause of obstruction.

Suspected large intestinal obstruction

There are two options to evaluate suspected large bowel obstruction: by retrograde barium contrast studies of the colon or by flexible sigmoidoscopy. The absence of retrograde filling or obvious areas of luminal narrowing are diagnostic for obstruction of the large bowel.[1,4]

In conclusion, to diagnose all possible obstruction sites, contrast studies of the small and large bowel are needed in all patients who are being considered for surgical intervention.

Nasogastric suction was started after a supine and erect plain X-ray showed dilated loops of small bowel within the air–fluid interface (Figure 13.2). Clinical examination revealed palpable abdominal masses, but no ascites. The presence of constipation

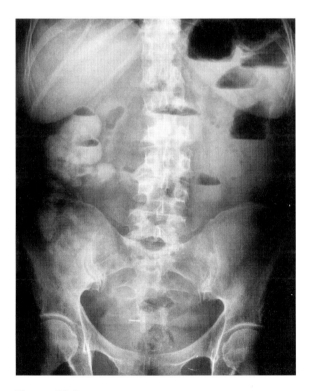

Figure 13.2
Plain erect abdominal X-ray showing 'fluid levels' typical of intestinal obstruction.

was excluded. The ECOG (see Appendix 3) perform-ance status was 1. A small bowel contrast study with barium was performed. An extramucosal mass with some deformity of the ileum was found, and an incomplete obstruction in the ileum was suspected. Transit time was nearly normal. A flexible sigmoi-doscopy was performed, but no obstruction was found. Nasogastric suction for three days provided no relief of the symptoms.

A laparotomy was performed, which revealed diffuse involvement of the intestines by tumour. It was possible to perform a bypass procedure, and three weeks later chemotherapy with a platinum–paclitaxel combination was started.

What is the pathogenesis and incidence of intestinal obstruction?

Several mechanisms may be involved in the onset of intestinal obstruction:

1. Mechanical obstruction by extrinsic or intra-luminal occlusion due to primary tumour mass, metastases, tumour recurrence, or malignant adhesions.
2. Motility disorders caused by infiltration by the tumour in the mesentery or involvement of the coeliac plexus.
3. Obstruction by benign causes such as benign adhesions, postradiation fibrosis, biochemical disorders such as hypercalcaemia or hypokalaemia, or faecal impaction due to opiates or chemotherapeutic agents.[4,13]

In the literature, figures about the incidence of intestinal obstruction in patients treated previ-ously for ovarian cancer vary considerably, ranging from 5% to 51%.[1,11,13–18] The difference in incidence between studies may be explained by the heterogeneity of the study population as well as by variation in the type of intervention. The only conclusion that can be drawn from the available data is that intestinal obstruction is an important and common problem in patients with ovarian cancer.

Table 13.1 Obstruction sites in all patients or during laparotomy for intestinal obstruction

Ref	No. of patients	Small bowel (%)	Large bowel (%)	Combined (%)
19	49	61	33	6
15	23	36	40	24
7	19	36	32	32
20	98	54	21	25
6[a]	41	56	32	12
5	52	44	33	22
13[a]	127	52	33	15
11	38	42	16	42
Total	447	51	28	21

[a] Obstruction sites in conservative and surgically treated patients.

Patients with a high obstruction will present with different symptoms from those with a low obstruction. A proximal obstruction in the small intestine is frequently accompanied by vomiting. Pain will be absent unless a perforation has occurred. Distal obstruction of the small intestine causes nausea, vomiting, abdominal distension, and colicky or diffuse pain. The absence of evacuation of faeces and flatus, abdominal distension, and colicky pain are characteristic of large bowel obstruction.

In Table 13.1, the relative incidence of the sites of obstruction observed in all patients or at laparotomy is presented. It is clear from this table that in half of the ovarian cancer patients, ileus is caused by small bowel obstruction.

Which patients benefit from surgery?

When surgical treatment of intestinal obstruction is considered in patients with recurrent ovarian cancer, it should be borne in mind that the perioperative mortality rate (i.e. death within 30 days of surgery), the major operative complication rate, and inoperability (i.e. the inability to carry out a definitive procedure for obstruction) are high. In the studies listed in Table 13.2, inoperability ranges from 0% to 24% (mean 10%), the major complication rate ranges from 5% to 49%

Table 13.2   Inoperability, major operative complications, and perioperative deaths in patients with ovarian cancer and intestinal obstruction after surgery[a]

Ref	No. of patients	Inoperability (%)	Major operative complications (%)	Perioperative deaths (%)
15	23	0	28	12
13	90	0	NS	14
21	60	18	31	18
14	21	0	20	4
20	98	22	12	22
19	49	0	49	14
11	26	8	42	15
5	52	21	NS	17
22	19	0	NS	16
6	25	24	32	32
23	30	0	NS	NS
7	19	11	16	11
17	22	5	5	9
Total/Mean	534	10	24	18

[a] Inoperability: the inability to carry out a definitive procedure for obstruction. Perioperative deaths: deaths within 30 days of surgery. NS, not stated.

(mean 24%), and the mean perioperative mortality is 18% (range 9–32%).

Surgery is arbitrarily considered to be beneficial if a patient survives for at least two months after the laparotomy.[15] Krebs and Goplerud[20] were the first to propose the use of a prognostic index score (Table 13.3). On the basis of this prognostic index, they reported a 'benefit' from surgery in 84% of patients with a low score (≤6) and in 20% of those with a higher score (>6). Table 13.4 shows comparable results of Larson et al[22] and Gadducci et al,[17] who used the same risk score system. However, there are many other selection criteria that have been used by other authors.[2,3,7,8,12,13,17,19,20,22–25] There is, however, room for improvement in this scoring system:

Table 13.3 Prognostic criteria used by Krebs and Goplerud[20]	
Parameters	Assigned risk score
Age (years):	
<45	0
45–65	1
>65	2
Nutritional impairment:	
None or minimal	0
Moderate	1
Severe	2
Tumour status:	
No palpable intra-abdominal masses	0
Palpable intra-abdominal masses	1
Liver involvement or distant metastases	2
Ascites:	
None or mild (asymptomatic, abdomen not distended)	0
Moderate (abdomen distended)	1
Severe (symptomatic, requires frequent paracentesis)	2
Previous chemotherapy:	
None, or no adequate trial	0
Failed single-drug therapy	1
Failed combination drug therapy	2
Previous radiotherapy:	
None	0
Radiotherapy to pelvis	1
Radiotherapy to whole abdomen	2

Table 13.4   Survival in surgically treated patients related to the Krebs–Goplerud risk score (see Table 13.3)

	Risk score ≤6				Risk score >6			
Ref	No. of patients	60d surv (%)	180d surv (%)	365d surv (%)	No. of patients	60d[a] surv (%)	180d surv (%)	365d surv (%)
20	83	84	—	—	35	20	—	—
22	21	81	43	38	12	50	8	0
17	16	88	56	19	6	17	0	0

[a] 60d surv, 60-day survival, etc.

1. Potential confounding factors are not eliminated by using logistic regression analysis.[19]
2. Radiation therapy is now rarely used as primary therapy for ovarian cancer. However, in patients who have previously received whole abdominal radiation, the risk of developing a benign cause of obstruction due to adhesions is high.[2,18] Krebs advised strongly against surgery in patients who have been treated with radiation therapy.[20] He based his opinion on the data of four patients, who developed a dehiscence of the intestinal anastomosis after surgery. They were all previously treated with radiation therapy, and were responsible for 33% of fatal surgical complications. Castaldo et al[15] reported a major complication rate of 56% in nine patients who received prior radiation therapy. This is in contrast with our own series, which did not find any major complications in all six patients in the same category.[7] Previous radiation therapy is, in our opinion, not an absolute contraindication for surgery, although increased morbidity can be expected in these patients.
3. Failure of an inadequate trial of previous chemotherapy is an important diagnostic criterion, but rarely an issue now since most patients will have received platina-containing chemotherapy.
4. There is uncertainty about the importance of age as a prognostic factor. In two studies (with a total of 180 patients), it was related to survival, while in three studies (with a total of 120 patients), it was not.[2,17,20,22,24]
5. Nutritional status has been regarded as a prognostic factor. However no clear definition of nutritional status is given. This is in contrast to performance status, which has been defined accurately by the ECOG. Performance status is also related to nutritional status. We therefore feel that it is more rational to use performance status as a prognostic factor.

In conclusion, several of the Krebs criteria are no longer valid, partly owing to insufficient data and changes in treatment policy.

Table 13.5 summarizes the data about prognostic factors and their relationship to survival. We conclude from these data that tumour status (absence of palpable masses), ascites (not rapidly accumulating and less than two or three litres),

Table 13.5   Prognostic factors related or not related to survival[a]

Prognostic factor	Related to survival	Not related to survival	Refs
No. of previous chemotherapy regimens		××	8, 17
Interval since last treatment <6 months	×		23
Previous radiation therapy	×	×××	2, 7, 20, 24
Interval initial diagnosis–obstruction	××	××	2, 17, 22, 24
Tumour status	×××××		2, 3, 12, 20, 24, 25
Ascites	×××××××		2, 3, 7, 20, 23–25
Nutritional status	××××		2, 12, 20, 24
Age	××	×××	2, 17, 20, 22, 24
Motility disorder/carcinomatosis	××		3, 13
No multiple obstruction sites	××		13, 24
Degree of obstruction		××	13, 24
Elevated alkaline phosphatase level	×		2
Elevated blood urea nitrogen level	×		2

[a] The number of crosses indicates the number of times the prognostic factor is mentioned in the literature.

and performance status (ECOG 0–2) are the most important prognostic factors in the initial selection of patients who might benefit from surgery.

What surgery should be performed?

Intestinal obstruction in the group of patients with which we are dealing in this chapter occurs as a result of tumour recurrence or progression after platina-containing chemotherapy. Common findings are diffuse intestinal tumour involvement, with multiple loops of small bowel matted together by tumour on peritoneal surfaces, and oedematous or fibrotic bowel with a poor blood supply. A primary resection and re-anastomosis of bowel under these circumstances is usually not possible. Since survival is not influenced by tumour resection in these heavily pretreated patients, it is better in the majority of cases to perform an intestinal bypass using a side-to-side anastomosis.[13,15,19,20]

Obstruction of the colon is usually treated by colostomy. In most instances, a transverse loop colostomy is performed, and less often a sigmoid loop colostomy.[13,15,19–21] Owing to inadequate bowel preparation and intestinal distension, a primary resection and re-anastomosis of the bowel is usually not feasible.[1]

The role of total parenteral nutrition as an adjunct to surgery in a patient with ovarian cancer who has bowel obstruction remains unclear, since it has not been established that the correction of a nutritional deficit will have an impact on long-term survival.[19] Rubin et al[5] reported that the likelihood of accomplishing a definitive procedure was unrelated to the use of perioperative total parenteral nutrition.

The administration of postoperative chemotherapy depends mainly on the type of agents previously used, the duration of remission, and the treatment-free interval. Furthermore, the postoperative performance status needs to be taken into account, as well as the wishes of the patient and her family.

Which conservative modalities should be considered in patients who are not suitable for surgery?

The median survival time for patients with recurrent and inoperable disease treated with drugs after the onset of intestinal obstruction ranges from 30 to 92 days.[6,7,11,13,22] The aim of conservative treatment is to relieve distressing symptoms.

We advise against the administration of further chemotherapy, since in heavily pretreated patients, restoration of intestinal function rarely occurs.[26]

When treating symptoms of intestinal obstruction pharmacologically, the following issues are important. Firstly, as vomiting is frequent, the oral administration of drugs should be discouraged. Secondly, it is important to limit the numbers of drugs used, so that one can establish whether a drug is working and assess its side-effects (see also Chapter 19).

Pharmacological therapy for colicky pain

The causes of colicky pain are constipation, intestinal distension, pressure due to peritumoural oedema, organ infiltration, and nerve compression. Recommendations for treating colicky pain are given in Table 13.6.

Enemas are often effective for pain caused by constipation, which is a common feature in patients with intestinal obstruction due to immobility, dehydration, and use of opioids. Intestinal distension pain can be treated by scopolamine (hyoscine) or scopolamine butylbromide.[27] It has an analgesic as well as an antiemetic effect. Scopolamine butylbromide is a drug with anticholinergic activity, decreasing tone and peristalsis in smooth muscle. It also reduces the production of gastrointestinal fluids.

Colicky pain due to pressure from peritumoural oedema, organ infiltration, and nerve compression may be reduced by dexamethasone or other steroids. These drugs may also improve appetite and induce well-being[27] and help in the management of nausea and vomiting.[28]

If these drugs do not relieve pain, opioids should be given. Fentanyl given by transdermal patch is the drug of choice. It may also be given

Table 13.6   Pharmacological therapy for colicky pain

Drug	Dosage
Scopolamine (hyoscine) butylbromide or hyoscine hydrobromide	Starting 80–120 mg/day subcutaneously 800–2400 µg/day
Dexamethasone	16–24 mg p.o. once or twice a day; after 5 days reduce dose by 2 mg/day to the lowest that will control symptoms
Fentanyl patches	Starting 25 µg every 3 days, transdermally

Table 13.7   Pharmacological therapy for relief of nausea and vomiting

Mechanism	Drug	Dosage
Mechanical	Domperidone	30–60 mg 8-hourly suppository
	Metoclopramide	60–240 mg/day s.c. infusion
	Octreotide	0.2–0.9 mg/day s.c. infusion
Chemical	Levomepromazine (methotrimeprazine)	12.5–200 mg/day s.c.
	Haloperidol	5–15 mg/day s.c.
Vagal stimulation	Scopolamine (hyoscine) butylbromide	80–120 mg/day s.c.
	Hyoscine hydrobromide	800–2400 µg/day s.c. infusion
	Scopolamine	1.5 mg every 3 days transdermally
	Cyclizine	100–250 mg/day s.c. or 50 mg 8-hourly suppository
Anxiety	Methotrimeprazine	50–100 mg 8-hourly suppository

by subcutaneous continuous infusion. If these drugs are ineffective, a coeliac block with alcohol, or spinal or epidural analgesia should be considered.

Pharmacological therapy to relieve nausea and vomiting

Nausea and vomiting can be caused by three mechanisms:[27]

1. Mechanical, due to gastric distension caused by gastrointestinal fluid obstruction.
2. Chemical, due to drugs like opioids, antibiotics, tricyclic antidepressants, uraemia, hypercalcaemia and bacterial toxins.
3. Vagal stimulation, due to stretched liver capsule by metastases, or bowel distension, due to intestinal obstruction or constipation.

The drugs commonly used for relief of nausea and vomiting related to these mechanisms are summarized in Table 13.7. Metoclopramide and domperidone are antiemetic drugs that increase gastric motility. These drugs are recommended in patients with incomplete intestinal obstruction and in patients who do not have an upper gastrointestinal obstruction.[28] Octreotide, an analogue of somatostatin, is the second-line drug of choice when symptom control fails with conventional antiemetics. It reduces gastrointestinal fluid production by decreasing gastric acid secretion, bile flow, and splanchnic blood flow. In addition, intestinal motility is reduced. In most patients, vomiting is controlled within two to three days of starting treatment. In patients with a nasogastric tube, drainage has been shown to decrease from 2000 ml/day to under 100 ml/day after starting octreotide treatment.[29,30] Octreotide is an expensive but highly effective drug.

Levomepromazine (methotrimeprazine) and haloperidol are neuroleptic drugs. Nausea,

Table 13.8   Results of percutaneous endoscopic gastrostomy (PEG) in patients with intestinal obstruction

Ref	No. of patients	Type of patients	Technical success rate[a] (%)	Complication rate (%)	Effective procedure[b] (%)	Death[c] (%)
35	45	Malignant ascites	98	9	93	2
36	28	Gynaecological cancer	93	0	93	0
37	10	Ovarian	100	30	80	0
38	12	Malignant ascites	100	33	100	0
39	46	Intraperitoneal cancer	89	4	88	2
32	34	Gynaecological cancer	94	6	85	0
33	12	Intraperitoneal cancer	92	8	92	0
Total/Mean	187		92	9	89	1

[a] The rate of procedures in which placing of a PEG is successful.
[b] The rate of PEG catheters that are functioning.
[c] Death due to complication resulting in death after procedure.

particularly when due to the adverse effect of opioids, responds well to these drugs. The combination morphine–levomepromazine is superior to the combination morphine–haloperidol, owing to a reinforcing analgesic, antiemetic, and anxiolytic effect.[31]

If anxiety is prominent, methotrimeprazine is a very effective antiemetic and sedative drug.[4]

Percutaneous endoscopic gastrostomy

Prolonged nasogastric suction and intravenous fluids for symptomatic treatment of inoperable patients are not recommended. During long-term drainage, a nasogastric tube can interfere with coughing to clear pulmonary secretions, and may be associated with nasal cartilage erosion, otitis media, aspiration pneumonia, oesophagitis, and bleeding. It is sometimes more uncomfortable for the patient than the basic condition itself.[29,32]

A percutaneous endoscopic gastrostomy (PEG) can be placed during laparotomy when a patient turns out to be inoperable, or under local anaesthesia. The latter approach results in a lower morbidity and mortality and a shorter hospital stay.[33] The use of ultrasound imaging at the time of endoscopy allows rapid localization of an appropriate area for PEG placement and reduces the risk of inadvertently entering adjacent organs or metastatic foci.[34]

Table 13.8 shows the results of PEG in patients with intraperitoneal malignancies. The technical success rate (i.e. the rate of procedures in which placing of a PEG is successful) is high, although the rate of an effective procedure (i.e. the rate of well-functioning catheters) is somewhat lower (88–100%). The complications are dislodgement, leakage of gastric fluid causing wound infection and excoriation, peritonitis, and haemorrhage.

The presence of ascites is regarded as a relative contraindication to PEG, because the stomach may be displaced from the anterior abdominal wall by fluid, making stomach puncture difficult. This may result in pericatheter leakage of ascitic fluid.[38] The problem can be managed by paracentesis before the procedure and gastropexy to prevent catheter dislodgement.[35,38] Ryan et al[35] recommended additional serial paracentesis after the procedure when reaccumulation of ascites close to the site of gastrostomy catheter is detected, in order to prevent pericatheter leakage.

A PEG should be considered in all inoperable patients who need nasogastric decompression.

Total parenteral nutrition

For long-term total parenteral nutrition, it is necessary to insert a central venous cannulation, usually through the subclavian vein. Although not common, complications of total parenteral nutrition include mechanical, catheter-placement problems, as well as metabolic, fluid electrolyte, hydration, and septic complications. There is little evidence of any major improvement in survival with nutritional support.[40] However, in a retrospective study, King et al[41] stated that home parenteral nutrition in patients with inoperable mechanical intestinal obstruction resulted in significant palliation and an improved quality of life. In this study of 61 patients who received home parenteral nutrition, only 15% of hospital admissions were related to parenteral nutrition complications.

In contrast to King et al,[41] Abu-Rustum et al[26] and August et al[42] stated that the value of total parenteral nutrition in patients with end-stage ovarian cancer was limited. In 11 patients who received chemotherapy and total parenteral nutrition, median survival was 18 days longer in patients with chemotherapy and total parenteral nutrition compared with patients without total parenteral nutrition.[26]

In the light of possible complications, costs

and increase in home supportive care, we believe that total parenteral nutrition in ovarian cancer patients who present with concomitant inoperable intestinal obstruction cannot be supported. However, there may be room for such therapy in a few selected patients.

LEARNING POINTS

✳ Intestinal obstruction in ovarian cancer is in most cases due to malignant obstruction.
✳ After an initial period of conservative management, patients should undergo evaluation to assess their suitability for surgery.
✳ The rates of inoperability, major complications, and perioperative mortality after surgery for intestinal obstruction are high.
✳ The primary selection criteria for surgery are:
  – performance score (ECOG 0, 1, or 2),
  – tumour (absence of palpable masses),
  – ascites (not rapidly reaccumulating and <2 or 3 litres).
✳ The secondary selection criteria for surgery are the absence of paralytic ileus (transit time) and the absence of multiple sites of obstruction (determined by radiological examination of the small and large bowel).
✳ Conservative treatment with drugs or percutaneous endoscopic gastrostomy is an effective alternative in patients who are not eligible for surgery, and in inoperable patients.

REFERENCES

1. Krebs HB, Helmkamp BF, Management of intestinal obstruction in ovarian cancer. *Oncology* 1989; **3**: 25–31.
2. Fernandes JR, Seymour RJ, Suissa S, Bowel obstruction in patients with ovarian cancer: a search for prognostic factors. *Am J Obstet Gynecol* 1988; **158**: 244–9.
3. Gallick HL, Weaver DW, Sachs RJ, Bouwman DL, Intestinal obstruction in cancer patients.

An assessment of risk factors and outcome. *Am Surg* 1986; **52**: 434–7.

4. Ripamonti C, Management of bowel obstruction in advanced cancer. *Curr Opin Oncol* 1994; **6**: 351–7.

5. Rubin SC, Hoskins WJ, Benjamin I, Lewis JL, Palliative surgery for intestinal obstruction in advanced ovarian cancer. *Gynecol Oncol* 1989; **34**: 16–19.

6. Lund B, Hansen M, Lundvall F et al, Intestinal obstruction in patients with advanced carcinoma of the ovaries treated with combination chemotherapy. *Surg Gynecol Obstet* 1989; **169**: 213–18.

7. Bais JM, Schilthuis MS, Slors FJ, Lammes FB, Intestinal obstruction in patients with advanced ovarian cancer. *Int J Gynecol Cancer* 1995; **5**: 346–50.

8. Jong P, Sturgeon J, Jamieson CG, Benefit of palliative surgery for bowel obstruction in advanced ovarian cancer. *Can J Surg* 1995; **38**: 454–7.

9. Wittich G, Salomonowitz E, Szepesi T et al, Small bowel double-contrast enema in stage III ovarian cancer. *Am J Roentgenol* 1984; **142**: 299–304.

10. Yuhasz M, Laufer I, Sutton G et al, Radiography of the small bowel in patients with gynecologic malignancies. *Am J Roentgenol* 1985; **144**: 303–7.

11. Redman CW, Shafti MI, Ambrose S et al, Survival following intestinal obstruction in ovarian cancer. *Eur J Surg Oncol* 1988; **14**: 383–6.

12. Clarke-Pearson DL, DeLong ER, Chin N et al, Intestinal obstruction in patients with ovarian cancer. Variables associated with surgical complications and survival. *Arch Surg* 1988; **123**: 42–5.

13. Tunca JC, Buchler DA, Mack EA et al, The management of ovarian-cancer-caused bowel obstruction. *Gynecol Oncol* 1981; **12**: 186–92.

14. Solomon HJ, Atkinson KH, Coppleson JV et al, Bowel complications in the management of ovarian cancer. *Aust NZ J Obstet Gynaecol* 1983; **23**: 65–8.

15. Castaldo TW, Petrilli ES, Ballon SC, Lagasse LD, Intestinal operations in patients with ovarian carcinoma. *Am J Obstet Gynecol* 1981; **139**: 80–4.

16. Donato D, Angelides A, Irani H et al, Infectious complications after gastrointestinal surgery in patients with ovarian carcinoma and malignant ascites. *Gynecol Oncol* 1992; **44**: 40–7.

17. Gadducci A, Iacconi P, Fanucchi A et al, Survival after intestinal obstruction in patients with fatal ovarian cancer: analysis of prognostic variables. *Int J Gynecol Cancer* 1998; **8**: 177–82.

18. Whelan TJ, Dembo AJ, Bush RS et al, Complications of whole abdominal and pelvic radiotherapy following chemotherapy for advanced ovarian cancer. *Int J Radiat Oncol Biol Phys* 1992; **22**: 853–8.

19. Clarke-Pearson DL, Chin N, DeLong ER et al, Surgical management of intestinal obstruction in ovarian cancer. Clinical features, postoperative complications, and survival. *Gynecol Oncol* 1987; **26**: 11–18.

20. Krebs HB, Goplerud DR, Surgical management of bowel obstruction in advanced ovarian carcinoma. *Obstet Gynecol* 1983; **61**: 327–30.

21. Piver MS, Barlow JJ, Lele SB, Frank A, Survival after ovarian cancer induced intestinal obstruction. *Gynecol Oncol* 1982; **13**: 44–9.

22. Larson JE, Podczasju ES, Manetta A et al, Bowel obstruction in patients with ovarian carcinoma: analysis of prognostic factors. *Gynecol Oncol* 1989; **35**: 61–5.

23. Zoetmulder FA, Helmerhorst ThJ, van Coevorden F et al, Management of bowel obstruction in patients with advanced ovarian cancer. *Eur J Cancer* 1994; **30**: 1625–8.

24. Krebs HB, Goplerud DR, Mechanical intestinal obstruction in patients with gynecologic disease: a review of 368 patients. *Am J Obstet Gynecol* 1987; **157**: 577–83.

25. Ooijen B van, Van der Burg ME, Planting AS et al, Surgical treatment or gastric drainage only

for intestinal obstruction in patients with carcinoma of the ovary or peritoneal carcinomatosis of other origin. *Surg Gynecol Obstet* 1993; **176**: 469–74.

26. Abu-Rustum NR, Barakat RR, Venkatraman E, Spriggs D, Chemotherapy and total parenteral nutrition for advanced ovarian cancer with bowel obstruction. *Gynecol Oncol* 1997; **64**: 493–5.

27. Regnard CF, Tempest S, *A Guide to Symptom Relief in Advanced Cancer*, 3rd edn. Manchester: Haigh & Hochland, 1992: 18, 26–7.

28. Fainsinger RL, Spachynski K, Hanson J, Bruera E, Symptom control in terminally ill patients with malignant bowel obstruction. *J Pain Sympt Manage* 1994; **9**: 12–18.

29. Mangili G, Franchi M, Mariani A et al, Octreotide in the management of bowel obstruction in terminal ovarian cancer. *Gynecol Oncol* 1996; **61**: 345–8.

30. Mercadante S, The role of octreotide in palliative care. *J Pain Sympt Manage* 1994; **9**: 406–11.

31. van Dongen DJ, Keizer HJ, Welvaart K, Cleton FJ, Palliatieve behandeling van darmobstructie bij patienten met kanker. *NtvG* 1993; **137**: 1871–4.

32. Campagnutta E, Cannizzaro R, Gallo A et al, Palliative treatment of upper intestinal obstruction by gynecological malignancy: the usefulness of percutaneous endoscopic gastrostomy. *Gynecol Oncol* 1996; **62**: 103–5.

33. Adelson MD, Kasowitz MH, Percutaneous endoscopic drainage gastronomy in the treatment of gastrointestinal obstruction from intraperitoneal malignancy. *Obstet Gynecol* 1993; **81**: 467–71.

34. Vargo JJ, Germain MM, Swenson JA, Harrison CR, Ultrasound-assisted percutaneous endoscopic gastrostomy in a patient with advanced ovarian carcinoma and recurrent intestinal obstruction. *Am J Gastroenterol* 1993; **88**: 1946–8.

35. Ryan JM, Hahn PF, Mueller PR, Performing radiologic gastrostomy or gastrojejunostomy in patients with malignant ascites. *Am J Roentgenol* 1998; **17**: 1003–6.

36. Marks WH, Perkal MP, Schwartz PE, Percutaneous endoscopic gastrostomy for gastric decompression in metastatic gynecologic malignancies. *Surg Gynecol Obstet* 1993; **177**: 573–6.

37. Malone JM Jr, Koonce T, Larson DM et al, Palliation of small bowel obstruction by percutaneous gastrostomy in patients with progressive ovarian carcinoma. *Obstet Gynecol* 1986; **68**: 431–3.

38. Lee MJ, Saini S, Brink JA et al, Malignant small bowel obstruction and ascites: not a contraindication to percutaneous gastrostomy. *Clin Radiol* 1991; **44**: 332–4.

39. Herman LL, Hoskins WJ, Shik M, Percutaneous endoscopic gastrostomy for decompression of the stomach and small bowel. *Gastrointest Endosc* 1992; **38**: 314–18.

40. Henshaw EC, Schloerb PR, Nutrition and the cancer patient. In: *Clinical Oncology: A Multidisciplinary Approach for Physicians and Students* (Rubin P, McDonald S, Qazi R, eds). Philadelphia: Saunders, 1992: 691–7.

41. King LA, Carson LF, Konstantinides N et al, Outcome assessment of home parenteral nutrition in patients with gynecologic malignancies: What have we learned in a decade of experience? *Gynecol Oncol* 1993; **51**: 377–82.

42. August DA, Thorn D, Fisher RL, Welchek CM, Home parenteral nutrition for patients with inoperable malignant bowel obstruction. *J Parenter Enteral Nutr* 1991; **15**: 323–7.

14

Management of an isolated recurrent pelvic mass

Michelle R Scurr, Michael L Friedlander, Neville F Hacker

INTRODUCTION

When a patient with epithelial ovarian cancer develops evidence of recurrent disease, one question that must be addressed is whether to start chemotherapy immediately or to attempt surgical cytoreduction. If the patient can undergo successful cytoreduction, she may be more likely to have a sustained remission with additional chemotherapy. On the other hand, an unsuccessful surgical procedure does not benefit the patient. Multiple factors must be considered when making such a decision. These factors include prior response to chemotherapy, duration of disease-free interval, and findings of imaging studies. Following the decision about secondary cytoreduction, the oncologist must consider additional therapy (chemotherapy, radiotherapy, and hormonal therapy) or close follow-up without additional therapy. The following case histories and discussions address the issue of recurrent ovarian cancer and secondary therapy.

CASE HISTORY 1

A 33-year-old female with no past medical history and a family history of breast cancer presented to another institution with pelvic pain. Pelvic ultra-sonography revealed bilateral ovarian masses 5–6 cm in diameter and a CA125 titre performed at the time was not elevated. She underwent a hysterectomy and bilateral salpingo-oophorectomy at a community hospital, with no formal surgical staging undertaken. The pathology revealed bilateral grade II serous cystadenocarcinoma. She then had 12 cycles of chlorambucil, at the end of which she clinically remained disease free. She did not undergo second-look surgery.

Fourteen years later, at the age of 47, she was referred to our institution with fatigue and a recently elevated CA125 titre of 82 U/ml. Vaginal examination revealed a mass between the vagina and the rectum, which was confirmed on a computed tomographic (CT) scan. There was no associated ascites or other evidence of recurrence. After a full bowel preparation, she underwent a laparotomy, at which a 7 cm × 5 cm mass was found involving the sigmoid mesentery (Figure 14.1). She underwent a sigmoid colectomy with primary reanastomosis. At the end of the procedure, there was no evidence of macroscopic residual disease. The pathology on this occasion was a grade I serous papillary adenocarcinoma. The patient received carboplatin, AUC ('area under the concentration–time curve') 5, and remains free of disease eight years later.

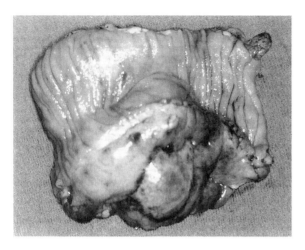

Figure 14.1
Isolated recurrence in the sigmoid mesocolon, completely resected with sigmoid colectomy and primary reanastomosis.

Is this delayed relapse of an (occult) advanced tumour or development of a new one?

This patient had apparent stage IB disease at diagnosis, although formal staging was not undertaken. The five-year survival rate of patients with stage I ovarian cancer ranges from 60% to 90%; this wide range is almost certainly due to differences in staging in various centres. The techniques and requirements for staging in 'apparent' early ovarian cancer are well established, and there are widely published guidelines for staging. There have been several studies assessing whether patients with ovarian cancer are being appropriately staged. McGowan et al[1] found that only 35% of patients who were surgically treated by a general surgeon, and 52% of those treated by a specialist gynaecologist, underwent complete surgical staging. Munoz et al[2] recently reported a random retrospective review of 785 women with ovarian cancer registered on the US National Cancer Institute (NCI) Surveillance, Epidemiology and End Results (SEER) programme, and found that only 10% of women

with presumptive stage I or II ovarian cancer had recommended staging and treatment. The most common cause of incomplete staging was the omission of a lymphadenectomy. It has been known for many years that a rigorous staging laparotomy will upstage a significant number of patients with apparently localized ovarian cancer. Young et al[3] reported on a series of 100 patients who underwent repeat staging procedures. Of these women, 31% were upstaged, and most of these had stage III disease. Further studies have shown that up to 27% of patients with 'stage I' disease will have microscopic pelvic and/or para-aortic lymph node metastases at time of diagnosis, upstaging them to FIGO stage III. Zanetta et al[4] retrospectively reviewed data on 350 women with a presumptive stage I ovarian cancer, and found that only 30% had complete surgical staging. In this group with early-stage disease, the only independent variables for overall and disease-free survivals were tumour grade and the completeness of staging.

Had this patient been referred following her initial surgery, thorough surgical staging may have obviated the need for chemotherapy, if the appropriate staging biopsies had been negative. The patient, however, received 12 months of chlorambucil, which is associated with an approximately 8.5% actuarial risk of developing leukaemia at 10 years.[5]

An alternative explanation for late relapse is the development of a new tumour. This may be due to 'field cancerization'. This interesting concept is accepted in cancers of the head and neck, colon, and breast, and yet there is little information in the ovarian cancer literature. The principle of 'field cancerization' is that there is an intrinsic instability in the genotype of tissue of the same embryonic derivation, in this case the coelemic-derived tissue such as ovary and peritoneum, and that so-called late recurrences are in fact new primaries. This has been suggested by

Buller et al,[6] who assessed chromosomal and allelic heterogeneity in ovarian cancer cells of women who presented with late relapse (median 42.7 months). In 77% of cases, the original tumour and the 'relapsed' tumour were significantly different. Although this could be explained by a polyclonal tumour origin, Buller et al proposed that, in some cases, the late recurrence may in fact be a new primary. There are implications with respect to treatment in these patients, since it may be that in fact they have a better prognosis than those with a true relapse.

What is the role of secondary cytoreductive surgery in recurrent ovarian cancer?

The role of secondary cytoreductive surgery is contentious. Interpretation of the published results is difficult, since most studies have been retrospective, with small and heterogeneous study populations, and variations in surgical techniques and methods of assessing outcome. However, despite these limitations, there does appear to be evidence for a role for secondary cytoreductive surgery in a select group of women with recurrent ovarian carcinoma.

In 1983, Berek et al[7] showed a significant survival benefit for patients who had optimal (<1.5 cm) secondary cytoreduction compared with those who did not (median survival 20 months versus 5 months). Since then, several studies have assessed the variables that are associated with this improved survival. The two most important and constant independent prognostic variables are:

1. The disease-free interval after the primary treatment.
2. Optimal debulking of the tumour at the time of secondary cytoreductive surgery.

Janicke et al[8] published a retrospective study of 30 patients undergoing secondary cytoreductive surgery after a median disease-free interval of 16 months. Complete resection was achieved in 47% of patients, and 40% of patients had less than 2 cm of residual disease. Patients with a disease-free interval of more than 12 months had a significantly better survival (29 months versus 8 months). Furthermore, those patients with complete resection of tumour had a median survival of 29 months, compared with 9 months for those with less than 2 cm of residual tumour. Vaccarello et al,[9] in 1995, retrospectively analysed 57 patients with recurrent ovarian cancer who had a previous negative second-look laparotomy. Thirty-eight of the 57 (67%) underwent surgery; 14 of these had residual tumour less than 0.5 cm at the end of the procedure. The median survival for those patients who had not undergone surgery was 9 months, compared with 23 months for suboptimal debulking. The median survival for those with less than 0.5 cm had not been reached by the close of the study ($p < 0.0001$), and this group had a 75% probability of being alive at 41 months. Eisenkop et al[10] published the results of a small prospective study of 36 patients. The goal of the study was to achieve complete resection of all macroscopic disease and assess the variables that made this possible. In 30 patients, they were able to achieve no residual macroscopic disease (25 required multiple operations and 14 a modified posterior extenteration). The median survival for those having no residual disease was 43 months, compared with 5 months for those with any residual disease. In an unpublished report, we have retrospectively reviewed our experience with 46 patients undergoing secondary cytoreductive surgery for recurrent epithelial ovarian carcinoma at the Royal Hospital for Women, Sydney. In 41% of cases, complete macroscopic excision was achieved, while 42% had less than 2 cm and 17% greater than 2 cm of residual tumour. The median survival for patients with residual tumour less than 2 cm following secondary debulking was not significantly different from that of patients with greater than 2 cm, but in those who had no macroscopic residual disease, the median survival had not been reached with a median follow-up of 63 months. This study again confirmed that the duration of the disease-free interval prior to recurrence was highly significant, patients with a disease-free interval of 24 months or greater having a median survival of 80 months, compared with 17 months if the disease-free interval was less than 24 months.

Complete resection therefore appears to be necessary in order for secondary cytoreductive surgery to provide a significant survival benefit. It is therefore important to be able to determine in which patients complete surgical cytoreduction is likely to be achievable. Eisenkop et al[10] found that none of the variables associated with the primary tumour, such as tumour grade, stage, histology, size of the largest metastasis, or location of the metastases, was significant. The prognostic factors at secondary debulking surgery that predicted outcome were the Gynecologic Oncology Group (GOG) performance status (0–2) and the size of the tumour (<10 cm). Five patients in this study had a solitary metastasis, and complete resection was possible in all of these patients. In our own study (Tay, unpublished data), 54% of the patients had clinically localized disease on preoperative assessment. At the end of surgery, patients with localized tumour recurrence were more likely to have no residual disease compared with those with disseminated disease, again suggesting that apparently localized disease is associated with a better prognosis.

What is the role of chemotherapy or hormonal therapy in recurrent disease?
Chemotherapy
Unlike the patient described in the above case history, who was treated initially with a single alkylating agent, most patients with ovarian cancer are treated with platinum-based combination chemotherapy following surgery. Until relatively recently, patients were treated with platinum (either cisplatin or carboplatin) and cyclophosphamide, but since the GOG III study[11] was published in 1996, most now receive platinum and paclitaxel. Despite the improvement associated with platinum-based chemotherapy, the majority of patients with advanced ovarian cancer will relapse and subsequently die of progressive disease. The treatment options depend on a number of factors, including the initial response to chemotherapy and the treatment-free interval, which can help to predict whether the tumour will respond to further chemotherapy. Patients whose tumours recur within six months of completing chemotherapy tend to have a poor prognosis and a low likelihood of response to reintroduction of platinum, in contrast to those patients, such as the case described above, who have a long disease-free interval and who are more likely to respond to further chemotherapy.[12] Markman and Hoskins[13] reported the results of a retrospective analysis of 72 patients who had received at least two cisplatin–carboplatin-based regimens that provides the basis for treatment decisions in this setting. In those patients with a platinum-free interval (PFI) of 5–12 months, the response rate was 27%, while those with a 13–24 month PFI had a response rate of 53%. Of the patients with a platinum-free interval of greater than 24 months, 51% responded to the reintroduction of platinum. Similar findings have been reported by others, yet a precise definition of the minimum required duration of the 'treatment-free interval' to determine potential resistance versus chemosensitivity to platinum agents is still contentious. The patient under discussion had a particularly long (14-year) interval between initial diagnosis and relapse. This is very uncommon, and clearly reflects the indolent biology of the tumour in this patient.

Our policy is to treat patients with single-agent carboplatin (AUC 5–7) at relapse, providing they have a treatment-free interval of greater than six months, since there is no evidence to suggest that combination chemotherapy is superior to single agents in patients with recurrent ovarian cancer.[14] While it could be argued that this patient should possibly have received combination chemotherapy in view of the long disease-free interval, we were concerned about further exposure to alkylating agents and the increased risk of leukaemia, and therefore treated her with single-agent carboplatin.

There are a number of other chemotherapeutic agents that are active in patients with recurrent ovarian cancer and may play a role in its management (see Chapter 11). These include paclitaxel,[15,16] topetecan,[17] oral etoposide,[18] gemcitabine, liposomal doxorubicin, vinorelbine, hexamethylmelamine, and ifosfamide.[19] The response rates range from 13% to 35% and the response duration is usually measured in months. The response rates tend to be higher in patients with 'platinum-sensitive' disease (i.e. those with a prior response to platinum and a treatment-free interval of greater than six months), but responses are also observed in patients with platinum-resistant ovarian cancer. In general, most patients with recurrent ovarian cancer will have reintroduction of carboplatin if they previously responded to platinum, and will go on to receive one of the other agents at relapse. However, there is a small group of patients who may be successfully retreated with carboplatin if once again they respond to treatment and have a prolonged treatment-free interval. Eisenhauer et al[20] have recently analysed the factors predicting response to paclitaxel in patients with recurrent ovarian cancer following platinum-based chemotherapy. In their analysis, serous histology, tumour bulk, and hemoglobin, but surprisingly not treatment-free interval, were all important predictors of response. They went on to extend these observations, and analysed the results of treatment with a variety of agents in over 1200 platinum-pretreated patients. In a multivariate analysis, only three factors remained as significant predictors of response; these were serous histology, number of disease sites, and tumour size. The time from last treatment when evaluated as a continuous variable was not of prognostic significance, but correlated with tumour size.

It would be of great value to be able to identify patients with recurrent ovarian cancer who are likely to benefit from further treatment. Hoskins et al[21] have recently developed a prognostic model for survival after first relapse in women with advanced ovarian cancer based on a prediction-tree analysis. The good-prognosis group (time to recurrence/progression more than 18 months with a grade I or II tumour, or time to recurrence of more than 24 months with a grade III tumour) had a median survival of 18 months. In contrast, they could identify a poor-prognosis group with a poor performance status and short disease-free interval who had a median survival of one month. The majority formed an intermediate-prognosis group with a median survival of six months. Although this model has its limitations, further refinement may help determine which patients should go on to receive second and third chemotherapy at relapse.

Hormonal therapy

Hormonal therapy appears to have a limited role in the management of patients with recurrent ovarian cancer. There are a series of phase II trials that report objective response to tamoxifen in approximately 10% of patients and stable disease in 20% of patients.[22] Although there are no specific data to help in selecting those patients most likely to respond, tamoxifen seems to be more likely to be active in those patients who do not have truly chemoresistant disease or a poor performance status. We have observed a response rate in about 18% of patients,[23] and in practice tend to use tamoxifen in patients who are asymptomatic but have rising CA125 levels consistent with progressive disease. Tamoxifen is generally very well tolerated, with few side-effects, and may benefit a subset of patients with recurrent ovarian cancer. Other hormonal agents have been tried, and include progestogens and luteinizing-hormone-releasing hormone (LHRH) agonists.

Is there a role for radiotherapy?

There are data to support the use of whole-abdominal radiotherapy as primary treatment following surgery for selected patients with ovarian cancer. This would include those patients with stage I, II, or III ovarian cancer with no or small-volume macroscopic residual disease following surgery.[24,25] However, this approach has not found widespread acceptance. Similarly, there may be a role for either localized (involved-field or pelvis) or whole-abdominal radiotherapy for selected patients with recurrent ovarian cancer. These would include patients with no or small-volume macroscopic residual disease following debulking surgery.[26,27] The problem is that these patients would have had at least two prior surgical procedures, and the risk of whole-abdominal radiotherapy is significantly increased if there is evidence of multiple adhesions. There have not been studies comparing radiotherapy with chemotherapy in the recurrent setting, and although most patients are treated with chemotherapy, there is a role for radiotherapy.

Should a patient be observed after removal of all macroscopic unifocal disease?

Observation alone is a reasonable treatment option in selected patients with recurrent ovarian cancer (see Chapter 15). It is, however, probably not appropriate in the case discussed here, in view of her young age, localized disease amenable to

surgery, and limited exposure to chemotherapy. While few would argue against observation in those patients who are asymptomatic with slowly rising CA125 levels and no clinical or radiographic evidence of recurrence, we have also opted for this approach in selected patients following surgical excision of solitary metastases. These are usually patients who have had a lot of prior chemotherapy or have relatively indolent tumours and have a localized solitary metastasis such as a splenic metastasis amenable to surgery.

CASE HISTORY 2

A 64-year-old female presented with an acute abdomen. At laparotomy, she was found to have bilateral ovarian tumours, and underwent a total abdominal hysterectomy, bilateral salpingo-oophorectomy, and omentectomy at a community hospital. The pathology revealed a stage IC, grade 3 bilateral serous cystadenocarcinoma. She was referred to our unit, but refused a staging laparotomy. She underwent four cycles of adjuvant cisplatin and cyclophosphamide according to our protocol at the time. On routine follow-up two years later, a right pelvic mass was noted, despite a normal CA125 titre. Pelvic ultrasonography revealed a 5 cm complex cystic mass in the right fornix. At laparotomy she had a 6 cm × 6 cm right pelvic sidewall mass, which was resected, and a right pelvic lymphadenectomy was performed. At the end of the operation, there was no evidence of residual macroscopic disease. The pathology revealed a poorly differentiated serous carcinoma with associated residual normal ovarian tissue, and there were no lymph node metastases.

What is the origin of an apparent ovarian cancer in a patient previously thought to have had a bilateral salpingo-oophorectomy?

This patient presents with an interesting problem. She has had a previous bilateral salpingo-oophorectomy for stage IC cystadeno-carcinoma of the ovary, yet two years later re-presents with a right pelvic sidewall mass that proves to be an epithelial ovarian cancer in an ovarian remnant.

The literature describes two differing possibil-ities for persistent ovarian tissue after bilateral oophorectomies.

1. *Supernumerary ovaries* – where there is extra ovarian tissue that has developed during embryogenesis and is not removed during surgery. This is obviously a rare occurrence.
2. *Ovarian remnant* – where there has been inad-vertent incomplete excision of one or both ovaries during a bilateral oophorectomy. This usually occurs when there are a lot of adhe-sions, making simple clamping of the infundibulo-pelvic ligaments difficult, but basically reflects poor surgical technique. An ovarian remnant typically occurs when mul-tiple operations have occurred to remove the uterus, fallopian tubes, and ovaries, such as in a patient with endometriosis where attempts are made to preserve the reproductive capabil-ity of the woman. Theoretically, re-implantation of small amounts of ovarian tissue at the time of surgery could occur, as was shown by the experiments of Shemwell and Weed.[28]

The concept of ovarian remnants has been known since the late 1950s. Ovarian remnant syndrome has been well documented in the liter-ature. It is a clinical condition of pelvic pain occurring in the setting of previous ovarian abla-tion due to functional ovarian remnant tissue undergoing cystic changes, with or without haemorrhage. Much of the literature relates to benign conditions, but there are several case reports of patients developing typical epithelial ovarian cancers in an ovarian remnant.[29–31] This problem may well assume greater import-ance, since laparoscopic bilateral salpingo-oophorectomy is being more commonly used as an adjuvant therapy for premenopausal women with early breast cancer. The problem may also apply to carriers of *BRCA1* and *BRCA2* gene mutations undergoing prophylactic bilateral oophorectomy. Despite undergoing an apparent bilateral oophorectomy, approximately 10% develop ovarian cancer at a later date. This may be attributable to the 'field effect', but another possibility is incomplete removal of all of the ovarian tissue. What role this latter hypothesis has in these women is not known.

SUMMARY

A pelvic mass in a patient previously treated for ovarian cancer may represent recurrent cancer (field effect). The decision as to whether or not to attempt secondary cytoreduction depends on the treatment-free interval and the appearance of the mass on imaging studies. In general, those patients with an apparently isolated mass are good candidates for secondary surgical resection. Most of these patients will be candidates for additional treatment, and such therapy will depend on the success of the surgical procedure, the treatment-free interval, and whether or not the recurrent or new disease was confined to the pelvis.

LEARNING POINTS

❋ It is important to stage patients appropriately with early-stage ovarian cancer.
❋ A patient who has undergone bilateral salpingo-oophorectomy (for ovarian cancer or benign disease) who presents with a pelvic mass should be considered for surgical explo-ration.
❋ It is possible that the recurrence after a long disease-free interval is actually a new primary

Table 14.1   Treatment options in recurrent ovarian cancer
Surgery
Secondary debulking
Palliative (e.g. for bowel obstruction)
Chemotherapy
Reintroduction of platinum
Paclitaxel
Topetecan
Gemcitabine
Oral etoposide
Liposomal doxorubicin
Vinorelbine
Hormonal therapy
Tamoxifen
LHRH agonists
Radiotherapy
Observation

tumour due to 'field cancerization', although the true significance of this is not yet established.

❋ Secondary cytoreductive surgery is indicated for recurrent ovarian cancer when the disease-free interval is at least 12 months and the recurrence appears amenable to complete resection. These are the two independent prognostic variables associated with a better overall and relapse-free survival.

❋ Patients with recurrent ovarian cancer should usually be offered chemotherapy. The choice of treatment depends on several factors, in particular the (platinum) treatment-free interval. If this is greater than six months, the probability of a response to single-agent carboplatin is quite high. Other agents may be active, but there is little evidence to suggest

that combination chemotherapy, which has a higher incidence of side-effects, is superior to single active agents.

❋ Whole-abdominal or pelvic radiotherapy may have a role in the small group of patients who have no residual tumour, or only small-volume localized disease, after surgery.

❋ Table 14.1 summarizes treatment options in recurrent ovarian cancer.

REFERENCES

1. McGowan L, Patterns of care in carcinoma of the ovary. *Cancer* 1994; 71(Suppl 2): 628–33.
2. Munoz KA, Harlan LC, Trimble EL, Patterns of care for women with ovarian cancer in the United States. *J Clin Oncol* 1997; **15**: 3408–15.
3. Young RC, Decker DG, Wharton JT et al, Staging laparotomy in early ovarian cancer. *JAMA* 1983; **250**: 3072–6.
4. Zanetta G, Rota S, Chiari S et al, The accuracy of staging: an important prognostic determinator in stage I ovarian carcinoma. A multivariate analysis. *Ann Oncol* 1998; **9**: 1097–101.
5. Perry MC (ed), *The Chemotherapy Source Book*, 2nd edn. Baltimore: Williams & Wilkins, 1997.
6. Buller RE, Skilling JS, Sood AK et al, Field cancerization: why late 'recurrent' ovarian cancer is not recurrent. *Am J Obstet Gynecol* 1998; **178**: 641–9.
7. Berek JS, Hacker NF, Lagasse LD, Nieberg RK, Alashoff RM, Survival of patients following secondary cytoreductive surgery in ovarian cancer. *Obstet Gynecol* 1983; **61**: 189–93.
8. Janicke F, Holsher M, Kuhn W et al, Radical surgical procedure improves survival time in patients with recurrent ovarian cancer. *Cancer* 1992; **70**: 2129–36.
9. Vaccarello L, Rubin SC, Vlamis V et al, Cytoreductive surgery in ovarian carcinoma patients with a documented previously complete surgical response. *Gynecol Oncol* 1995; **57**: 61–5.

10. Eisenkop SM, Friedman RL, Wang H, Secondary cytoreductive surgery for recurrent ovarian cancer. A prospective study. *Cancer* 1995; **76**: 1606–14.

11. McGuire WP, Hoskins WJ, Brady MF et al, Cyclophosphamide and cisplatin compared with paclitaxel and cisplatin in patients with stage III and stage IV ovarian cancer. *N Engl J Med* 1996; **334**: 1.

12. Gore ME, Fryatt I, Wiltshaw E et al, Treatment of relapsed carcinoma of the ovary with cisplatin or carboplatin following initial treatment with these compounds. *Gynecol Oncol* 1990; **36**: 207–11.

13. Markman M, Hoskins PJ, Response to salvage chemotherapy in ovarian cancer: a critical need for precise definitions of the treated population. *J Clin Oncol* 1992; **10**: 413–14.

14. Bolis G, Parazzini F, Scarfone G et al, Paclitaxel vs. epidoxorubicin plus paclitaxel as second line therapy for platinum-refractory and -resistant ovarian cancer. *Gynecol Oncol* 1999; **72**: 60–4.

15. Eisenhauer EA, ten Bokkel Huinink WW, Swenerton KD et al, European–Canadian randomised trial of paclitaxel in relapsed ovarian cancer: high dose versus low dose and long versus short infusion. *J Clin Oncol* 1994; **12**: 2654–66.

16. Phillips KA, Friedlander MF, Olver F et al. Australasian multicentre phase II study of paclitaxel (Taxol) in relapsed ovarian cancer. *Aust NZ Med* 1995; **25**: 337–43.

17. ten Bokkel Huinink W, Gore M, Carmichael J et al, Topetecan versus paclitaxel for the treatment of recurrent epithelial ovarian cancer. *J Clin Oncol* 1997; **15**: 2183–93.

18. Rose PG, Blessing JA, Mayer AR et al, Prolonged oral etoposide as second line therapy for platinum resistant (PLATR) and platinum sensitive (PLATS) ovarian carcinoma: a Gynecologic Oncology Group study. *Proc Am Soc Clin Oncol* 1996; **15**: 282.

19. Ozols RF, Treatment of recurrent ovarian cancer: increasing options – 'recurrent' results. *J Clin Oncol* 1997; **15**: 2177–80.

20. Eisenhauer EA, Vermorken JB, Van Glabbeke M, Predictors of response to subsequent chemotherapy in platinum pretreated ovarian cancer: a multivariate analysis of 704 patients. *Ann Oncol* 1997; **8**: 963–8.

21. Hoskins P, Tu D, James K et al, Factors predictive of survival after first relapse or progression in advanced epithelial ovarian carcinoma: a prediction tree analysis-derived model with test and validation groups. *Gynecol Oncol* 1998; **70**: 224–30.

22. Hatch KD, Beecham JB, Blessing JA, Creasman WT, Responsiveness of patients with advanced ovarian carcinoma to tamoxifen. *Cancer* 1991; **68**: 269–71.

23. van der Velden J, Gitsch G, Wain GV et al, Tamoxifen in patients with advanced epithelial ovarian cancer. *Int J Gynecol Cancer* 1995; **5**: 301–5.

24. Weiser EB, Burke TW, Heller PB et al, Determinants of survival of patients with epithelial ovarian carcinoma following whole abdominal irradiation (WAR). *Gynecol Oncol* 1988; **30**: 201–8.

25. Fuller DB, Sause WT, Plenk HP, Menlove RL, Analysis of postoperative radiation therapy in stage I through III epithelial ovarian carcinoma. *J Clin Oncol* 1987; **5**: 897–905.

26. Carey M, Dembo AJ, Fyles AW, Simm J, Testing the validity of a prognostic classification in patients with surgically optimal ovarian carcinoma: a 15-year review. *Int J Gynecol Cancer* 1993; **3**: 24–35.

27. Dembo AJ, Bush RS, Current concepts in cancer: ovary – treatment of stages III and IV. Choice of postoperative therapy based on prognostic factors. *Int J Radiat Oncol Biol Phys* 1982; **8**: 893–7.

28. Shemwell RE, Weed JC, Ovarian remnant syndrome. *Obstet Gynecol* 1970; **36**: 299–303.

29. Hamid R, May D, Ovarian malignancy in remnant ovarian tissue. *Int J Gynecol Obstet* 1997; **58**: 319–20.

30. Weber AM, Hewitt WJ, Gajewski WH, Curry

SL, Serous carcinoma of the peritoneum after oophorectomy. *Obstet Gynecol* 1992; **80**: 558–60.

31. Bruhwiler H, Luscher KP, Ovarialkarzinom bei ovarian remnant syndrome. *Geburtshilfe und Frauenheilkunde* 1991; **51**: 70–1.

15

Symptomless rise in CA125

Maria EL van der Burg

INTRODUCTION

Elevation of CA125 is found in more than 90% of patients with relapsed ovarian cancer. A rising CA125 during follow-up is thought to be the first indication of relapse in about 70% of patients. A rise in serum CA125 may predate clinical relapse by several months. Knowledge that the CA125 is rising in a patient who is well creates a clinical dilemma and anxiety for the patient. At what point is the patient deemed to have relapsed? Should investigations be performed once the CA125 has risen, or should chemotherapy be instituted on the basis of an abnormal CA125 alone?

The case presented in this chapter illustrates a common problem facing clinicians following patients with ovarian cancer. As chemotherapy at relapse is not curative, it is important to examine the reasons for or against the early institution of treatment. The possibility of prolonging the symptom-free period, or even survival, has to be balanced against the toxic effects of chemotherapy in a patient who is well. As different policies are being pursued by clinicians, there is a need to examine the value of CA125 follow-up and timing of treatment in randomized controlled trials.

CASE HISTORY

An epithelial ovarian carcinoma, FIGO stage IIIC, was diagnosed in a 40-year-old woman in February 1997. A bilateral oophorectomy, hysterectomy, omentectomy and tumour debulking were performed. After debulking surgery, residual lesions of less than 2 cm remained. The preoperative serum CA125 level was 12 245 U/ml, falling postoperatively to 2472 U/ml prior to chemotherapy. The patient was treated with six cycles of weekly paclitaxel (Taxol) and cisplatin induction chemotherapy, followed by five cycles of three-weekly paclitaxel and cisplatin. During chemotherapy, the serum CA125 decreased, and became normal (<30 U/ml) by July 1997. Physical, general and pelvic examination, transvaginal ultrasonography, and a computed tomography (CT) scan confirmed a clinically complete remission. In September 1997, at the end of treatment, the patient was still in complete remission. The follow-up protocol was explained to the patient and her husband. At each visit, a physical and pelvic examination, and transvaginal ultrasound would be performed, and the serum CA125 values would be measured. We agreed that the serum CA125 values would not be discussed, to prevent unnecessary anxiety due to small, insignificant, rises in serum CA125. If, however, the serum

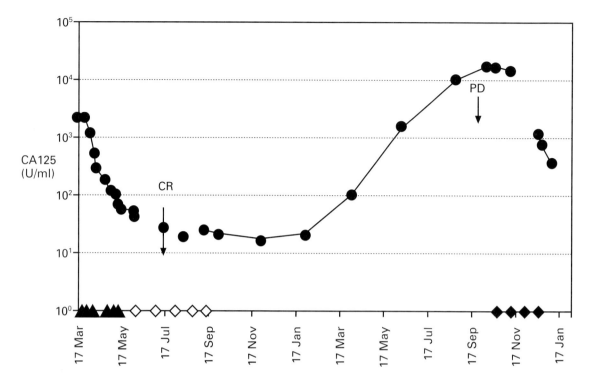

Figure 15.1

The course of serum CA125 during treatment and follow-up in a patient with advanced-stage ovarian cancer: —●—, CA125; ▲, weekly paclitaxel–cisplatin; ◇, three-weekly paclitaxel–cisplatin; ◆, three-weekly paclitaxel–carboplatin; CR, complete remission; PD, progressive disease.

CA125 level increased significantly, action would be taken to detect an early recurrence. Both agreed with this policy.

From September 1997, the patient was monitored every two months. In April 1998, the serum CA125 level rose to 114 U/ml; the value two months earlier had been 22 U/ml. At the time of the increase in CA125, the patient had no symptoms, and physical and pelvic examination and transvaginal ultrasonography were normal. The course of disease and serum CA125 is shown in Figure 15.1.

The increase in CA125 from 22 to 114 U/ml was significant. A tumour recurrence had occurred as defined by a number of different criteria that have been reported in the literature.[1–6] If a second sample confirms the increase in CA125, the likelihood that this is due to recurrent disease is greater than 98%.

The options for management of this patient who had no sign of disease were as follows:

1 Ignore the serum increase in CA125 and wait until symptoms developed or there were clinical signs of recurrent disease.
2 Perform more extensive investigations, such as CT scan or laparoscopy, to demonstrate recurrent disease and then start chemotherapy if the recurrence was confirmed.

3 Initiate chemotherapy just on the basis of the increased CA125.

It was decided not to take immediate action, but to wait till the next outpatient visit in June, at which time the serum CA125 and clinical examinations would be repeated. At this visit, the serum CA125 value had increased to 1690 U/ml. The patient still had no signs or symptoms of recurrence. The physical and pelvic examination and transvaginal ultrasonography were normal. A spiral CT scan was performed, which did not show any sign of recurrent disease. The patient had no evidence of a benign disease that could explain the rise in CA125.[6,7] The results were discussed with the patient and her husband. The uncertainty about the best management and the benefit of initiating chemotherapy based only on an increased CA125 were outlined. Because of the lack of any clinical signs or symptoms of recurrent disease, the patient and her husband decided not to start treatment but to wait until she became symptomatic. She and her family went on summer holidays, and had a wonderful time together.

At the beginning of October 1998, she complained of some abdominal discomfort. The physical and pelvic examinations were normal, but now the transvaginal ultrasonography and CT scan showed a small amount of intraperitoneal fluid. The cytology was positive for ovarian tumour cells. By this time, the serum CA125 had increased to 17 913 U/ml, although only a small amount of ascites and some small peritoneal lesions were observed on the CT scan. The therapy-free interval had now been more than one year. The chance to respond to platinum and paclitaxel combination therapy was high. The patient had two small children at home. She therefore preferred outpatient therapy. In October, treatment with three-weekly paclitaxel and carboplatin was started. After the second cycle, all her symptoms had disappeared. After the third cycle, the clinical examination,

transvaginal ultrasonography and CT scan were normal. The serum CA125 level had decreased to 897 U/ml. Treatment was continued, and after the fifth cycle, serum CA125 fell to 50 U/ml.

How should a patient with an asymptomatic rise in serum CA125 be managed?

This is a case of the everyday practice of a physician treating ovarian cancer patients. The knowledge that the patient has a rising CA125 level and yet remains clinically very well without any evidence of disease presents a major management dilemma in the follow-up of ovarian cancer patients.[8,9] In each case where the CA125 rises in a patient with no evidence of disease, there is the dilemma of what to do. Should the patient be called to the outpatient clinic for extra clinical examinations? Should she be informed that her CA125 is rising, which will cause strong emotional pressure for her and her family? What additional examinations should be done when the physical and pelvic examination and transvaginal ultrasonography are normal? Should treatment be started just on the basis of an increased CA125, and is this of therapeutic benefit to the patient?

Ovarian cancer is a chemosensitive tumour. Although most patients respond to first-line chemotherapy, the majority will eventually experience a recurrence.[10–12] A recurrence, like the primary tumour, often lacks specific signs and symptoms. It is therefore difficult to detect recurrence at an early stage. At the time of clinical signs or symptoms, the tumour is often large, widespread and difficult to treat.

Conventional examinations in the follow-up

In a retrospective study, the value of the different conventional examinations to detect progressive disease was investigated.[13] In this study, a positive pelvic examination was found in 67% of patients with progressive disease, the physical

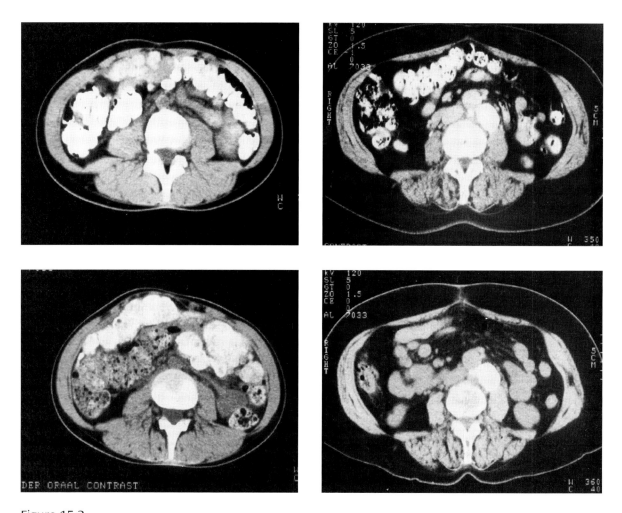

Figure 15.2
CT scans of two patients with recurrent ovarian cancer. The recurrences, intraabdominal and in the para-aortic lymph nodes, were initially missed on the CT scans with contrast because of the calcifications in the tumour due to psammoma bodies (top scans). On the CT scans (bottom) without contrast, the calcified tumours are well presented.

examination and CT scan were positive in 30% each, and surgery was positive in 14%. The CT scan is the best examination to detect metastases in the liver, spleen and para-aortic lymph nodes. Small lesions in the mesentery and omentum and on the diaphragm, liver surface and pelvic peritoneum are frequently missed.[14–16] Also, tumours with calcifications are often difficult to detect with CT scans when contrast is used (Figure 15.2). The false-positive rate of the conventional examinations in patients with no evidence of disease was 2% for pelvic examination, 4% for physical examination and 14% for CT scan. The CT scan was most likely to give false-positive results for mesenteric, omental and nodal involvement.[15]

Serum marker CA125

The serum marker CA125 is a reliable tumour marker to monitor the response to treatment in ovarian cancer and to detect early progression. In more than 90% of the patients with advanced epithelial ovarian carcinoma, CA125 is increased (>35 U/ml).[6,7,17] During treatment and follow-up, a rising CA125 level is, in the majority of patients, the first indication of relapse.[1,3] A retrospective study has shown that when CA125 was used in combination with conventional examinations, progressive disease was diagnosed in 73% of patients by serum CA125 alone and in 92% by combined use of CA125 and pelvic and physical examination.[13]

However, the serum CA125 antigen is not specific for ovarian cancer. Increased serum CA125 levels are observed in patients with malignancies of the breast or gastrointestinal tract and in other gynaecological tumours. Increased serum CA125 levels are also found in patients with benign diseases of the liver, gastrointestinal tract, pleura and peritoneum, and with non-malignant ascites or pleural effusions.[6,7,18,19]

Despite this lack of specificity, serum CA125 has been shown to be a reliable marker for the early detection of recurrent disease in ovarian cancer. A great number of retrospective studies have reported on the excellent correlation between the course of CA125 levels and progression in the follow-up of ovarian cancer patients.[4,6,7,13,20,21] Only 2% of the serum CA125 samples taken during follow-up of patients with no evidence of disease rose above the upper limit of normal (35 U/ml).[4,13] A persistently rising CA125 level was always associated with recurrent disease, except in rare cases of benign ascites or pleural fluid or other benign diseases.[13] CA125 frequently rose several months before the clinical evidence of recurrence. The median lead-time of the rise of CA125 and recurrence was 4.5 months, with a range of 1 month to 2.5 years.

Two prospective follow-up studies confirmed the positive predictive value of CA125 in diagnosing recurrence.[2,22] In a large prospective longitudinal study, 311 patients with no evidence of disease were monitored by serial CA125 measurement. In 176 patients with recurrent disease, an increase in serum CA125 preceded the recurrence, and of 126 patients with no evidence of disease, only 6 had increased CA125 values. One of these patients had a benign serous cystadenoma and 4 others had elevated human antimurine antibodies (HAMA) due to prior immunoscintigraphy.

Hoberg and Kagedal[2] followed 33 patients by means of standard conventional examinations and monthly serum CA125. Patients with a serum CA125 above 40 U/ml were asked to come for a pelvic examination under anaesthesia. If an abnormality was found, a fine-needle puncture was performed. If the examination was normal, a CT scan and finally a laparoscopy or laparotomy were performed. A symptomless rise in CA125 was observed in 19 cases. A recurrence was diagnosed by pelvic examination under anaesthesia in 7 patients, and by CT scan and surgery in 6 patients each. During the follow-up period, of the 649 samples from the patients with no evidence of disease, 6 samples (0.9%), from four patients, rose incidentally just above 35 U/ml.

These two prospective studies have established that all symptomless increases in CA125 above 40 U/ml, confirmed by a second sample, correlated with recurrent disease. These data are consistent with the data found at a second-look operation. All patients in clinically complete remission but with increased CA125 prior to second-look surgery had residual tumour at surgery or developed a recurrence shortly after surgery.

Conclusion

Based on these data, we may conclude that an increase in CA125 in patients with no evidence of disease does correlate with a recurrence if the increase is established with a second sample and a benign cause of the increase can be excluded. In these patients, invasive diagnostic examinations to confirm the recurrence are no longer obligatory.

What level of serum CA125 defines a recurrence?

There is not yet an agreed definition for recurrence. The different criteria for recurrence used are:

1. An increase of CA125 above the upper limit of normal;[5,13]
2. A doubling of the CA125 value above the normal range;[17]
3. An increase in CA125 above 65 U/ml or 100 U/ml;[3–5]
4. An increase in CA125 above two times the normal cut-off level.[4]

For all criteria, the serum CA125 increases should be confirmed by a second serum sample to exclude sampling error, and benign diseases or other malignancies that could be responsible for a CA125 increase should be excluded.

The false-positive rate is comparable for all the different criteria. The explanation for this might be that when a recurrence occurs, the rise in CA125 is usually substantial: the mean CA125 increase in patients with a recurrence is 75 U/ml/month, in contrast to 4 U/ml/month in patients with no evidence of disease.[22]

What are the chemotherapeutic options at relapse?

Salvage therapy in patients with recurrent ovarian cancer is based on whether the patient is platinum-resistant or platinum-sensitive.[23–26] As a general guide, patients with a recurrence within six months of the last first-line platinum administration are considered resistant to platinum-based drugs. This early recurrence reflects either an intrinsic or an acquired resistance. In these patients, the response to platinum-containing therapy as well as to different new drugs such as paclitaxel, topotecan, etoposide, liposomal doxorubicin or gemcitabine is low and varies between 9% and 20%, with a median time to progression of about four months.[27–30] For a more detailed description, see Chapter 12. It is possible that platinum resistance is a relative phenomenon and might be overcome with an increase in platinum dose density. In studies with weekly cisplatin, the response rate increases to 56%.[31–33]

Patients with a platinum-free interval of more than six months are likely to respond again to platinum-based therapy. The response rate in these patients is strongly related to the platinum-free interval, varying from 33% to 98%, and there is a median response duration of 15 months[23–25,31,32] (see Chapter 11). There are also data that in these good-prognosis patients, survival might be increased by salvage debulking surgery.[34]

Should patients with an asymptomatic rise in serum CA125 be treated?

No curative salvage therapy is available for recurrent ovarian cancer. It therefore remains questionable whether patients with an asymptomatic rise in CA125 should be treated at the first indication of recurrent disease or whether it is appropriate to delay treatment until the patient has clinical signs or symptoms.

Theoretically, chemotherapy is most effective in patients with the smallest tumour burden. In a large study of second-line therapies, Eisenhauer et al[35] demonstrated that in patients with recurrent disease, the performance status, history, tumour size and number of tumour lesions were independent prognostic factors for response to therapy, and progression-free and overall survival. These data argue in favour of early treatment with chemotherapy, although a bias, based on unavoidable selection, cannot be excluded. Serum CA125 can detect subclinical recurrent disease. Therefore, if effective therapy is available, the asymptomatic rise in CA125 should be the best moment to start therapy. Hoberg and Kagedal[2] followed patients with no evidence of disease prospectively with CA125, and started treatment in patients with subclinical disease. In this group of patients, the five-year survival rate was 73%. It is possible that the early detection of the recurrence by CA125 contributed to these good results of second-line therapy, but selection bias cannot be excluded.

Although the median time from a rise in CA125 to clinically detectable tumour is four months, some patients will remain without signs or symptoms for more than two years. Riedinger et al[36] investigated the relation between tumour growth rate and CA125 doubling-time during follow-up of non-treated patients. The median doubling-time of CA125 was 64 days, with a range of 5–375 days. In a multivariate analysis with early clinical, histological, biological and therapeutic parameters of the primary tumour, the CA125 doubling-time was the major predictive parameter for the lead-time between CA125 rise and clinical and/or radiological signs of recurrence. More importantly, the CA125 doubling-time was the most important prognostic factor for survival. The survival for patients with a doubling-time of less than 120 days was a median of 14 months, in contrast to 40 months ($p = 0.001$) in patients with doubling-time greater than 120 days. Moreover, about 40% of the patients with a long CA125 doubling-time were still alive after five years, while all patients with a short doubling-time died within three years. If these data can be confirmed, the CA125 doubling-time might become an important selection criterion for early or delayed treatment of recurrent disease or for the selection of the type of treatment regimen.

A platinum-free interval of more or less than six months is an important selection criterion for therapy sensitivity or resistance. If treatment is started on the basis of a rise in CA125 alone, it should be remembered that the median lead-time of the CA125 rise and the clinical recurrence is 4.5 months. Consequently, the dividing line for therapy sensitivity, which is currently six months, might have to be reduced to three months.

The optimum duration of treatment and method of evaluating response of subclinical disease is unknown. Should a standard number of cycles (e.g. six cycles) be given, or should treatment be continued with three cycles after the normalization of CA125? It should, however, be remembered that although there is a good correlation between the course of CA125 and the response to platinum-based treatment, discrepancies have been observed between the clinical response and the course of CA125 in patients treated with second-line paclitaxel monotherapy. Several patients with progressive disease had a significant fall in CA125, and other patients with a response showed a significant rise in CA125 (Figure 15.3).[37,38]

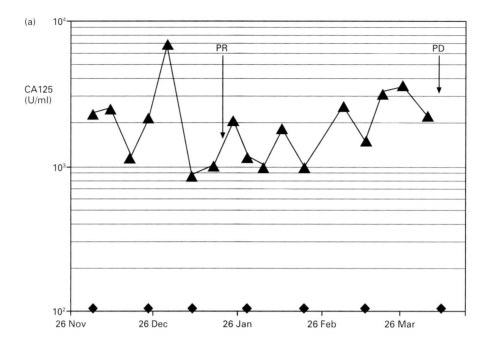

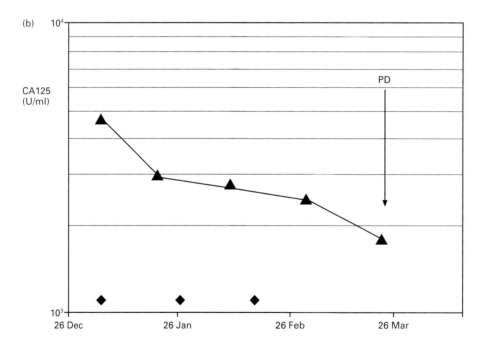

Figure 15.3

(a) Discrepancy between the course of CA125 and the clinical response in a patient with a partial response (PR) to paclitaxel monotherapy. (b) Discrepancy between the course of CA125 and the clinical response in a patient with progressive disease (PD) under paclitaxel monotherapy. ▲, CA125; ◆, paclitaxel.

What is current policy?

At present, there is no evidence that either searching for the site of relapse or early treatment by surgery or chemotherapy is of any survival benefit. The contrary has not been proven either! Therefore both approaches – the 'active' and 'passive' – can be justified for the individual patient. In decision-making, the psychological pressure of the knowledge of a recurrence, the loss of a therapy-free period and the toxicity of the therapy must be considered and balanced against the potential increase in symptom-free and overall survival and the quality of life with and without treatment.

Currently, there are several policies being pursued in the follow-up of ovarian cancer patients. Many clinicians measure serum CA125, and start salvage therapy only when recurrent disease is clinically detected or ignore a rising level unless the patient has symptoms. Others just reintroduce chemotherapy based on an increase in CA125 alone. Only a minority of the clinicians do not measure CA125 at all.

In an international consensus workshop in 1993, and at the consensus meeting of the Gynecologic Oncology Group (GOG) in the USA in 1994, it was concluded that CA125 is the only marker that should be applied routinely in the clinical setting for monitoring tumour response. No consensus could be reached about early treatment based only on an increase in serum CA125.[8,9] At an international consensus workshop in 1998, five years later, the only consensus reached was that the benefit of the measurement of CA125 and early treatment based on a CA125 rise should be investigated in a prospective randomized study.[39]

Recently a large Intergroup study of the UK Medical Research Council (MRC) and the Gynecological Cancer Cooperative Group of the European Organization for Research and Treatment of Cancer (EORTC)/GCCG has commenced to investigate the therapeutic benefit of the monitoring with serum CA125 on survival and quality of life of patients with no evidence of disease (Figure 15.4).

In this study, patients in clinical complete remission and with a normal serum CA125 after first-line platinum-based chemotherapy are registered at the data centre. The patients are monitored according to the standard policy with conventional examinations and serum CA125.

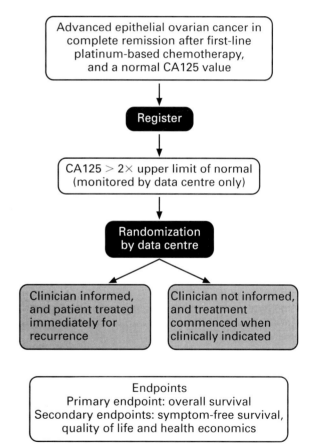

Figure 15.4
A randomized trial in relapsed ovarian cancer: early treatment based on CA125 level alone versus delayed treatment based on conventional clinical indicators. An Intergroup study: EORTC/GCCG 55955 and MRC OV05.

The value of the serum CA125, however, is blinded from the treating physician and is sent for monitoring to the data centre. If there is an increase in CA125, the patient is randomized between the clinician being informed and immediate treatment with chemotherapy versus the clinician not being informed and delayed treatment. The endpoints of the study are overall survival, symptom-free interval, quality of life and health economics.

This very important study will finally determine the value of the follow-up controls and of the early treatment of patients with a complete remission.

LEARNING POINTS

❋ Serum CA125 is a reliable marker in the follow-up of patients with no evidence of disease after first-line chemotherapy. It detects subclinical disease in 98% of recurrences. The lead-time between rise in CA125 and clinical signs or symptoms is a median of 4.5 months (range 0.5–29.5 months).

❋ A CT scan and surgery are of little additional value in the detection of recurrent disease.

❋ Although more effective second-line therapy is available, cure and long-term responses remain rare. Nor is there any evidence that early treatment with more effective therapy, based on a rise in CA125, increases symptom-free and overall survival or the quality of life. However, the contrary has not been demonstrated either.

❋ Only a prospective randomized study will answer the question of whether intensive monitoring with serum CA125 and early treatment of recurrences is superior to treatment based on clinical signs and symptoms in regard to symptom-free survival, overall survival and quality of life.

REFERENCES

1. Van der Burg MEL, Lammes FB, Verweij J, The role of CA 125 in the early diagnosis of progressive disease in ovarian cancer. *Ann Oncol* 1990; **1**: 301–2.
2. Höberg T, Kågedal B, Long-term follow-up of ovarian cancer with monthly determinations of serum CA 125. *Gynecol Oncol* 1992; **46**: 191–8.
3. Rustin GJS, Van der Burg MEL, Berek JS, Tumour markers. *Ann Oncol* 1993; 4(Suppl 4): 71–7.
4. Koelbl H, Schieder K, Neunteufel W, Bieglmayer C, CA 125 in the follow-up of patients with ovarian cancer. *Eur J Gynecol Reprod Biol* 1988; **27**: 335–42.
5. Van der Burg MEL, Lammes FB, Verweij J, Review: CA 125 in ovarian cancer. *Netherlands J Med* 1992; **40**: 36–51.
6. Jacobs I, Bast RC, Clinical review. The CA 125 tumour-associated antigen: a review of the literature. *Hum Reprod* 1989; **4**: 1–12.
7. Markman M, Follow-up of the asymptomatic patient with ovarian cancer. *Gynecol Oncol* 1994; **55**: 134–7.
8. Allen DG, Baak J, Belpomme D et al, Advanced epithelial ovarian cancer. *Ann Oncol* 1993; 4(Suppl 4): 583–8.
9. Neijt JP, ten Bokkel Huinink WW, van der Burg MEL et al, Long-term survival in ovarian cancer. *Eur J Cancer* 1991; **27**: 1367–72.
10. Rubin SC, Hoskin WJ, Saigo PE et al, Recurrence after negative second-look laparotomy for ovarian cancer: analyses of risk factors. *Am J Obstet Gynecol* 1988; **159**: 1094–8.
11. Rubin SC, Randall TC, Armstrong KA et al, Ten-year follow-up of ovarian cancer patients after second-look laparotomy with negative findings. *Obstet Gynecol* 1999; **93**: 21–4.
12. Van der Burg MEL, Lammes FB, Verweij J, The role of CA 125 and conventional examinations in diagnosing progressive carcinoma of the ovary. *Surg Gynecol Obstet* 1993; **176**: 310–14.

13. Duk LM, Kauer FM, Fleuren GJ, de Bruijn HW, Serum CA 125 levels in patients with a provisional diagnosis of pelvic inflammatory disease. Clinical and theoretical implications. *Acta Obstet Gynecol Scand* 1989; **68**: 637–41.

14. Kimura K, Ezoe K, Yokozeki H et al, Elevated serum CA 125 in progressive systemic sclerosis with pleural effusion. *J Dermatol* 1995; **22**: 28–31.

15. Shiels RA, Peel KR, MacDonald HN et al, A prospective trial of computed tomography in the staging of ovarian malignancy. *Br J Obstet Gynaecol* 1985; **92**: 407–12.

16. Nelson BE, Rosenfield AT, Schwartz PE, Preoperative abdominopelvic computed tomographic prediction of optimal cytoreduction in epithelial ovarian carcinoma. *J Clin Oncol* 1993; **11**: 166–72.

17. Razzaq R, Carrington BM, Hulse PA, Kitchener HC, Abdominopelvic CT scan findings after surgery for ovarian cancer. *Clin Radiol* 1998; **53**: 820–4.

18. Bast RC, Klug TL, John ES et al, A radioimmunoassay using a monoclonal antibody to monitor the course of epithelial ovarian cancer. *N Engl J Med* 1983; **309**: 883–7.

19. Rustin GJS, Nestrop AE, Tuxen MK, Lambert HE, Defining progression of ovarian cancer during follow-up according to CA 125: a North Thames Ovary Group study. *Ann Oncol* 1996; **7**: 361–4.

20. Niloff JM, Knapp RC, Lavin PT et al, The CA 125 assay as a predictor of clinical recurrence in epithelial cancer. *Am J Obstet Gynecol* 1986; **155**: 55–60.

21. Meier W, Stieber P, Fateh-Moghadam A et al, CA 125 in gynecological malignancies. *Eur J Cancer* 1987; **23**: 713–17.

22. Meier W, Baumgartner L, Stieber P et al, CA 125 based diagnosis and therapy in recurrent ovarian cancer. *Anticancer Res* 1997; **17**: 3019–20.

23. Blackledge G, Lawton R, Redman E et al, Response of patients in phase II studies of chemotherapy in ovarian cancer: implications for patient treatment and the design of phase II trials. *BMJ* 1989; **59**: 650–3.

24. Markman M, Rothman R, Hakes T et al, Second-line platinum therapy in patients with ovarian cancer previously treated with cisplatin. *J Clin Oncol* 1991; **9**: 389–93.

25. Chauvergne J, Chinet-Charrot P, Stockle E et al, Carboplatin and etoposide combination for treatment of recurrent epithelial ovarian cancer. *Bull Cancer* 1996; **83**: 315–23.

26. Trimble EL, Salvage chemotherapy for epithelial ovarian cancer. *Gynecol Oncol* 1994; **55**: 143–50.

27. Eisenhauer EA, ten Bokkel Huinink WW, Swenerton KD et al, European–Canadian randomised trial of paclitaxel in relapsed ovarian cancer: high dose versus low dose and long versus short infusion. *J Clin Oncol* 1994; **12**: 2654–66.

28. ten Bokkel Huinink WW, Gore M, Carmichael J et al, Topotecan versus paclitaxel for the treatment of recurrent epithelial ovarian cancer. *J Clin Oncol* 1997; **15**: 2183–93.

29. Muggia FM, Hainsworth JD, Jeffers S et al, Phase II study of liposomal doxorubicin in refractory ovarian cancer: antitumor activity and toxicity modification by liposomal encapsulation. *J Clin Oncol* 1997; **15**: 987–93.

30. Lund B, Hansen OP, Theilade K et al, Phase II study of gemcitabine (2',2'-difuorodeoxycytidine) in previously treated ovarian cancer patients. *J Natl Cancer Inst* 1994; **86**: 1530–3.

31. Van der Burg MEL, Logmans A, de Wit R et al, Weekly high dose cisplatin and daily oral vepesid: a highly active salvage regimen for progressive or recurrent ovarian cancer after platinum therapy. *Eur J Cancer* 1997; **33**(Suppl 8): 118 (Abst 529).

32. Van der Burg MEL, de Wit R, Logmans A et al, Phase I study of weekly cisplatin and four weekly or weekly Taxol in patients with advanced epithelial ovarian cancer. *Eur J Cancer* 1997; **33**(Suppl 8); 245 (Abst 1108).

33. Zanaboni F, Scarfone G, Presti M et al, Salvage

chemotherapy for ovarian cancer; weekly cisplatin in combination with epirubicin or etoposide. *Gynecol Oncol* 1991; **43**: 24–7.

34. Kuhn W, Schmalfekdt B, Pache L et al, Disease-adapted relapse therapy for ovarian cancer: results of a prospective study. *Int J Oncol* 1998; **13**: 57–63.

35. Eisenhauer EA, Vermorken JB, van Glabecke M, Predictors of response to subsequent chemotherapy in platinum pretreated ovarian cancer: a multivariate analysis of 740 patients. *Ann Oncol* 1997; **8**: 963–8.

36. Riedinger JM, Coudert B, Buffenoir G et al, Intérêt clinique de l'estimation de la vitesse de croissance des récidives ovariennes premières par le temps de doublement du CA 125. *Bull Cancer* 1997; **84**: 855–60.

37. Van der Burg, Myles JD, Hoskin PJ et al, CA 125 is an unreliable marker for monitoring response to Taxol therapy in patients with relapsed ovarian cancer. In: *Seventh European Conference on Clinical Oncology and Cancer Nursing*, Jerusalem, 1993; S133 (Abstr 723).

38. Davelaar EM, Bonfer JMG, Verstraeten RA et al, Is CA 125 a valid marker in ovarian carcinoma patients treated with paclitaxel? *Cancer* 1996, **78**: 118–27.

39. Berek JS, Bertelsen K, Du Bois A et al, Advanced epithelial ovarian cancer: 1998 Consensus Statements. *Ann Oncol*, 1999; **10**: 587–92.

SECTION 4: Diagnostic Aspects in Ovarian Cancer

16

Interpretation of asymptomatic elevation of CA125

Hans-Gerd Meerpohl

CASE HISTORY

A 36-year-old woman was admitted because of fatigue, mild dyspnea and coughing of about two months' duration. On clinical examination, she had left pleural effusion. The serum CA125 level was elevated (150 U/ml). Combined vaginal and rectal examinations were negative. Radiologic and ultra-sonographic examinations revealed bilateral pleural effusions and ascites. No pelvic masses were identified by transvaginal sonography. Cytologic studies of pleural effusions and ascites were all negative. The pleural fluid was an exudate with high lymphocyte counts and elevated CA125 (450 U/ml). Tuberculous pleuritis was diagnosed, based on findings of sputum culture and of pleural biopsies. Antituberculous chemotherapy was started, and the patient responded well. Both pleural effusions and ascites decreased; the levels of CA125 also decreased to the normal range in about two months.

What is the significance of a raised CA125 in this setting?

In women with elevated serum CA125 (>65 U/ml) non-malignant conditions constitute approximately 10–15% of diagnoses. Non-cancerous conditions that can cause elevated CA125 serum levels include endometriosis, pelvic inflammatory disease, any condition that inflames the pleura, pancreatitis, peritonitis and liver diseases.

In asymptomatic premenopausal women, menstruation and pregnancy can cause increases in CA125 serum levels. Asymptomatic post-menopausal women with elevated CA125 serum levels are more likely to have a past history of breast cancer. These women are at increased risk to develop gynecologic cancer in the future.

Background

Since the discovery of the OC125 monoclonal antibody in 1983 by Bast et al,[1] substantial progress has been made in the understanding and the limitations of the CA125 assay.

CA125, first found to be elevated in more than 80% of epithelial ovarian carcinomas, is not elevated exclusively in the blood of these patients. CA125 levels can also be raised in sera from patients with other malignancies, such as metastatic breast cancer, and cancers of the uterus, cervix, pancreas, liver, colon, lung and digestive tract.[2–4] Non-cancerous conditions that can cause elevated CA125 serum levels include endometriosis, fibroids, pelvic inflammatory disease, any condition that inflames the pleura,

Table 16.1   Conditions other than ovarian cancer that can cause elevated CA125

Non-cancerous conditions
- Endometriosis
- Adenomyosis uteri
- Fibroids
- Pelvic inflammatory disease
- Peritonitis
- Inflammatory conditions of the pleura
- Chronic liver disease (e.g. cirrhosis)
- Peritoneal dialysis patients
- Ovarian hyperstimulation syndrome
- Benign ovarian cysts
- Pregnancy
- Menstrual cycle
- False-positive-unknown

Cancerous conditions
- Cervical carcinoma
- Endometrial carcinoma
- Metastatic breast cancer
- Gastrointestinal and peritoneal malignancies

pancreatitis, peritonitis, various liver diseases and renal failure (Table 16.1).

In healthy *premenopausal women*, elevation of CA125 serum levels predominantly occurs during pregnancy and during menstrual phases. During pregnancy, CA125 is found in maternal serum, in amniotic fluid and in placental tissues.[5] In women with regular menstrual cycles, fluctuations of serum CA125 levels have been observed throughout the cycle, with peak levels during menstrual phases.[6,7] In *postmenopausal* women, the reasons for elevated CA125 serum values (>65 U/ml) differ from those in premenopausal women. Postmenopausal patients show more often at the time of first elevated CA125 mea-

surement a history of antecedent breast cancer, a higher incidence of synchronous gynecologic and non-gynecologic cancer, and a lower incidence of benign conditions.[38]

Tissue distribution and CA125 expression

Tissue distribution and expression of CA125 have been extensively studied with immunohistochemical techniques based on the OC125 monoclonal antibody. A wide distribution of the antigen in cancerous tissues as well as in placental tissue, amnion, derivatives of the fetal müllerian duct, adult pleura and peritoneum has been demonstrated. Apart from being present in different tissues, CA125 is also present in pleural effusions, ascites and mucus of different origin.[9] Many factors influence the level of circulating CA125. In benign ovarian cysts, the basement membrane and the peritoneum are believed to be a natural border preventing CA125 access to the circulation.[10] This explains why in most (but not all) benign ovarian tumors, CA125 serum levels are within a normal range, despite high CA125 levels in benign ovarian cyst fluid.[11] Malignant tumor growth will disturb these natural borders, thus leading to increased CA125 serum levels. However, also in physiologic events, it seems likely that increased tissue production of CA125 coincides with a rise in serum CA125 only in such situations where changes of surface barriers simultaneously occur (e.g. decidua in the first trimester of pregnancy).

The CA125 antigen is also expressed in peritoneal tissue, particularly in areas of inflammation and adhesion.[12] Mesothelial cells are capable of producing CA125 in cell culture supernatant. As a result, CA125 levels correlate with the extent of peritoneal inflammation.[13]

The CA125 antigen

Data on the nature of the CA125 epitope are still contradictory. The OC125 monoclonal antibody reacts with an antigenic determinant (CA125) expressed on a high-molecular-weight glycoprotein complex composed of a protein and predominantly O-linked carbohydrate side-chains. The CA125 molecule is heterogeneous with regard to size and charge. Discrepancies in the biochemical properties of the CA125 glycoprotein complex may lie in different origins of the CA125 preparations as well as in different methods of isolation of these complexes. For the core CA125 subunit, molecular masses in excess of 200 kDa have been reported.[14,15] Smaller subunits are thought to result from breakdown or cleavage of the high-molecular-weight antigen complex. To characterize the various CA125 species, different sources have been used, including ovarian cancer cell cultures, supernatant serum and ascites fluid of ovarian cancer patients, human seminal plasma, human milk, and amniotic fluid. Further enlightment about the CA125 molecule will probably not come until the gene encoding the peptide component has been cloned.

Apart from OC125, various other monoclonal antibodies have been found to react with epitopes expressed on the CA125-bearing glycoprotein complex.[16,17] When using hereologous double-determined assays based on a combination of OC125 and other antibodies (e.g. NS19.9, B72.3, DF3, Mov8 and OC3632) in serum, a gain in specificity for ovarian cancer was only reached at the expense of a marked decrease in sensitivity compared with the OC125 homologous double-determined assay. Interestingly, the number of falsely elevated CA125 serum levels in healthy controls can be reduced by using serum assays recognizing distinct CA125 epitopes. Therefore comparison of alternative heterologous double-determined assays with the conventional OC125-based homologous double-determined assay deserves further attention when one is aiming at a reduction in false-positive CA125 elevations or false-negative CA125 test results.

Recently, a second-generation immunoradiometric method (IRMA II) has been introduced to determine CA125 serum levels. Statistically significant differences were observed when comparing the values obtained with IRMA CA125 II and IRMA CA125 I assays in different groups of patients.[18] Consequently, it is important, especially in the follow-up of patients, that CA125 serum values be obtained using kits of the same generation.

Release of CA125

Release of secretion of CA125 appears to be directly linked to the epidermal growth factor (EGF) receptor signal transduction pathway.[15] Prior to its release from cultured cells, CA125 is phosphorylated at either or both serine and threonine, and dephosphorylated when released.

In vitro experiments have demonstrated that CA125 production in endometrial stromal cell cultures is inhibited by medroxyprogesterone acetate (MPA), the effect of which can be blocked by estradiol or progesterone antagonists.[19] No inhibition of CA125 expression by hormones was observed in ovarian cancer cell lines, except for glucocorticosteroids.[20] The data presented demonstrate that hormonal regulatory mechanisms for CA125 release in vivo are not yet fully understood.

CA125 expression is also a dynamic process.[20] In vitro experiments on cancer cells have shown that sometimes either suppression or enhancement of CA125 expression occurs after administration of glucocorticosteroids or interferon-γ.[21,22] The effects of cytotoxic drugs on serum antigen levels in ovarian cancer patients remain largely unknown. It seems that tissue expression of CA125 is not seriously altered after chemotherapy.[23] In some cases of patients with elevated CA125 levels but CA125-negative tumors, reactive mesothelial cells may explain such findings. In other cases, poor perfusions and local fibrosis might prevent elevated CA125 serum levels.

CA125 serum levels in healthy women

The cut-off level of the CA125 immunoradiometric assay IRMA I is set at 35 U/ml, which is exceeded in approximately 2% of healthy women.[1] When using an upper limit of 65 U/ml, only 0.2% of 888 controlled subjects showed elevated CA125 serum levels. Other studies have reported positivity in healthy controls ranging from 0% to 5% at a cut-off of 35 U/ml, and from 0% to 1.7% at the higher 65 U/ml cut-off level (Table 16.2).

More recent data demonstrated lower normal values for females with increasing age.[24] These data might be explained by the probability that younger age groups included a substantial portion of menstruating women or women with subclinical endometriosis.

Benign conditions causing CA125 elevations in premenopausal women
Endometriosis

CA125 serum levels are elevated in about 30% of patients with endometriosis, and more so during menstruation[7] (Table 16.3). In patients being treated for endometriosis, pretreatment CA125 serum levels appear to correlate with the severity

Table 16.2 Elevated CA125 levels in healthy subjects

| No. of patients | Cut-off level of CA125 | | Ref |
	>35 U/ml (%)	>65 U/ml (%)	
888	1.0	0.2	1
56	0	0	49
67	4.5	—	50
226	1.8	0.44	51
58	5.0	1.7	52
60	1.7	—	53
150	1.0	—	54
61	4.9	1.6	55
68	—	0	56
915	3.9	0.76	57
50	4.0	—	58
323	4.6	0.93	39
1082	3.3	1.0	59
258	0.39	0.39	60
780	4.2	0.8	24
5550	2.5	—	41
10 592	288/10 524 2.7%	50/4715 1.1%	

Table 16.3   CA125 serum levels in endometriosis and endometriotic cysts

No. of patients	Cut-off level of CA125		Ref
	>35 U/ml (%)	>65 U/ml (%)	
10	—	0/10	61
10	2/10	0/10	62
15	9/15	—	63
30	25/30	11/30	64
8	7/8	—	65
60	10/60	—	66
37	5/37	—	67
31	13/31	—	68
10	7/10	—	55
19	15/19	10/19	69
15	4/15	—	70
21	11/21	—	71
11	9/11	6/11	72
20	0/20	0/20	73
54	8/54	—	74
39	9/39	—	75
67	12/67	—	76
61	29/61	—	77
44	14/44	10/44	78
22	—	16/22	79
6	5/6	2/6	80
15	0/15	—	81
605	194/563	55/172	
	34.4%	31.9%	

and course of disease.[25,26] Also, a correlation between CA125 serum levels and response to therapy has been described. CA125 levels were significantly higher in the poor-response group than in the good-response group, with a sensitivity of 86% and a specificity of 100% in predicting recurrent or persistent endometriosis.[27] Other groups have reported, despite a correlation with the American Fertility Society (AFS) score at diagnosis, no correlation of CA125 serum levels and AFS score at second-look laparoscopy after treatment. They have suggested that mechanisms other than the change in the extent of the disease are involved in the CA125 decrease during therapy.[28] Although patients responded to various treatment regimens such as danazol, gonadotropin-releasing hormone (GnRH) analogs and MPA, as indicated by AFS score, only those patients treated with danazol or GnRH analogs had a significant decrease in serum CA125 levels.[29] From these observations, it has been concluded that decrease of serum CA125 levels is mediated by suppression of ovarian activity, implying that CA125 is not a useful marker for monitoring the course of endometriosis.[27] There are preliminary data available indicating that patients with uterine adenomyosis may have a higher CA125-positive rate than those with leiomyomas or normal controls.[30]

Pregnancy

CA125 elevations in maternal serum occur especially in the first trimester of pregnancy and after delivery.[31,32] Serum levels mostly drop down to non-pregnancy levels in the second and third trimesters of pregnancy. There are some reasons to support the concept that tubal reflux explains the rise and fall of serum concentrations of CA125 in pregnancy.

The predictive value of maternal serum CA125 measurement was investigated in cases of threatened abortion. Some reports indicate that in patients with vaginal bleeding for three days or longer and high maternal serum CA125 activity, the abortion risk is extremely high.[33] These findings suggest that the maternal serum CA125 level is directly related to decidual destruction, and determines the outcome of pregnancy. In contrast, evaluation of CA125 median values of amniotic fluids in pregnancies affected by Down's syndrome and in normal controls have shown that CA125 has no role to play in Down's syndrome screening.[34]

To prevent misinterpretation of tumor marker values during pregnancy (CA125, CA19.9 and CA15.3) further investigation is needed to find normal values for each trimester, paying attention to parity and fetal sex.

Menstruation

In theory, the intermenstrual rise in CA125 seems to be due to retrograde menstruation. The effect of the menstrual cycle on CA125 levels has been investigated in a population study.[35] Elevated serum CA125 levels (>35 U/ml) were present in 5.2% of the premenopausal women (77/1478 patients). This study suggests that in the population as a whole, the effect of the menstrual cycle on serum CA125 is not clinically significant. The theory of retrograde menstruation is challenged by observations by others, who have described elevated CA125 serum concentrations during menstruation also in patients with tubal obstructions.[36]

Benign ovarian neoplasms

Benign ovarian cystic neoplasms are a frequent source of CA125 elevation, with 17.6% of all patients showing elevated CA125 serum levels (Table 16.4). However, there are no significant differences concerning the CA125 serum level between benign and malignant lesions of the ovary. As a consequence, the value of CA125 as a potential non-invasive procedure to differentiate benign from malignant lesions is limited.[37] In clinical practice, a single CA125 elevation in a healthy person should be interpreted with caution, since intercurrent benign conditions might interfere with CA125 serum levels. The diagnostic value of measuring CA125 levels in peritoneal fluid from women with non-malignant gynecologic disorders has also been investigated. The data clearly show that measurement of CA125 levels in peritoneal fluids is not useful. The CA125 levels observed are comparable to the reported lower range of levels observed in patients with intraperitoneal malignancies.

Table 16.4   CA125 serum levels in patients with benign ovarian neoplasms

| No. of patients | Cut-off level of CA125 | | Ref |
	>35 U/ml (%)	>65 U/ml (%)	
25	—	0/25	61
10	0/10	0/10	50
10	1/10	1/10	82
32	6/32	4/32	83
64	16/64	—	68
41	2/41	—	62
50	10/50	—	63
95	—	15/95	64
40	10/42	—	55
27	9/27	—	84
36	—	5/36	85
68	20/69	12/68	69
69	11/69	—	70
63	8/63	—	58
31	3/31	0/31	72
10	0/10	0/10	86
32	8/32	3/32	87
51	6/51	—	88
46	9/46	8/46	89
15	1/15	—	90
29	—	8/29	79
38	6/38	—	81
12	1/12	—	91
46	5/46	—	92
103	17/103	13/103	93
48	11/48	—	94
1069	160/909	69/527	
1099	17.6%	13%	

Other benign disorders

A plethora of conditions, including irritated or inflamed peritoneal tissue, pelvic inflammatory disease, pancreatitis, hepatitis, or diseases such as liver cirrhosis and congestive heart failure, inducing benign ascites or pleural effusions may cause elevated CA125 serum levels (Table 16.1). Renal failure is also associated with elevated

CA125 serum levels. Elevated CA125 measured in the effluent of peritoneal dialysis patients has been suggested as a marker for the mesothelial cell mass. In patients with vanishing of the mesothelial cell layer, the decrease of CA125 in the effluent may reflect the change in peritoneal transport properties and the development or manifestation of peritoneal sclerosis.[38]

Elevated CA125 serum levels in asymptomatic postmenopausal women

Postmenopausal ovarian cysts
In postmenopausal women, the normal range of CA125 is much lower than that of cycling women. In women with raised CA125 in the menopause, transvaginal sonography may sometimes be helpful to separate those with normal sonomorphology of the ovaries who are not at increased risk of ovarian cancer and those with suspect findings who are at substantial risk of developing ovarian cancer. Laparoscopic surgery may be considered in patients with multilocular sonographic findings and normal CA125 serum levels

CA125 in screening
Randomized controlled clinical trials designed to determine the impact of ovarian cancer screening on mortality are currently in progress.[39–42] Results have not been reported to date. On the basis of available data, it cannot be assumed that a screening program for ovarian cancer using CA125 as marker will save lives. A number of important factors that may limit the impact of screening have been discussed extensively elsewhere. CA125 lacks both sensitivity and specificity and ultrasound lacks sufficient specificity. Well-defined risks of screening are associated with false-positive results. To overcome these deficits, multimodality approaches using both CA125 and ultrasound in a sequential fashion are in progress. Nevertheless, guidelines in clinical practice for the use of screening are urgently needed – at least to assist women at high risk, such as members of families with genetic predisposition.

Cervical cancer
Levels of CA125 are more likely to be elevated with adenocarcinoma than squamous cell carcinoma of the uterine cervix.[43] Most frequently, elevated CA125 levels are found in cervical adenocarcinomas (27%). Most authors agree that the number of patients with elevated CA125 levels increases with the stage of disease. About 40% of all stage III–IV patients show elevated CA125 serum levels (>35 U/ml). An interesting correlation has also been found with blood vessel invasion: only 19% of low-stage patients without evidence of vascular-spread disease had positive CA125 levels.[44] When a multivariate analysis was performed, age, stage and elevated CA125 were of prognostic significance.[45] In 21 patients with benign cervical disease, none has been described with positive CA125 serum level.[43] Elevated CA125 levels, however, were described in normal cervical mucus and endocervical mucosa during the menstrual cycle.[46]

Endometrial cancer
Elevated CA125 serum levels have been reported for patients with endometrial cancer, especially tumors of the serous papillary type. CA125 serum levels correlate with stage of disease, and more than 50% of all patients with advanced disease (FIGO stage III/IV) have elevated levels exceeding 35 U/ml. The circulating marker, however, appears to have only limited utility in monitoring the effect of adjuvant therapy in this disease, and may not predict recurrences in the absence of other clinical findings except for individuals with papillary serous carcinomas of the endometrium.[47]

Metastatic breast cancer

CA125 serum levels are elevated in 8% of patients with lung metastases, in 89% of patients with pleural metastases and in 94% of patients showing both sites of metastases. In patients with pleural metastases, CA125 serum levels follow the course of disease. Therefore CA125 can be considered as a relatively selected marker for the diagnosis and follow-up of pleural metastases in breast cancer patients.[48]

CONCLUSIONS

Over the last 15 years, substantial progress has been made in understanding the potential and the limitations of the CA125 assay. A common factor in all pathologic and physiologic events associated with elevation of serum CA125 levels seems to be the occurrence of a process that alters normal tissue barriers in relation to tissues known to produce CA125. When increased tissue production of CA125 coincides with changes in surface barriers, a rise in serum CA125 is usual. CA125 is most consistently elevated in patients with advanced-stage epithelial ovarian cancer. The most well-established application of the CA125 assay is in monitoring these cancer patients.

In defined clinical situations, CA125 levels can aid in distinguishing malignant from benign pelvic masses. When aiming to predict either the malignant or the benign nature of a pelvic mass, menopausal status plays an important role.

CA125 levels are also elevated in healthy women as well as in patients with numerous benign conditions. In pregnancy, CA125 is released in maternal serum and in amniotic fluid, and is detected in placental tissues. CA125 is detected in fetal müllerian duct derivatives, fallopian tube, endometrium, endocervix, pleura, pericardium and mesonephric duct. Most benign CA125 elevations occur in premenopausal patients owing to age-related conditions such as menses, endometriosis or pelvic inflammatory disease. In the postmenopausal group, the incidence of ovarian cancer and most other relevant malignancies is higher.

Within the context of screening, most benign/physiologic causes of an elevated serum CA125 are either clinically apparent or uncommon in the age group most likely to be selected for screening. Elevations of CA125 in malignancies other than ovarian cancer are largely associated with advanced-stage clinically apparent disease, and monitoring by CA125 is not a useful clinical tool.

LEARNING POINTS

✣ CA125 is produced by a variety of cell populations. Mean values decrease with increasing age, but do not vary across ethnic groups.
✣ Most physiologic and pathologic events associated with elevation of serum CA125 levels are induced by a process that alters normal tissue barriers in relation to tissues known to produce CA125.
✣ Elevated serum levels of CA125 (>65 U/ml) are associated with non-malignant conditions in approximately 10% of cases:
  – in *asymptomatic premenopausal women*, elevated CA125 serum levels occur mostly at the time of menstrual and follicular/luteal phases and during pregnancy;
  – in *asymptomatic postmenopausal women*, elevated CA125 is more often associated with a past history of breast cancer;
  – postmenopausal women with elevated serum levels of CA125 are at substantially increased risk of developing gynecologic cancer in the future.

REFERENCES

1. Bast RC, Klug TL, St John E et al, A radioimmunoassay using monoclonal antibody to monitor the course of epithelial ovarian cancer. *N Engl J Med* 1983; **309**: 883–9.

2. Jacobs IJ, Bast RC, The CA 125 tumour associated antigen: a review of the literature. *Hum Reprod* 1989; **4**: 1–12.

3. Eltabbakh GH, Belinson JL, Kennedy AW et al, Serum CA 125 measurements >65 U/ml. Clinical value. *J Reprod Med* 1997; **43**: 635–6.

4. Omar Y, Al Naquep N, el Nas S et al, Serum levels of CA 125 in patients with gastrointestinal cancers. *Tumor Biol* 1989; **10**: 316–23.

5. Barbati A, Anceschi MM, Alberti P et al, Ontogeny of CA 125 in pregnancy: immunoradiometric determination in amniotic fluid and immunohistochemical localisation in fetal membranes. *Am J Obstet Gynecol* 1989; **160**: 514–18.

6. Kan YY, Yeh SH, Ng HAT, Lou CM, Effect of menstruation on serum CA 125 levels. *Asia Oceania J Obstet Gynecol* 1992; **18**: 3339–43.

7. Imai A, Horibe S, Takagi A et al, Drastic elevation of serum CA 125, CA 72-4 and CA 19-9 levels during menses in a patient with probable endometriosis. *Eur J Obstet Gynecol Reprod Biol* 1998; **78**: 79–81.

8. Menton U, Talaat A, Jeyarajah AR et al, Ultrasound assessment of ovarian cancer risk in postmenopausal women with CA 125 elevation. *Br J Cancer* 1999; **80**: 1644–7.

9. Metzger J, Haussinger K, Wilmanns W et al, CA 125 Serumspiegel bei benignem Ascites oder Pleuraerguß. *Geburtshilfe und Frauenheilkunde* 1987; **47**: 463–5.

10. Fleuren G, Nap M, Aalders J et al, Explanation of the limited correlation between tumour CA 125 content and serum CA 125 antigen levels in patients with ovarian tumours. *Cancer* 1987; **60**: 2437–42.

11. Boerman O, Makking W, Thomas C et al, Monoclonal antibodies that discriminate between human ovarian carcinomas and benign ovarian tumors. *Eur J Cancer* 1990; **26**: 117–27.

12. van Niekerk C, Jap P, Thomas C et al, Marker profile of mesothelial cells versus ovarian carcinoma cells. *Int J Cancer* 1989; **43**: 275–85.

13. Duk J, Kauer F, Fleuren G, deBruijn H, Serum CA 125 levels in patients with a provisional diagnosis of pelvic inflammatory disease. *Acta Obstet Gynecol Scand* 1989; **68**: 637–41.

14. Nagata A, Hirota N, Sakai T et al, Molecular nature and possible presence of a membranous glycan phosphatidylinositol anchor of CA 125 antigen. *Tumor Biol* 1991; **12**: 279–86.

15. O'Brien TJ, Tanimoto H, Konoshi I et al, More than 15 years of CA 125: what is known about the antigen, its structure and its function. *Int J Biol Markers* 1998; **13**: 188–95.

16. Nap M, Vitali A, Nustad A et al, Immunohistological characterization of 22 monoclonal antibodies against the CA 125 antigen. 2nd report from the ISOBMnTD-1 Workshop. *Tumor Biol* 1996; **17**: 325–31.

17. Yu Y, Schlossman D, Harrison C et al, Coexpression of different antigenic markers on moieties that bear CA 125 determinants. *Cancer Res* 1991; **51**: 468–75.

18. Cioffi M, Fratta M, Gazzerro P et al, OVCA (CA125) second generation: technical aspects and serum levels in controls, patients with liver disease, pregnant women and patients with ovarian disease. *Tumori* 1997; **83**: 594–8.

19. Bischof P, Tseng L, Brioschi P, Hermann W, Cancer antigen CA 125 is produced by human endometrial stromal cells. *Hum Reprod* 1986; **1**: 423–6.

20. Berchuk A, Olt G, Soisson A et al, Heterogeneity of antigen expression in advanced epithelial ovarian cancer. *Am J Obstet Gynecol* 1990; **162**: 883–8.

21. Karlan BY, Amin W, Casper SE, Littlefield BA, Hormonal regulation of CA 125 tumor marker expression in human ovarian carcinoma cells: inhibition by glucocorticoids. *Cancer Res* 1988; **48**: 3502–6.

22. Marth C, Fuith L, Böck G, Daxenbichler G et

al, Modulation of ovarian carcinoma tumor marker CA 125 by gamma-interferon. *Cancer Res* 1989; **49**: 3502–6.

23. Rubin S, Hoskins W, Hakes T et al, Serum CA 125 levels and surgical findings in patients undergoing secondary operations for epithelial ovarian cancer. *Am J Obstet Gynecol* 1989; **160**: 667–71.

24. Verstraeten A, Kenemans P, Bon G et al, Normal values of serum tumor marker levels in relation to age. In: *Proceedings of XIXth International Society for Oncodevelopmental Biology and Medicine Meeting 13–17 October 1991 Siena, Italy*: 385.

25. Mastropaolo W, Fernandez Z, Miller E, Pronounced increases in the concentration of an ovarian tumor marker, CA 125, in serum of a healthy subject during menstruation. *Clin Chem* 1986; **32**: 2110–11.

26. Pittaway D, The use of serial CA 125 concentrations to monitor endometriosis in infertile women. *Obstet Gynecol* 1990; **163**: 1032–7.

27. Franssen A, van der Heijden P, Thomas C et al, On the origin and significance of serum CA 125 concentrations in 97 patients with endometriosis before, during and after buserelin acetate, nafarelin, or danazol. *Fertil Steril* 1992; **57**: 974–9.

28. Marana R, Muzii L, Muscatello P et al, Gonadotropin releasing hormone agonist (buserelin) in the treatment of endometriosis: changes in the extent of the disease and in CA 125 serum levels after 6-month therapy. *Br J Obstet Gynaecol* 1990; **97**: 1016–19.

29. Kaupilla A, Telimass S, Ronnberg L et al, Placebo controlled study on serum concentrations of CA 125 before and after treatment on endometriosis with danazol or high-dose medroxyprogesterone acetate alone or after surgery. *Fertil Steril* 1988; **49**: 37–41.

30. Zhou Y, Wu B, Li H, The value of serum CA 125 assays in diagnosis of uterine adenomyosis. *Chung Hua Fu Chan Ko Tsa Chih* 1996; **31**: 590–3.

31. Seki K, Kikuchi Y, Uesatom T, Kato K,

Increased serum CA 125 levels during the first trimester of pregnancy. *Acta Obstet Gynecol Scand* 1986; **65**: 583–5.

32. Kobayashi F, Sagawa N, Nakamura K et al, Mechanism and clinical significance of elevated CA 125 levels in the sera of pregnant women. *Am J Obstet Gynecol* 1989; **160**: 563–6.

33. Ocer F, Bese T, Saridogan E et al, The prognostic significance of maternal serum CA 125 measurement in threatened abortion. *Eur J Obstet Gynecol Reprod Biol* 1992; **23**: 137–42.

34. Spencer K, Muller F, Aitken DA, Amniotic fluid and maternal serum levels of CA 125 in pregnancies affected by Down syndrome: a reevaluation of the role of CA 125 in Down syndrome screening. *Prenat Diagn* 1997; **17**: 701–6.

35. Grover S, Koh H, Weidemann P, Quinn MA, The effect of the menstrual cycle on serum CA 125 levels: a population study. *Am J Obstet Gynecol* 1992; **167**: 1379–81.

36. Bon GG, Kenemans P, Dekker JJ et al, Fluctuations in CA 125 and CA 15-3 serum concentrations during spontaneous ovulatory cycles. *Hum Reprod* 1999; **14**: 566–70.

37. Bodor D, CA 125 concentrations in malignant and nonmalignant disease. *Clin Chem* 1991; **37**: 1968–74.

38. Lai KN, Lai KB, Szeto CC et al, Dialysate cell population and cancer antigen 125 in stable continuous peritoneal dialysis patients: their relationship with transport parameters. *Am J Kidney Dis* 1997; **29**: 699–705.

39. Zurawski VR, Orjaseter H, Andersen A, Jellum E, Elevated serum CA 125 levels prior to diagnosis of ovarian neoplasia; relevance for early detection of ovarian cancer. *Int J Cancer* 1988; **42**: 677–80.

40. Jacobs IJ, Oram DH, Bast RC, Strategies for improving the specificity of screening for ovarian cancer with tumor-associated antigens CA 125, CA 15-3 and Tag 72.3. *Obstet Gynecol* 1992; **80**: 396–9.

41. Einhorn N, Sjovall K, Knapp RC et al,

Prospective evaluation of serum CA 125 levels for early detection of ovarian cancer. *Obstet Gynecol* 1992; **80**: 14–18.

42. Helzlsouer KJ, Bush TL, Alberg AJ et al, Prospective study of serum CA 125 levels as markers of ovarian cancer. *JAMA* 1993; **269**: 1123–6.

43. Gocze PM, Vahrson HW, Freeman DA, Serum levels of squamous cell carcinoma antigen and ovarian carcinoma antigen (CA 125) in patients with benign and malignant diseases of the uterine cervix. *Oncology* 1994; **51**: 430–4.

44. Massuger LF, Koper NP, Thomas CM et al, Improvement of clinical staging in cervical cancer with serum squamous cell carcinoma antigen and CA 125 determinations. *Gynecol Oncol* 1997; **64**: 473–6.

45. Ngan HY, Cheung AN, Lauder IJ et al, Tumor markers and their prognostic value in adenocarcinoma of the cervix. *Tumor Biol* 1998; **19**: 439–44.

46. Crombach G, Scharl A, Wuerz H, CA 125 in normal tissues and carcinomas of the uterine cervix, endometrium and fallopian tube. *Arch Gynecol Obstet* 1989; **244**: 113–22.

47. Abramovich D, Markman M, Kennedy A et al, Serum CA 125 as a marker of disease activity in uterine papillary serous carcinoma. *J Cancer Res Clin Oncol* 1999; **125**: 697–8.

48. Kramer S, Jäger W, Lang N, CA 125 is an indicator for pleural metastases in breast cancer. *Anticancer Res* 1997; **17**: 2967–70.

49. Klug TL, Blast RC, Niloff JM et al, Monoclonal antibody immunoradiometric assay for an antigen determinant (CA 125) associated with human epithelial ovarian carcinoma. *Cancer Res* 1984; **44**: 1048–53.

50. Ricolleau G, Chatal JF, Fumoleau P et al, Radioimmunoassay of the CA 125 antigen in ovarian carcinoma: advantages compared with CA 19-9 and CEA. *Tumour Biol* 1984; **5**: 151–9.

51. Rubial A, Alvares Moro FJ, Comet R et al, Creatine phototransferase B subunit, as a tumor marker: preliminary results. *Rev Esp Oncol* 1984; **31**: 415–20.

52. Crombach G, Zippel HH, Würz J, Experiences with CA 125, a tumor marker for malignant epithelial ovarian tumors. *Geburtshilfe Frauenheilk* 1985; **45**: 205–12.

53. Kawahara M, Terasaki PI, Chia D et al, Use of four monoclonal antibodies to detect tumor markers. *Cancer* 1986; **58**: 2008–12.

54. Dokia B, Canney PA, Pectasides D et al, A new immunoassay using monoclonal antibodies HMFG1 and HMFG2 together with an existing marker CA 125 for selective detection and management of epithelial ovarian cancer. *Br J Cancer* 1986; **54**: 891–5.

55. Negishi Y, Furukawa T, Oka T et al, Clinical use of CA 125 and its combination assay with other tumor markers in patients with ovarian carcinoma. *Gynecol Obstet Invest* 1987; **23**: 200–7.

56. Sevelda P, Haider F, Spona J, Immunosuppressive acid protein (IAP) — improvement in tumor marker diagnosis in epithelial ovarian cancer. *Geburtshilfe Frauenheilk* 1987; **47**: 452–5.

57. Zurawski VR, Broderick SF, Pickens P et al, Serum CA 125 levels in a group of nonhospitalized women: relevance for the early detection of ovarian cancer. *Obstet Gynecol* 1987; **69**: 606–11.

58. Knauf S, Bast RC, Tumor antigen NB/70K and CA 125 levels in the blood of preoperative ovarian cancer patients and controls: a preliminary report of the use of the NB12123 and Ca 125 radioimmunoassay alone and in combination. *Int J Biol Markers* 1988; **3**: 75–81.

59. Zurawski VR, Slovall K, Schoenfeld DA et al, Prospective evaluation of serum CA 125 levels in a normal population, phase I: the specificities of single and serial determinations in testing for ovarian cancer. *Gynecol Oncol* 1990; **36**: 299–305.

60. Westhoff C, Gollub E, Patel J et al, CA 125 levels in menopausal women. *Obstet Gynecol* 1990; **76**: 428–31.

61. Niloff JM, Knapp RC, Schaetzl E et al, CA 125 antigen levels in obstetric and gynecologic patients. *Obstet Gynecol* 1984; **64**: 703–7.

62. Einhorn N, Bast RC, Knapp RC et al, Preoperative evaluation of serum CA 125 levels in patients with primary ovarian cancer. *Obstet Gynecol* 1986; **67**: 414–16.

63. Pasini F, Bellinazzi A, Rainaldi V et al, Serum CA 125 in ovarian pathology and its variation in ovarian carcinoma after integrated therapy. *Gynecol Obstet Invest* 1986; **21**: 47–51.

64. Fioretti P, Gadducci A, Ferdeghini M et al, Combined evaluation of some tumor associated antigens in the monitoring of integrated surgical and chemotherapeutic treatment of epithelial ovarian cancer. *Eur J Gynaecol Oncol* 1986; 7: 200–5.

65. Giudice LC, Jacobs AJ, Bell CE, Lippmann L, Serum levels of CA-125 in patients with endometriosis. *Gynecol Oncol* 1986; **25**: 256–8.

66. Barbieri RL, Niloff JM, Bast RC et al, Elevated serum concentrations of CA 125 in patients with advanced endometriosis. *Fertil Steril* 1986; **45**: 630–4.

67. Patton PE, Field CS, Harms RW et al, CA-125 levels in endometriosis. *Fertil Steril* 1986; **45**: 770–3.

68. Malkasian GD Jr, Podratz KC, Stanhope CR et al, CA 125 in gynecologic practice. *Am J Obstet Gynecol* 1986; **155**: 515–18.

69. Chen DX, Schwartz PE, Li XG, Yang Z, Evaluation of CA 125 levels in differentiating malignant from benign tumors in patients with pelvic masses. *Obstet Gynecol* 1988; **72**: 23–7.

70. Patsner B, Mann WJ, The value of preoperative serum CA 125 levels in patients with a pelvic mass. *Am J Obstet Gynecol* 1988; **159**: 873–6.

71. Malkasian GD Jr, Knapp RC, Lavin PT et al, Preoperative evaluation of serum CA 125 levels in premenopausal and postmenopausal patients with pelvic masses: discrimination of benign from malignant disease. *Am J Obstet Gynecol* 1988; **159**: 341–6.

72. Vasilev SA, Schlaerth JB, Campeau J, Morrow CP, Serum CA 125 levels in preoperative evaluation of pelvic masses. *Obstet Gynecol* 1988; **71**: 751–6.

73. Moretuzzo RW, DiLauro S, Jenison E et al, Serum and peritoneal lavage fluid CA-125 levels in endometriosis. *Fertil Steril* 1988; **50**: 430–3.

74. Fedele L, Arcaini L, Vercellini P et al, Serum CA 125 measurements in the diagnosis of endometriosis recurrence. *Obstet Gynecol* 1988; **72**: 19–22.

75. Fedele L, Vercellini P, Arcaini L et al, CA 125 in serum, peritoneal fluid, active lesions, and endometrium of patients with endometriosis. *Am J Obstet Gynecol* 1988; **158**: 166–70.

76. Dawood MY, Khan-Dawood FS, Ramos J, Plasma and peritoneal fluid levels of CA 125 in women with endometriosis. *Am J Obstet Gynecol* 1988; **159**: 1526–31.

77. Masahashi T, Matsuzawa K, Ohsawa M et al, Serum CA 125 levels in patients with endometriosis: changes in CA 125 levels during menstruation. *Obstet Gynecol* 1988; **72**: 328–31.

78. Moloney MD, Thornton JG, Cooper EH, Serum CA 125 antigen levels and disease severity in patients with endometriosis. *Obstet Gynecol* 1989; **73**: 767–9.

79. Chen DX, Schwartz PE, Li FQ, Saliva and serum CA 125 assays for detecting malignant ovarian tumors. *Obstet Gynecol* 1990; **75**: 701–4.

80. Soper JT, Hunter VJ, Daly L et al, Preoperative serum tumor-associated antigen levels in women with pelvic masses. *Obstet Gynecol* 1990; **75**: 249–54.

81. Suzuki M, Sekiguchi I, Tamada T et al, Clinical evaluation of tumor-associated mucin-type glycoprotein CA 54/61 in ovarian cancers: comparison with CA 125. *Obstet Gynecol* 1990; **76**: 422–7.

82. Heinonen PK, Tontti K, Koivula T et al, Tumor-associated antigen CA 125 in patients with ovarian cancer. *Br J Obstet Gynaecol* 1985; **92**: 529–31.

83. Sevelda P, Salzer H, Dittrich C et al, Clinical

significance of the tumor marker CA-125 for the preoperative management of patients with malignant ovarian cancers. *Geburtshilfe Frauenheilkd* 1985; **45**: 769–73.

84. Geyer H, Kleine W, Tumor markers in gynecologic diseases. *Geburtshilfe Frauenheilkd* 1987; **47**: 168–72.

85. Sevelda P, Wagner G, Diagnosis of the recurrence of epithelial ovarian cancer with the tumor marker CA 125. *Wien Klin Wochenschr* 1987; **99**: 768–70.

86. Gocze PM, Szabo DG, Than GN et al, Occurrence of CA 125 and CA 19-9 tumor-associated antigens in sera of patients with gynecologic, trophoblastic, and colorectal tumors. *Gynecol Obstet Invest* 1988; **25**: 268–72.

87. Yedema C, Massuger L, Hilgers J et al, Preoperative discrimination between benign and malignant ovarian tumors using a combination of CA125 and CA15.3 serum assays. *Int J Cancer Suppl* 1988; **3**: 61–7.

88. Mogensen O, Mogensen B, Jakobsen A, CA 125 in the diagnosis of pelvic masses. *Eur J Cancer Clin Oncol* 1989; **25**: 1187–90.

89. Bartel U, Johannsen B, Elling D, The value of CA 125 determination in the serum of patients with ovarian cancer. *Zentralbl Gynaekol* 1989; **111**: 301–9.

90. Mogensen O, Mogensen B, Jakobsen A et al, Preoperative measurement of cancer antigen 125 (CA 125) in the differential diagnosis of ovarian tumors. *Acta Oncol* 1989; **28**: 471–3.

91. Stigbrand T, Riklund K, Tholander B et al, Placental alkaline phosphatase (PLAP)/PLAP-like alkaline phosphatase as tumour marker in relation to CA 125 and TPA for ovarian epithelial tumours. *Eur J Gynaecol Oncol* 1990; **11**: 351–60.

92. Mogensen O, Mogensen B, Jakobsen A, Tumor-associated trypsin inhibitor and cancer antigen 125 in pelvic masses. *Gynecol Oncol* 1990; **38**: 170–4.

93. Tholander B, Taube A, Lindgren A et al, Pretreatment serum levels of CA-125, carcinoembryonic antigen, tissue polypeptide antigen, and placental alkaline phosphatase, in patients with ovarian carcinoma, borderline tumors, or benign adnexal masses: relevance for differential diagnosis. *Gynecol Oncol* 1990; **39**: 16–25.

94. McGuckin MA, Layton GT, Bailey MJ, Evaluation of two new assays for tumor-associated antigens, CASA and OSA, found in the serum of patients with epithelial ovarian carcinoma — comparison with CA 125. *Gynecol Oncol* 1990; **37**: 165–71.

17
Ovarian cancer with a family history

Elizabeth A Poynor, Kenneth Offit

INTRODUCTION

Hereditary ovarian cancer accounts for approximately 10% of ovarian cancer. Proper identification of women at risk is important in order to allow appropriate screening and, in some cases, prophylactic surgery. The major risk groups are those individuals belonging to breast–ovarian families (*BRCA1* and *BRCA2* mutations) and hereditary non-polyposis colon cancer (HNPCC) families (mismatch-repair gene mutations). This chapter addresses both types of hereditary ovarian cancer.

CASE HISTORY 1

A 52-year-old patient presented to her gynecologist with right-sided abdominal pain, abdominal bloating, and urinary frequency. Her past medical history was notable for breast cancer diagnosed at the age of 45, two full-term deliveries, and a benign ovarian cyst removed at age 23. Her family history was notable for a father diagnosed with prostate cancer at age 57, two paternal aunts diagnosed with breast cancer at the ages of 45 and 50, a paternal grandmother diagnosed with ovarian cancer at age 55, and a maternal grandmother diagnosed with colon cancer at age 75. Figure 17.1 details the patient's cancer family history. The patient's physical examination showed a normal breast examination status post right lumpectomy, abdominal distension with shifting dullness to percussion, and 2+ pitting bilateral lower-extremity edema. A pelvic examination showed normal external genitalia and normal vagina and cervix. She was found to have a firm, fixed right-sided pelvic mass. Bimanual examination revealed a palpable nodularity in the cul de sac. Her laboratory values included a high CA125 serum level of 3245 U/ml. Additionally, a solid, cystic pelvic mass was noted on an ultrasound (USG) examination of the abdomen and pelvis.

The patient underwent an exploratory laparotomy for presumed ovarian cancer. Following total abdominal hysterectomy and debulking, pathology revealed a stage IIIC, grade 3 papillary serous epithelial ovarian cancer. The patient was started on a regimen of carboplatin and paclitaxel (Taxol). The CA125 serum level rapidly normalized, and she remains free of disease four years later. The patient continues to be followed with CA125 measurement and pelvic examination on a six-monthly basis.

At the completion of therapy, the patient's oncologist recommended genetic counseling. Because the patient has two daughters, for whom the test results would have medical implications, she opted to

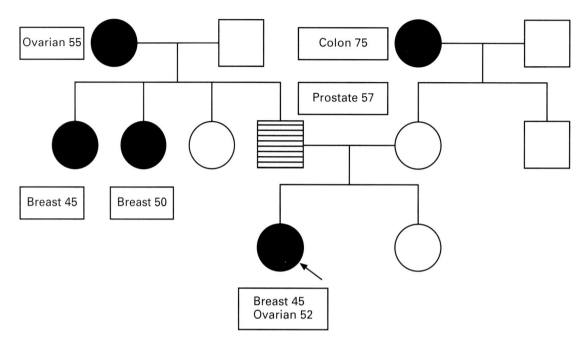

Figure 17.1
The cancer family history for Case 1. The numbers in the boxes give the age at diagnosis of the indicated cancer. The patient discussed is indicated by the arrow.

undergo testing. She was tested for a BRCA mutation, and was found to carry a germline mutation of the BRCA1 gene.

The etiology of ovarian cancer is poorly understood. At this time, there appears to be a correlation between the number of ovulatory cycles and the risk of ovarian cancer. Factors that decrease the number of total lifetime ovulatory cycles also decrease a woman's risk of developing the disease. The strongest risk factor for the development of ovarian cancer is a family history of the disease.

What is the risk of inherited ovarian cancer?

A woman who has one first-degree relative with ovarian cancer has a 5% lifetime risk of developing epithelial ovarian cancer, compared with the general population risk of 1.8%.[1] For a woman with one first-degree relative and one second-degree relative with ovarian cancer, this risk may be as high as 7%.[2] These clusterings of ovarian cancer within a family are described as 'familial' ovarian cancer, and are believed to be due to a combination of genetic and environmental factors. If a woman has two first-degree relatives with ovarian cancer, her risk may be increased to as high as 50%. These cases may be due to a mutation in a cancer disposition gene such as BRCA1 or BRCA2, and are described as 'hereditary' ovarian cancer.

Hereditary ovarian cancer was first recognized and described in the 1950s. Such cancers are characterized by an autosomal dominant transmission of the disease from generation to generation, and comprise approximately 5–10% of ovarian cancers.[3] Epithelial ovarian cancer occurs as a component of three hereditary cancer syndromes: hereditary breast and ovarian cancer (HBOC), hereditary site-specific ovarian cancer (HSSOC), and the hereditary non-polyposis colorectal cancer syndrome (HNPCC). The most common form of hereditary ovarian cancer is as a component of the HBOC syndrome, which is characterized by an autosomal dominant transmission of breast and ovarian cancer. The second most common form of hereditary ovarian cancer is HSSOC, in which ovarian cancer is transmitted in a hereditary nature. Kindreds in which three cases of ovarian cancer have been diagnosed meet the criteria for this condition.

The identification of families in which an elevated risk is transmitted in an autosomal dominant fashion provides the oncologist with the opportunity to intervene in these patients' care and possibly help to prevent a lethal malignancy. The oncologist should obtain a detailed family history on each patient, including medical information for at least three generations. Counseling sessions should be provided for individuals at an elevated risk for hereditary cancer, and should include information on risk assessment, genetic testing opportunities, and risk-reduction strategies.

BRCA1 and BRCA2

The majority of hereditary breast and ovarian cancers are caused by mutations in the BRCA1 and BRCA2 tumor suppressor genes. Cloned in 1994, the BRCA1 gene is located on chromosome 17q. A large gene, it consists of over 100 000 nucleotides, and encodes for a protein consisting of 1863 amino acids.[4] The BRCA2 gene is located on chromosome 13q. It also consists of over 100 000 nucleotides and encodes for a 3418-amino-acid protein.[5] Both BRCA1 and BRCA2 are thought to be tumor suppressor genes, involved in the repair of double-strand breaks of DNA. Recently, the BRCA1 protein was found to interact with p53, and stimulates tran-

scription from the p21/WAF1/CIP1 promoter.[6]

Mutations in the BRCA1 gene were initially thought to explain up to 90% of HBOC kindreds and about 40% of families affected only by hereditary breast cancer.[7–9] Mutations in BRCA2 were estimated to account for a smaller proportion of HBOC families and about 30% of hereditary breast cancers.[10,11] More recent analysis based on full sequencing has shown that, in fact, the proportion of hereditary breast cancer and HBOC families attributable to other genes may be as high as 30–70%.[12] Table 17.1 details the risks of developing cancer based on the presence of a BRCA1 or BRCA2 mutation.[13] A woman's lifetime risk of developing ovarian cancer is estimated to be 28–44% if she is a BRCA1 heterozygote and to be 27% if she is a BRCA2 heterozygote.[9,14,15] For carriers of BRCA1 mutations, initial estimates for ovarian cancer risk were 67%, with a risk of up to 85% for breast cancer.[8,9] However, these initial studies were based on large families with multiple cases of breast and ovarian cancer, resulting in an overestimation. For families in which there are multiple cases of breast and ovarian cancer, it is reasonable to use these initial risk assessments. Another set of estimates, derived from a population-based study of selected mutations, revealed a breast cancer risk of 56% by age 70 and an ovarian cancer risk of 16%.[16] Mutations in the BRCA1 gene are also associated with a smaller increase in risk for colon cancer and prostate cancer. Individuals who are BRCA2 heterozygotes also have an elevated risk for pancreatic and male breast cancer. Mutations have been found throughout these genes, and no one 'hotspot' for mutations has been demonstrated. Thus, full-length sequencing is necessary in most cases in order to detect mutations.

Founder mutations

In populations such as those of Ashkenazi Jewish origin, founder mutations exist. 'Founder effect'

Table 17.1   Risk of developing cancer, based on a mutation in *BRCA1* or *BRCA2*[a]

Gene mutation	Site	Cancer risk
BRCA1	Ovary	16–44% by age 70
	Breast	56–87% by age 70 33–50% by age 50
	Contralateral breast cancer	64% by age 70 25% within 5 years
	Colon	3.3-fold elevated risk
	Prostate	3-fold elevated risk
BRCA2	Ovary	27% by age 70
	Breast	56–87% by age 70 33–50% by age 50
	Contralateral breast cancer	64% by age 70 25% within 5 years
	Prostate	3-fold elevated risk
	Male breast cancer	6%
	Pancreas	Increased

[a] Adapted with permission from Frank TS, Hereditary risk of breast and ovarian carcinoma: the role of the oncologist. *Oncologist* 1998; 3: 403–12.

refers to a high frequency of a specific mutation in ancestors of a common descendant. This results from random genetic mutations in a small population that have become amplified after expansion and restricted breeding of a geographically or culturally isolated group. Founder mutations have been identified in the *BRCA1* and *BRCA2* genes in island populations, as well as in the Ashkenazi Jewish population. Approximately 2.5% of Ashkenazi Jewish women will harbor a *BRCA1* or *BRCA2* mutation.[17,18] The *BRCA1*

mutation 185delAG, which is a two-base-pair deletion in codon 22 of the gene, is found in 1.05% of Jewish women, while the *BRCA2* mutation 6174delT, a one-base-pair deletion in codon 1756, is found in 1.3% of Jewish women. Another *BRCA1* mutation, 5382insC, is also observed in this group. As many as 30% of Ashkenazi Jewish women with ovarian cancer will have one of the aforementioned mutations.[19] Some investigators have suggested that all women with ovarian cancer who are of Ashkenazi

Jewish descent should be tested for one of these *BRCA1* or *BRCA2* mutations.

Obtaining a family history

A detailed family history of at least three generations is crucial for an accurate assessment of an individual's risk of hereditary cancer. It is also important to attempt to document self-reported family histories by obtaining medical records. Table 17.2 outlines the probabilities for harboring a *BRCA1* or *BRCA2* mutation based on family history.[13] Important features of hereditary cancers that must be noted are young age at onset of the cancers (generally 10–15 years younger than in the general population), an excess of bilateral cancers in paired organs, multiple primary cancers, and an autosomal dominant mode of transmission of the cancers in families. Thus, when the clinician is obtaining the family history, it is of special importance to note the relationships of the affected family members, the ages of these members at the onset of disease, and the ages of the family members who do not have disease. The family of the patient presented demonstrates the young ages at the time of diagnosis of breast cancer; a woman without a mutation in a cancer predisposition gene has only a 2% chance of developing breast

---

Table 17.2 The probability of harboring a *BRCA1* or *BRCA2* mutation based on family history; the unaffected first-degree relative will have a 50% chance of having a mutation[a]

Any relative with breast cancer <50 years old?	Any relative with ovarian cancer?	Proband: bilateral breast cancer or ovarian cancer?	Proband: breast cancer <40 years old?	Modeled probability of mutation in *BRCA1*	Modeled probability of mutation in *BRCA2*
•				10.1%	14.5%
•			•	28.2%	11.6%
•		•		41.5%	9.5%
•		•	•	71.1%	4.7%
	•			22.9%	12.5%
	•		•	22.9%	12.5%
	•	•		65.0%	5.7%
	•	•	•	65.0%	5.7%
•	•			22.9%	12.5%
•	•		•	50.9%	7.9%
•	•	•		65.0%	5.7%
•	•	•	•	86.7%	2.2%

[a] Used with permission from Frank TS, Hereditary risk of breast and ovarian carcinoma: the role of the oncologist. *Oncologist* 1998; 3: 403–12.

cancer prior to the age of 50, while a woman with a mutation in the *BRCA1* gene has a 33–55% chance of developing the disease prior to the age of 50.[20,21] The average age of diagnosis of ovarian cancer in women with hereditary ovarian cancer is significantly younger than the median age in the population, 59 years; the median ages of onset in the HBOC, HSSOC, and HNPCC syndromes are 52 years, 49 years, and 45 years, respectively.[22] Hereditary cancers associated with the *BRCA2* gene may present at a later age.[23] This family also demonstrates the importance of obtaining a thorough paternal family history. Family history data may be confounded by the fact that men do not develop ovarian cancer and infrequently develop breast cancer. Other factors that may confound family history data include small family size, lack of female offspring/descendants, and early death of family members due to other, non-cancer causes. All of these factors must be considered when interpreting a patient's family data.

Are the stage of disease and prognosis of hereditary ovarian cancer different from those of sporadic cancer?

The patient here presented with an advanced-stage papillary serous tumor of the ovary. Most commonly, whether tumors are sporadic or hereditary, epithelial ovarian cancer presents at an advanced stage. In the general population, 75% of patients will present with stage III and stage IV disease, and approximately 50% of ovarian cancers will be papillary serous. Ovarian cancer occurring in a hereditary setting does not appear to differ significantly in stage at presentation, and the serous histopathologic subtype may be even more frequently found in hereditary ovarian cancer. In a study by Rubin and his colleagues,[24] 81% of patients with a documented *BRCA1* mutation presented with stage III and stage IV disease, and 80% of patients had serous

tumors. Other investigators have also documented a preponderance of serous tumors in women with hereditary ovarian cancers. The vast majority of hereditary ovarian cancers are grade 3; however, borderline tumors may also occur in these families.[25] The contribution of borderline tumors and their significance in a family history are unclear. These tumors have been found to comprise only a small proportion of hereditary ovarian cancer, and in a study of Jewish women with borderline ovarian cancers, only 2.2% were found to have one of the founder *BRCA1* or *BRCA2* mutations, compared with approximately 50% in Jewish women with invasive ovarian cancer.[26] Borderline ovarian cancers should thus be considered as part of the phenotypic spectrum in interpreting a patient's pedigree, but it should be noted that they occur in these families with a much lower incidence than invasive ovarian cancers.

The prognosis for women with a hereditary ovarian cancer may be improved compared with that for women with sporadic ovarian cancer; however, this remains controversial. Investigators have found that women with ovarian cancer associated with a *BRCA1* mutation enjoyed a prolonged survival compared with those who did not have a mutation.[24] Women with a *BRCA1* mutation had a median survival of 77 months for advanced-stage disease, compared with 29 months for controls who had ovarian cancer and did not harbor a gene mutation. These findings, however, were not confirmed in a smaller study from Sweden.[27] It has been suggested that ascertainment bias accounted for the original findings, and further prospective study is required to answer this important question. The standard treatment of ovarian cancer is applied to these women. Further studies are required to determine if these tumors have an increased sensitivity to chemotherapy regimens commonly employed in ovarian cancer. Preliminary data suggest that they do have an elevated sensitivity to platinum.[28]

What are the recommendations for genetic testing?

The patient discussed here opted to undergo genetic testing. This is appropriate based on her personal and family history, and the results will have direct medical implications for her siblings and offspring. Individuals to whom genetic testing should be offered include women with a family history of hereditary breast and ovarian cancer, and women who are likely to base further decisions regarding medical intervention on the results of the test. Genetic testing should also be offered to the family members of women affected with breast or ovarian cancer. If a mutation is not found in an individual, at least two explanations exist. The hereditary cancers in the family may not be due to mutations in one of the tested tumor suppressor genes. Alternatively, the test may be falsely negative and a mutation may exist in an area of the gene that is not analyzed or escaped detection. If only an unaffected member of the family is tested, her 'negative' results have little value. The negative results are less meaningful because the existence of a mutation has not been established to cause the cancers in this family; either a mutation exists and the tested individual has not inherited the faulty allele, or a mutation does not exist.

All genetic testing should be offered by a specialized healthcare provider within the context of a counseling session. Genetic counseling should include the construction of a comprehensive pedigree, counseling on the possible risks and benefits of knowing test results, and a discussion of special surveillance and prophylactic surgery options for the patient. Special concerns, such as potential insurance and employment discrimination, should be discussed with the patient, along with the psychological impact of knowing test results. Strict confidentiality should be maintained, and, in some US states, it may be required that test results be kept in a separate file, independent of the patient's general medical record. Special legislation has been passed in the USA in order to offer partial protection to individuals at risk for discrimination based on genetic test results. The Health Insurance Accountability and Portability Act contains provisions that provide protection for individuals with 'preexisting conditions' – including genetic risk factors – who seek to change insurance coverage. However, there are at present no Federal laws guaranteeing that an individual will be protected from insurance-based genetic discrimination. Potential psychological stresses that arise from positive test results are evident. However, women with negative results may also be at risk for both stress and guilt due to the feeling that they have 'been spared'. Finally, it is important for the clinician to keep in mind that women who decline genetic testing may also be at risk for depression.[29]

Because of the large size of both the *BRCA1* and *BRCA2* genes, genetic testing for mutations is challenging. Most mutations in these genes lead to a truncated protein product. For women who are of Ashkenazi Jewish descent, genetic testing may begin by investigating whether one of the common founder mutations is present. However, if one of these mutations is not present, more than likely, full-length gene sequencing will be required. Owing to the size of the genes, this can be technically challenging and time-consuming.

After an affected woman learns her test results, she may then elect to inform her siblings and offspring of these results. If they opt to be tested for the mutation, they also should be thoroughly counseled in a similar manner to the patient. Currently, options for medical interventions include increased surveillance in order to detect ovarian cancer at an earlier stage or, alternatively, prophylactic surgery. Methods recommended for epithelial ovarian cancer screening include pelvic examination, transvaginal ultrasound, and CA125 measurement every six months beginning at the age of 25–35 years.[30] The ultrasound (USG) examination should be a transvaginal ultrasound with color Doppler imaging. For premenopausal women, the USG should be performed in the first week of the menstrual cycle, in order to decrease the likelihood of detecting functional cysts. CA125 measurement is also recommended as part of the screening process. It should be noted that for a young woman, the CA125 level will be elevated in approximately 12% of cases. Also, CA125 may not be elevated in up to 50% of early-stage tumors.[31,32] Thus, CA125 may have a low specificity and sensitivity. Patients should also be aware that the positive predictive value of this type of ovarian cancer screening is not well known for high-risk populations, who therefore may be subjected to surgical evaluation for benign disease. Finally, women should be thoroughly counseled before embarking on a screening program. They should be informed that this type of ovarian screening has not been proven to detect cancers at an earlier stage or to decrease mortality from ovarian cancer, as have other screening modalities such as mammography and colonoscopy for breast and colon cancers, respectively. For ovarian cancer screening to have an impact on outcome, tumors should be detected at stage I, where the five-year survival rate is 95%. The long-term effects of ovarian cancer screening on mortality from ovarian cancer have not been proven. Optimally, these women should be evaluated on a prospective research protocol.

How should patients with a high risk of ovarian cancer be managed?
Prophylactic oophorectomy

Prophylactic oophorectomy is a prevention option for women heterozygous for a mutation in the *BRCA1* or *BRCA2* gene. It is generally recommended that these women be offered prophylactic removal of the ovaries at the age of 35 or after they have completed childbearing. This procedure is usually performed through the laparoscope. Some women may also opt to have the uterus removed at the time of prophylactic surgery if they currently have uterine pathology, a family history of uterine cancer, or are members of HNPCC kindreds.

Important questions concerning this procedure are (1) whether it protects against the development of ovarian cancer, and (2) whether it is safe to place these women on hormone replacement therapy. It has been reported that from 2% to 11% of women will develop primary peritoneal cancer after prophylactic oophorectomy. This tumor is indistinguishable from ovarian cancer in terms of its clinical behavior and treatment.[33,34] Subsequent case reports have confirmed these observations. The origin of primary peritoneal cancer after prophylactic oophorectomy is unclear. It has been suggested that women are at elevated risk to develop peritoneal cancers because of the common origin of the germinal epithelium of the ovary and the coelomic epithelium of the peritoneum, and both are at risk from *BRCA1* and *BRCA2* mutations. This is supported by the findings of one study of women with primary peritoneal cancer and a *BRCA1* mutation, which demonstrated that these tumors tend to be multifocal in origin.[35] Another hypothesis has been put forward that these peritoneal cancers result from micrometastases from ovarian cancers, which are present but missed on pathologic review, at the time of the initial surgery. Thus, ovaries should be carefully inspected after removal.

If a woman undergoes prophylactic oophorectomy at a young age, she will suffer the side-effects of estrogen deprivation. These include hot flushes, vaginal dryness, and increased risk of heart disease and osteoporosis. The safety of estrogen replacement therapy in these women has not been documented. It has been suggested that transdermal estrogen may be beneficial in these women, because it avoids the large swings in blood levels found after oral absorption.

Thus, when explaining the option of prophylactic surgery to the patient, a thorough discussion of the procedure should include the fact that she is still at risk to develop primary peritoneal cancer after prophylactic surgery and that the safety of estrogen replacement therapy has not been documented. The discussion should also inform the patient that there are no long-term prospective data concerning the efficacy of prophylactic oophorectomy and that there are options for management of the menopausal symptoms that may be incurred secondary to the surgery.

Chemoprevention/oral contraceptives

For very young women, for whom prophylactic surgery is not an option, chemoprevention is considered. It is well known that the use of oral contraceptives (OCP) may decrease a woman's chance of developing ovarian cancer by up to 60%.[36] The protective effect of oral contraceptives in a woman who has a *BRCA1* or *BRCA2* mutation has also been shown. For women who were at high risk for the development of ovarian cancer, oral contraceptives were found to be 60% protective,[37] similar as for non-carriers of mutations. This possible benefit for ovarian cancer protection in high-risk individuals should be weighed against the risk of increasing the chances of developing breast cancer with OCP use. In a small study of Jewish women with ovarian cancer, the use of OCPs was associated with an increased risk of developing breast

cancer.[38] Again, prospective data are required to address these issues.

Summary

It is essential to obtain a detailed family history from all patients who present for medical care. It is also important for clinicians to be aware of family cancer syndromes so that patients can be appropriately referred to specialists who can institute a discussion of cancer risk and medical interventions in order to prevent it from occurring. Mutations in the *BRCA1* and *BRCA2* genes account for the vast majority of hereditary epithelial ovarian cancers, and women who are members of kindreds with a hereditary breast/ovarian cancer syndrome should be offered a discussion of their risk, further quantification of risk, and risk-reducing interventions. Prospective studies are required to answer the important questions of the effective means of ovarian cancer screening with available technologies in this population, the safety of estrogen replacement therapy, and the effectiveness of prophylactic surgery and chemoprevention with oral contraceptive use. Further areas of research that will benefit these women are the development of more effective screening strategies and chemoprevention agents.

LEARNING POINTS

❋ The recognition of families that may harbor a cancer predisposition gene.
❋ The risk of cancer in a woman heterozygous for a *BRCA1* or *BRCA2* mutation.
❋ The appropriate management for individuals who are at risk to develop a hereditary ovarian cancer.

CASE HISTORY 2

A 52-year-old woman presented with postmenopausal bleeding. Her past medical history was unremarkable. Her family history was notable for a mother diagnosed with colon cancer at the age of 48, a maternal aunt with colon cancer with age of onset at 55, and a maternal grandmother with colon cancer diagnosed at the age of 60. Her physical examination showed a 9 cm complex solid and cystic pelvic mass. An endometrial biopsy was performed, and revealed a FIGO grade 1 endometrial adenocarcinoma. The patient underwent an exploratory laparotomy along with a total abdominal hysterectomy, bilateral salpingo-oophorectomy, and a surgical staging procedure after the frozen-section diagnosis revealed an endometrioid adenocarcinoma involving the ovary and superficial endometrioid carcinoma in the uterus. Findings were notable for the large right pelvic mass, tumor implants in the pelvis, and a negative upper abdomen. The permanent section revealed a well-differentiated endometrioid adenocarcinoma of the ovary and a synchronous primary tumor in the uterus.

The patient was staged as having a stage IIA ovarian cancer and stage IA uterine cancer. She was treated with six courses of carboplatin and paclitaxel, and remains free of disease at two years. She has undergone a colonoscopy for screening purposes, and her family members have been counseled to undergo colon cancer screening at regular intervals, along with screening for uterine cancer, ovarian cancer, and urinary tract cancers, with urine cytology at regular intervals.

Although hereditary ovarian cancer most commonly occurs as HBOC or HSSOC, discussed above, it may also occur as a component of the hereditary non-polyposis cancer syndrome (NHPCC), also referred to as the Lynch I and II syndromes. The Lynch syndromes are thought to account for up to 5% of all colon cancer cases.[39]

How does one identify HNPCC families?

The HNPCC syndrome is characterized by the autosomal dominant transmission of colon cancer within a family. The Amsterdam criteria were developed for research purposes in order to identify individuals who are at the highest risk for having a mutation in a cancer predisposition gene. Based on these criteria, for a family to be considered as an HNPCC kindred, it must have at least three family members affected with colorectal cancer in at least two successive generations, with at least one case diagnosed before the age of 50 years; one of the affected members should be a first-degree relative of the other two.[40] Families that have only colorectal cancer have been referred to as having the Lynch I syndrome. In addition to the colorectal cancers, kindreds may have other component cancers. These families are commonly referred to as having the Lynch II syndrome. The cancers from other sites that occur in the Lynch II syndrome include endometrial, ovarian, small bowel, stomach, brain, and hepatobiliary tract and urinary tract cancers.[41] The most common 'component' cancer within these families is endometrial cancer.

What genetic mutations are seen in HNPCC families?
Mismatch repair genes, *MLH1*, *MSH2*, *PMS1*, *PMS2*, and *MSH6*

Mutations in the mismatch repair genes *MLH1*, *MSH2*, *PMS1*, *PMS2*, and *MSH6* account for the cancers in these kindreds. Of the mutations that have been reported to date, almost all have been found in *MSH2* and *MLH1*; only three have been reported in *PMS1* and *PMS2*.[42] These genes encode for proteins in the pathways that are responsible for DNA repair. Thus, a defect in one of these proteins will allow an accumulation of mutations to develop. This rapid accumulation of mutations in oncogenes and tumor suppressor genes allows a tumor to develop and progress. For individuals with mutations in the *MSH2* or *MLH1* genes, the risk for developing colon cancer is 80% (compared with a population risk of 4%) and that for endometrial cancer is 40–50% (compared with a general population risk of less than 2%).[43] Women who are members of an HNPCC family have a 3.5-fold elevated risk of ovarian cancer over that of the general population. The mean age of diagnosis of ovarian cancer in these families is 45 years,[22] which is 20 years younger than in the general population. It also appears that extracolonic cancers develop at an increased rate in individuals who inherit a mutated *MSH2* allele, compared with those who inherit a mutated *MLH1* allele.[44] The colon cancers that develop in these families are characterized by a preponderance of right-sided colon cancers, early age of onset, and the presence of synchronous and metachronous colon cancers. The average age of diagnosis of colon cancer is 45 years; however, individuals as young as 20 may be diagnosed.[43] Although the colon cancers in these families have been extensively studied, the clinicopathologic features of the other component cancers have not been evaluated. Endometrial cancer developing in these families occurs 15

years earlier than in the general population, where the average age is 55–75 years.[44] It is important to recognize these kindreds, so that women may be offered the appropriate prevention and screening management.

How should patients with these mutations be managed?

The management of the gynecologic cancers that occur in these women is the same as for women without a mutation. Few data exist on the clinicopathologic features of these malignancies; thus, treatment and counseling concerning prognosis are not modified. Figure 17.2 outlines the most recent recommendations for the screening of members of families at high risk to develop a breast, ovarian, or colon cancer. Colonoscopy beginning at early age and repeated at frequent intervals is the mainstay of screening for HNPCC, and would be recommended for all of the relatives of the kindred presented above. Screening for uterine and ovarian cancers is also recommended, and some investigators recommend urine cytologic examination as a means to

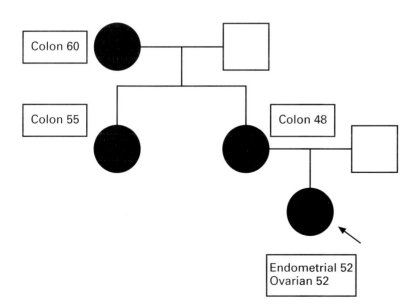

Figure 17.2
The cancer family history for Case 2. The numbers in the boxes give the age at diagnosis or onset of the indicated cancer. The patient discussed is indicated by the arrow.

Colon 60

Colon 55

Colon 48

Endometrial 52
Ovarian 52

screen for the urothelial tumors that are less frequently observed in these families.

What are the recommendations for genetic testing?

The Amsterdam criteria were developed in order to identify the families at highest risk for harboring a mutation in one of the aforementioned mismatch repair genes. It is estimated that 73% of families that meet the Amsterdam criteria will have mutations in one of the mismatch repair genes.[45] If a woman is a member of one of these kindreds, she should be referred to a genetic counselor, and appropriate screening should be instituted for colon, endometrial, and ovarian cancer. Genetic testing should be discussed with these individuals. For women who are members of families that may not meet the Amsterdam criteria, but are members of families with large numbers of colon cancers and other component cancers, the genetic testing recommendations need to be individualized. It is unknown how many of these families harbor a mutation in one of the known mismatch repair genes. As these kindreds are studied in greater depth, further genotype/phenotype associations will be made.

One option in the genetic evaluation of these families is to begin with testing of tumor material for the 'replication error repair' (RER) or 'microsatellite instability' phenotype that is associated with mutations of most of the genes associated with HNPCC. This phenotype can be detected by analysis of paraffin-embedded tumor material. If the RER phenotype is not detected, then the more costly analysis for mutations of the HNPCC-associated genes can generally be deferred.

As with *BRCA* testing, owing to genetic heterogeneity, the absence of detection of a mutation in a gene known to be associated with HNPCC is not a guarantee that an individual will not have a mutation in another as-yet-undiscovered gene associated with hereditary colon cancer. For this reason, as with families with hereditary breast and ovarian cancer, it is important to begin testing with the youngest affected member of the kindred.

LEARNING POINTS

❖ The identification of HNPCC kindreds.
❖ Knowledge of the 'component' cancers that occur in these families.
❖ Appropriate screening and prevention options for women who are members of these kindreds.

REFERENCES

1. Amos CI, Shaw GL, Tucker MA, Hartge P, Age at onset for familial epithelial ovarian cancer. *JAMA* 1992; **268**: 1896–9.
2. Lynch HT, Fitzcommons ML, Conway TA et al, Hereditary carcinoma of the ovary and associated cancers: a study of two families. *Gynecol Oncol* 1990; **36**: 48–55.
3. Claus EB, Shildkraut JM, Thompson WD et al, The genetic attributable risk of breast and ovarian cancer. *Cancer* 1996; **77**: 2318–24.
4. Miki Y, Swenson J, Shattuck-Eidens D et al, A strong candidate for the breast and ovarian cancer susceptibility gene BRCA1. *Science* 1994; **266**: 66–71.
5. Wooster R, Bignell G, Lancaster J et al, Identification of the breast cancer susceptibility gene BRCA2. *Nature* 1995; **378**: 789–92.
6. Chai YL, Cui J, Shao N et al, The second BRCT domain of BRCA1 protein interacts with p53 and stimulates transcription from the p21 WAF1/CAP1 promoter. *Oncogene* 1999; **18**: 263–8.
7. Narod SA, Ford D, Devilee P et al, Analysis of the genetic heterogeneity in 145 families with hereditary breast/ovarian cancer. *Am J Hum Genet* 1995; **56**: 254–64.
8. Easton DF, Bishop DT, Ford D, Crockford G

and the Breast Cancer Linkage Consortium, Genetic linkage analysis in familial breast and ovarian cancer: results from 214 families. *Am J Hum Genet* 1993; **52**: 678–701.

9. Whittemore AS, Gong G, Itnyre J, Prevalence and contribution of BRCA1 mutations in breast cancer and ovarian cancer: results from three US population based case control studies of ovarian cancer. *Am J Hum Genet* 1997; **603**: 496–504.

10. Wooster R, Neuhausen SL, Mangion J et al, Localization of a breast cancer susceptibility gene, BRCA2, to chromosome 13q12–13. *Science* 1994; **265**: 2088–90.

11. Narod SA, Ford D, Eyfjord JE et al, Genetic heterogeneity of breast and ovarian cancer revisited. *Am J Hum Genet* 1995; **57**: 957–8.

12. Frank TS, Manly SA, Olopade OI et al, Sequence analysis of BRCA1 and BRCA2: correlations of mutations with family history and ovarian cancer risk. *J Clin Oncol* 1998; **16**: 2417–25.

13. Frank TS, Hereditary risk of breast and ovarian carcinoma; the role of the oncologist. *Oncologist* 1998; **3**: 403–12.

14. Ford D, Easton DF, Bishop DT et al, Breast cancer linkage consortium: risks of cancer in BRCA1 mutation carriers. *Lancet* 1994; **343**: 692–5.

15. Ford D, Easton DF, Stratton M et al, Genetic heterogeneity and penetrance analysis of the BRCA1 and BRCA2 genes in breast cancer families. *Am J Hum Genet* 1998; **62**: 678–89.

16. Struewing JP, Hartge P, Wacholder S et al, The risk of cancer associated with specific mutations of the BRCA1 and BRCA2 among Ashkenazi Jews. *N Engl J Med* 1997; **33**: 1401–8.

17. Struewing JP, Abeliovich D, Peretz T et al, The carrier frequency of the BRCA1 185delAG mutation is approximately 1% in Ashkenazi Jewish individuals. *Nature Genet* 1995; **11**: 198–200.

18. Oddoux C, Struewing JP, Clayton CM et al, The carrier frequency of the BRCA2 6174delT mutation among Ashkenazi Jewish individuals is approximately 1%. *Nature Genet* 1996; **14**: 188–90.

19. Beller U, Halle D, Carane R et al, High frequency of BRCA1 and BRCA2 germline mutations in Ashkenazi Jewish ovarian cancer patients, regardless of family history. *Gynecol Oncol* 1997; **67**: 123–6.

20. Lu KH, Camer DW, Muto MG et al, A population based study of BRCA1 and BRCA2 mutations in Jewish women with epithelial ovarian cancer. *Obstet Gynecol* 1999; **93**: 34–7.

21. Easton DF, Ford D, Bishop DT, Breast Cancer Linkage Consortium: breast and ovarian cancer incidence in BRCA1 mutation carriers. *Am J Hum Genet* 1995; **56**: 265–71.

22. Lynch HT, Hereditary ovarian cancer: heterogeneity at age of onset. *Cancer* 1993; **71**: 573–81.

23. Takahashi H, Behbakht K, McGovern PE et al, Mutation analysis of the BRCA1 gene in ovarian cancers. *Cancer Res* 1995; **55**: 2998–3002.

24. Rubin SC, Benjamin I, Behbakht K et al, Clinical and pathological features of ovarian cancer in women with germ-line mutations of BRCA1. *N Engl J Med* 1996; **335**: 1413–16.

25. Narod S, Tonin P, Lynch H et al, Histology of BRCA1 associated ovarian tumors. *Lancet* 1994; **343**: 236–7.

26. Gotlieb WH, Friedman E, Bar-Sade RB et al, Rates of Jewish ancestral mutations in BRCA1 and BRCA2 in borderline ovarian tumors. *J Natl Cancer Inst* 1998; **90**: 995–1000.

27. Johannsson OT, Ranstam J, Borg A, Olsson H, Survival of BRCA1 breast and ovarian cancer patients: a population based study from southern Sweden. *J Clin Oncol* 1998; **16**: 397–404.

28. Husain A, He G, Venkatramen ES, Spriggs DR, BRCA1 up-regulation is associated with repair mediated resistance to *cis*-diamminedichloroplatinum(II). *Cancer Res* 1998; **58**: 1120–3.

29. Lerman C, Hughes C, Lemon SJ et al, What you don't know can hurt you: adverse psychologic effects in members of BRCA1 linked and BRCA2 linked families who decline genetic

testing. *J Clin Oncol* 1998; **16**: 1650–4.

30. Burke W, Daly M, Garber J et al, Recommendations for follow-up care of individuals with an inherited predisposition to cancer. II. BRCA1 and BRCA2. *JAMA* 1997; **277**: 997–1003.

31. Jacobs I, Bast RC, The Ca125 tumor associated antigen. *Hum Reprod* 1989; **4**: 1–12.

32. Muto MG, Ramer DW, Brown DL et al, Screening for ovarian cancer: the preliminary experience of a familial ovarian cancer center. *Gynecol Oncol* 1993; **51**: 12–20.

33. Piver MS, Jishi MF, Tsukada Y, Nava G, Primary peritoneal carcinoma after prophylactic oophorectomy in women with a family history of cancer. *Cancer* 1993; **71**: 2651–5.

34. Struewing JP, Watson P, Easton DF, Prophylactic oophorectomy in inherited breast/ovarian cancer families. *J Natl Cancer Inst Monogr* 1995; **17**: 33–5.

35. Schorge JO, Muto MG, Welch WR et al, Molecular evidence for multifocal papillary serous carcinoma of the peritoneum in patients with germline BRCA1 mutations. *J Natl Cancer Inst* 1998; **90**: 841–5.

36. Gross TP, Schlessman JJ, The estimated effect of oral contraceptive use on the cumulative risk of epithelial ovarian cancer. *Obstet Gynecol* 1994; **83**: 419–24.

37. Narod SA, Risch H, Moslehi R et al, Oral contraceptives and the risk of hereditary ovarian cancer. *N Engl J Med* 1998; **339**: 424–8.

38. Ursin G, Hendersen BE, Haile RW et al, Does oral contraceptive use increase the risk of breast cancer in women with BRCA1/BRCA2 mutations more than other women? *Cancer Res* 1997; **57**: 3678–81.

39. Rodriquez-Bigas MA, Boland CR, Hamilton SR et al, A National Cancer Institute Workshop on Hereditary Nonpolyposis Colorectal Cancer Syndrome: meeting highlights and Bethesda guidelines. *J Natl Cancer Inst* 1997; **89**: 1758–62.

40. Vasen HF, Mecklin JP, Khan PM, Lynch HT, The International Collaborative Group on Hereditary Nonpolyposis Colorectal Cancer (ICG–HNPCC). *Dis Colon Rectum* 1991; **34**: 424–5.

41. Watson P, Lynch HT, Extracolonic cancer in hereditary nonpolyposis colorectal cancer. *Cancer* 1993; **71**: 677–85.

42. Peltomaki P, Vasen HFA, International Collaborative Group on Hereditary Nonpolyposis Colorectal Cancer, Mutations predisposing to hereditary nonpolyposis colorectal cancer: database and results of a collaborative study. *Gastroenterology* 1997; **113**: 1146–58.

43. Vasen HFA, Winjen JT, Menko FH et al, Cancer risk in families with hereditary nonpolyposis colorectal cancer diagnosed by mutation analysis. *Gastroenterology* 1996; **110**: 1020–7 (Erratum: 1996; **111**: 1402).

44. Lynch HT, Smyrk TC, Hereditary nonpolyposis colorectal cancer (Lynch syndrome): an updated review. *Cancer* 1996; **78**: 1149–67.

45. Wijnen J, Khan PM, Vasen H et al, Hereditary nonpolyposis colorectal cancer families not complying with the Amsterdam criteria show extremely low frequency of mismatch repair mutations. *Am J Hum Genet* 1997; **61**: 329–35.

18

Living with ovarian cancer

Andrea B Hamilton

INTRODUCTION

Ovarian cancer presents circumstances that are particularly challenging to patients and their families. The disease represents a significant threat to mortality, the chances of recurrence are high, and episodic treatments are required to control tumor growth. Psychological sequelae, including but not limited to hopelessness, anticipatory anxiety, concerns about familial inheritance of the disease, loss of femininity, and sexual dysfunction, affect women as they proceed through phases of diagnosis, treatment, and recurrence. Not only is ovarian cancer a life-threatening challenge to those who have received a diagnosis, but it presents a threat to healthy family members who may be at increased risk of developing the disease owing to genetic factors. Physicians often encounter the patient who seeks treatment and the family member who seeks advice on surveillance options and prophylactic care. The two case reports presented here describe each of these scenarios, and provide recommendations for management of the psychological distress inherent to these conditions.

CASE HISTORY 1

A 36-year-old married woman with one child and a strong family history of breast and ovarian cancer was referred to an ovarian cancer surveillance program. She was highly anxious upon presenting for her initial screening evaluation. She had been unable to sleep the night before, and had been experiencing panic attacks. She continued to grieve for the loss of her sister, who had died of ovarian cancer several months previously. Feelings of guilt and helplessness, associated with her sister's death, interfered with her ability to concentrate at work and enjoy her life. She had become preoccupied with thoughts of dying of ovarian cancer. She had multiple questions and concerns. She and her husband planned to have another child, but she wondered whether she should have her ovaries and her breasts removed prophylactically. Should she have genetic testing? Should she explore alternative fertility options?

After the full range of risks and benefits of prophylactic surgery had been explained to the patient, she was referred to a genetic counselor and a consulting psychologist. She was diagnosed as having Panic Disorder, and began a course of anxiolytic and antidepressant therapy. In addition, she received weekly psychological counseling. After five weeks, her mood symptoms improved significantly. She remained in counseling to explore the personal consequences and benefits of genetic testing and prophylactic surgical procedures. She decided against genetic testing, because she believed that this information would not provide a substantial benefit, and she was worried about the potential negative impact this could have on her insurance coverage. She remained uncertain about prophylactic surgery, however. She continued to feel that cancer was a constant threat, and she became increasingly hypervigilant of all body aches and pains. After a careful review of the risks and benefits of prophylactic surgery, she decided to forgo the procedure until she had spoken to others who had had this experience. She also wanted more information about fertility options should she have her ovaries removed. She was referred to a fertility specialist to gather this information. She complied with her cancer surveillance program, and noted an acute increase in anxiety during the month of her scheduled screening visits. She learned to anticipate these periods, and prepared for them by limiting the stress in her life and practicing relaxation techniques on a daily basis during this period. After her second negative screening result, she became less focused on prophylactic surgery, and decided to pursue having a child naturally.

Are anxiety and or depression associated with screening programs for women with a family history?

Mutations of the *BRCA1* and *BRCA2* genes have recently been found to increase the lifetime risk of developing ovarian cancer to anywhere from 26% to 85%, depending upon the precise genetic factors involved.[1] As a result, recommendations for ovarian cancer surveillance for those at familial risk or genetic risk have been proposed by the Cancer Genetics Studies Consortium and the National Human Genome Research Institute.[2] Surveillance protocols typically include annual or biannual pelvic examinations, serum CA125 measurements, and transvaginal ultrasound.[3,4] These procedures may detect the disease at early stages, and, therefore, increase the chances of cure. The medical benefits versus the costs of such screening programs have yet to be defined, however. Because the screening process itself can be stressful, and is performed on a psychologically vulnerable population, the importance of assessing its potential risks and benefits to quality of life must be prioritized.

Women who attend ovarian cancer screening programs have higher rates of depression and anxiety than are found in the general population.[5] One study documented a 30% rate for clinical depression, which is six times greater than the prevalence of depression among women in community samples.[6] Screening centers seem to attract women with high levels of anxiety and depression, who may be motivated by their distress to seek professional help. In a study of a large sample of women attending a screening program, Wardel[7] documented that women who opt for screening tend to overestimate their risk and worry more about developing cancer than women who do not seek out screening.

What types of women are at greatest risk for psychological problems associated with an increased risk for ovarian cancer?

Recent studies have assessed the psychological impact of screening programs. These studies have identified women who may be especially vulnerable to psychological distress during the screening process. In addition to high rates of psychiatric morbidity, women at high risk for cancer experience a broad range of psychological reactions to the screening process, based on personality type and circumstance. Personality factors have been shown to moderate the level of distress experienced upon hearing screening results.[7] Information seekers, for example, experience more distress following positive results than patients who characteristically avoid information. Optimistic patients tend to be relieved of their anxiety after a negative result, but pessimistic patients remain worried even when screening results show no evidence of malignancy.[7] A number of psychosocial factors have been found to predict psychological distress in this setting.[5] Young women who have changed fertility plans based on their risk are especially vulnerable to high levels of anxiety and depression during the screening process. Poor social support, bereavement, family stress, and concerns about familial risk also increase the risk of psychological distress. Aspects of the screening process itself contribute to distress. Anticipatory anxiety prior to examinations is very common, and is often severe. In some cases, it may interfere with screening compliance. These issues warrant further research attention.

What types of counseling programs are appropriate for women at increased risk for ovarian cancer?

The high rates of psychiatric morbidity in this population suggest a need for supportive counseling and psychiatric evaluation to be an integral part of the screening process. Early identification of women at risk for psychiatric morbidity during screening may facilitate a more positive experience for these women. Valid and reliable brief screens for symptoms of depression and anxiety in medical settings are available for this purpose.[8,9] Once identified, women with psychiatric morbidity will benefit from receiving a referral to psychological counseling. Counseling helps the patient develop adaptive coping strategies. Counseling can help patients reason through difficult treatment decisions, and assists patients and families when challenging family conflicts emerge in the setting of genetic testing.

Patients with anxiety and depression may also require more time to process information. They need reassurance from their primary physicians and members of the medical staff. They may benefit from additional interventions to improve their understanding of complex medical issues. Medical staff can help by sitting down with patients when providing important information and encouraging patients to take notes and ask questions when they do not understand. Information presented in a slow, organized manner with the addition of simple visual aids (e.g. genograms), when appropriate, is more likely to be processed accurately and retained. After information is provided, it is important for the health professional to assess whether the patient has processed the information accurately. The health professional may state, for example, 'I know I have given you a lot of information, some of it may sound complicated. Based on what I have told you, what is your understanding of your situation?' Misunderstandings can be easily identified by medical staff when the health professional listens to the patient repeat information back to them in the patient's own words. Frequent educational sessions with genetic counselors or other medical staff may be necessary to clarify questions that emerge as the patient continues to process information after leaving the office. Further research is needed to help identify specific interventions that help patients cope with the multiple stress factors that arise in the context of living with the knowledge of being at high risk for developing ovarian cancer.

LEARNING POINTS

❈ Women with a family history of ovarian cancer are at high risk for anxiety and depression.

❈ Women benefit from receiving multimodal counseling, including genetic counseling, fertility counseling, and psychological counseling, in conjunction with disease screening protocols.

❖ Early identification of women in need of psychological counseling is important. This will prevent crises and facilitate decision-making and adaptive coping.

❖ Young women, women with a past history of psychiatric disorder, women who are facing difficult fertility decisions, and women with family/social stresses in addition to cancer-related concerns are at the greatest risk for psychological distress.

❖ The optimal treatment of moderate to severe symptoms of depression and anxiety in this population often includes psychotropic medication and psychotherapy.

❖ The long-term risk–benefit ratio incurred from ovarian cancer surveillance has yet to be determined, and warrants research attention.

❖ Specific psychological interventions aimed at improving the quality of life of women at high risk should be implemented and assessed for efficacy.

CASE HISTORY 2

A 58-year-old woman with ovarian cancer, initially diagnosed at stage IIIC, had recently been diagnosed with her first localized recurrence. She had undergone a hysterectomy and oophorectomy at age 56, which was followed by six cycles of carboplatin and paclitaxel therapy and second-look surgery, which was negative. She had been free of disease for 12 months. Fears of recurrence and fatigue – quite severe at the completion of chemotherapy – gradually waned. She and her husband had retired, and they were able to travel extensively, something they had always wanted to do but had never had the time. After her recurrence was confirmed, her mood deteriorated and she began to feel like a failure. She stopped planning for the future. She began to ruminate about death and loss of functioning. She felt

that she had let her husband, her family, and her oncologist down. She presented for her first chemotherapy treatment feeling hopeless and helplessly unmotivated. Her oncologist noted this to be a stark contrast to how she coped with her initial treatment, when she rallied him to help her 'beat this disease'. She reported that it was extremely difficult to meet the challenge of what she knew would be a rigorous course of chemotherapy that offered no hope for cure.

The patient and her husband received psychological counseling soon after her initial chemotherapy treatment for recurrence. Her main complaints were that she felt hopeless, out of control, and afraid of dying. Her husband expressed concerns that her negative thinking would cause her cancer to spread, and he noticed that she was withdrawing from him. They received several sessions of couples counseling, which focused on easing fears and re-establishing intimacy. They were told that negative thinking is a natural consequence of a cancer diagnosis, and research has not documented a link between negative thinking and the proliferation of disease. She was prescribed antidepressants, and she noticed a gradual improvement in her mood over several weeks. Subsequently, her depressive symptoms decreased in severity, and she experienced an increase in motivation to continue with chemotherapy. In counseling sessions, she developed a repertoire of distracting activities that she could rely on to block distressing thoughts of death as they emerged. She replaced thoughts of dying with thoughts concerning aspects of life over which she maintained control. Mild exercise, attending ovarian cancer advocacy groups, and taking walks with her husband were pleasurable, distracting activities that would help her reconnect to what she called her 'living self'. The couple were encouraged to communicate openly about how to meet each other's sexual needs and desire for intimacy. Distressing thoughts of death never disappeared, but they were 'turned down' to the point where she felt calm and in control of her life. The meaning of recurrent ovarian cancer was gradually re-defined. It was no longer a 'death sentence' but a chronic illness with episodic flare-ups that required intermittent treatment or maintenance therapy. She gradually began to feel as if she was able to face the future, despite her cancer. She and her husband began to plan activities again, but tailored them to her reduced endurance. They no longer took long vacations, but they planned small trips that required less effort. They went out to dinner and to the movies, and occasionally entertained friends. She maintained her antidepressant therapy, and discontinued psychotherapy after 12 sessions. She and her husband required episodic psychological consultation, thereafter, during periods of increased stress. They were able to maintain a satisfying level of activity and relationship intimacy, which helped them in coping with the uncertainty of the future.

Are there different patterns of psychological distress at diagnosis and at the time of recurrence of ovarian cancer?

Most women, upon hearing that they have ovarian cancer, go through a process of adaptation to crisis that begins with a period of despair and helplessness lasting for several weeks.[10,11] The initial response manifests in an acute fear of death, accompanied by intermittent tearfulness, anxiety, depressed mood, insomnia, and dissociation. Cancer patients show enormous resilience in the face of diagnosis, however. Though there is tremendous variability in patients' trajectory of adaptation, most women gradually adjust to their diagnosis over a period of several months.[12,13] Making treatment decisions usually facilitates coping, and moves patients out of this helpless state of mind. Most patients begin to utilize a healthy form of denial at this time, which allows them to replace their fears with the belief that the treatment will be successful. This period of adjustment usually lasts from several weeks to

several months, depending on the individual characteristics of the patient and the severity of the disease at diagnosis.

When the disease recurs, however, women experience more severe emotional distress than was experienced initially, and a longer period of adjustment is required. Research has shown that progression of ovarian cancer can be devastating to psychological well-being and quality of life.[14] In his study of advanced-stage ovarian cancer patients, Guidozzi found that patients with disease recurrence experienced a progressive deterioration of quality of life in areas of physical activity, daily living, health, outlook, and sexual activity. At this phase, there is a need to adapt to new goals of treatment and a shortened life-expectancy. The objective is no longer curing the disease but limiting the spread of cancer. Many women report that they feel reassured by hearing that there are several therapeutic options to try at this point. This gives them hope and assures them that their oncologist will not abandon them because their disease has recurred. At the same time, patients attempt to come to terms with the probability that they will die of their disease within months to years. Maintaining a satisfying quality of life in the face of severe existential crisis requires the ability to distract oneself from distressing thoughts of death and illness. This is impossible when symptoms of psychological distress or physical pain are severe. Therefore, the primary goal in helping women adjust to a disease recurrence is to establish adequate symptom relief.

Management of symptoms to reduce psychological distress

Women undergoing chemotherapy for ovarian cancer experience high rates of anxiety and depression,[14–16] physical discomfort,[16] and functional disability.[17] The management of acute psychological distress and physical pain is the primary goal in helping women adjust to their disease. Episodes of psychological distress will wax and wane in intensity over the course of the disease, and can be triggered by an increase in physical symptoms, side-effects of treatment, or psychosocial/existential concerns (see the discussion below).

Pain and physical discomfort are major contributors to treatment-related psychological distress.[17] While pain is reduced somewhat by cytoreductive surgery, over 40% of women with advanced-stage disease who are on treatment experience moderate to severe pain.[16] Pain related to peripheral neuropathy, a common side-effect of ovarian cancer chemotherapy regimens, is a frequently reported source of physical discomfort and disability. In addition to pain, fatigue, insomnia, and impaired role performance contribute significantly to decreased quality of life. Fortunately, patients report that pain responds to opiate and adjuvant analgesia. Adequate analgesia should result in significant improvements in level of distress and functional ability. Useful guidelines for achieving adequate management of cancer pain are available.[18]

The surgical procedures and chemotherapy regimens used to treat ovarian cancer are often accompanied by distressing sequelae that warrant attention. Management of these treatment-related side-effects is crucial to maintaining quality of life. Two treatment-related causes of distress are worth mentioning here: menopausal symptoms and steroid-induced mood dysregulation. For women who are pre- or perimenopausal before oophorectomy, the resulting abrupt depletion of estrogen and androgens occurring with the loss of ovarian function places these women at increased risk of depression, memory loss, and sexual dysfunction.[19] Women who have already reached menopause when they undergo oophorectomy are subject to an exacerbation of menopausal symptoms.

Hormone replacement therapy (HRT) is an effective means of enhancing quality of life after menopause. However, HRT is a controversial option for women with ovarian cancer.[2] Women are often concerned about the risk of developing breast cancer associated with HRT. Its safety with women who have ovarian cancer is not known. Women who receive estrogen replacement therapy (ERT) after oophorectomies have shown improvements in mood, memory function, and sexual functioning, and reduction in discomfort associated with hot flashes. The benefits of ERT, which include the prevention of cardiovascular disease and osteoporosis along with maintaining vaginal health, are also important factors to weigh in the decision-making process. There is evidence that HRT improves response to antidepressant therapy in postmenopausal depression.[20,21] The benefits of low-dose androgen and progesterone therapy alone or in combination with ERT to improve mood and sexual dysfunction in postmenopausal women have been documented.[20]

Because the safe and effective use of hormonal therapies for symptom relief in the ovarian cancer population has yet to be documented, the risks and benefits to the individual patient warrant careful review before these therapies are initiated. New methods of administering hormone replacement to decrease systemic absorption have been developed (e.g. Estring[22,23]), and may prove to be safer for women with cancer. Antidepressant and anxiolytic agents may provide adequate relief from postmenopausal emotional distress when hormone therapies are contraindicated. Low doses (12.5 mg twice daily) of the antidepressant venlafaxine have proven effective in the treatment of hot flashes, fatigue, and insomnia related to menopause in the cancer population.[24]

Mood disturbance is often a side-effect of adjuvant chemotherapy medications. Steroids, in particular, may cause mood disturbance severe enough to interfere with daily functioning. Dexamethasone, a corticosteroid given in conjunction with some chemotherapy regimens to prevent nausea and allergic reactions, has been shown to cause mood and behavioral disturbances. The biological and behavioral effects of exogenous corticosteroids have been reviewed.[25] Patients commonly report feeling irritable and restless on the days they take steroids. Most women endure mild to moderately severe symptoms without mentioning them to their oncologists. Severe symptoms such as panic attacks, crying jags, mood lability, euphoria, hypomania, or dangerous episodes of manic and psychotic behavior occur with unpredictable prevalence. The incidence of severe steroid-induced psychiatric morbidity ranges from 2% to 57%, depending upon the population studied.[25] Women, the elderly, and patients with a psychiatric history seem to be at greater risk for steroid-related mood disorders, but neither dose nor type of premorbid psychiatric problem can predict the specific behavioral response to steroids. Anxiolytic medications such as lorazepam, alprazolam, and clonazepam relieve mild to moderate anxiety, irritability, and restlessness. Neuroleptic medication is recommended for the treatment of severe mood lability, agitation, and psychosis.[26] Once symptoms become severe, psychotropic medication is needed to ensure patient safety and comfort. A psychiatric consultation is strongly indicated for these patients.

Helping patients cope with the psychological sequelae of recurrent ovarian cancer

In addition to the physiological determinants of distress discussed above, women with ovarian cancer face a number of stressful events and existential concerns, which cause them to experience increased anxiety and depressed mood. Mental health consultation is a useful way to introduce patients to behavioral interventions as means of controlling the psychological distress associated with the disease course and adjusting to changes in their lives brought on by illness. Behavioral techniques such as relaxation therapy and hypnosis can be used to distract patients from ruminative thoughts of death and illness. Patients often appreciate receiving professional support with respect to the making of wills, talking to their children about death, and preparing loved ones for a life without them. Additionally, exploring fears of death in psychotherapy can provide a context in which a patient's anxiety about future suffering can be calmed through reassurance that end-of-life pain and suffering will be treated adequately.

Psychological reactions at the time of disease recurrence can be complex. Some women experience a sense of relief, for example, having anticipated a recurrence since the cessation of primary chemotherapy.[27] Most patients report, however, that emotional distress, which had subsided during their initial disease-free period, peaks at the time of recurrence. Patients focus on issues of mortality, increased dependency, isolation, loss of control, financial concerns, body image, and concerns about relationship intimacy.

As patients approach the final weeks of a treatment course, they often experience an increase in psychological distress. By this point, most patients have come to view chemotherapy as a protective ally against disease progression. Fears of recurrence, therefore, become accentuated as patients perceive a loss of chemotherapy 'protection'. Anxiety wanes gradually as women see that their disease does not return immediately following cessation of treatment.[28] The intensity of post-treatment anxiety surprises most women, who anticipate feeling nothing but relief at the end of chemotherapy.

If the disease has been controlled by treatment, a gradual improvement in quality of life and psychological outlook has been reported to occur within the first year after treatment.[29–31]

Women continue to struggle, however, with several important post-treatment issues,[31–33] and the psychological effects of having had ovarian cancer persist, even during disease-free periods.[14] Multiple post-treatment issues have been described:[29,31,32,34,35] persistent fatigue, difficulty with self-concept, fear of recurrence, global uncertainty, and sexual dysfunction.[34,35] These are ongoing concerns for women recovering from ovarian cancer treatment. In addition, women are concerned about the risk of family members being diagnosed with the disease.

Fear associated with the uncertainty of the disease course is prominent, along with worry about death and future suffering. Because the rate of recurrence of ovarian cancer is so high, women have difficulty planning for the future, finding themselves unable to schedule future events outside the immediate future. Some are afraid to reconnect with children and partners owing to a fear of having to distance from them again when the disease recurs.

Treatment also leaves women feeling unattractive as the result of alopecia and changes in body shape and weight brought about by chemotherapy. Marked changes in appearance, particularly those brought about by steroids, cause marked disruptions in body image. Women become preoccupied with losing weight, and develop a negative self-concept. If body image problems existed before ovarian cancer, they persist and become more severe. The loss of reproductive function also forces a woman to adjust her sense of self-worth and feminine identity.

Financial losses, long-lasting side-effects such as peripheral neuropathy related to chemotherapy, and the uncertainty of recurrence add to a sense of loss of control. The sense of poor control over their disease course and daily routine leads many women to experience anticipatory anxiety prior to follow-up visits – at which a recurrence may be found by clinical examination or by changes in CA125 level. Many women begin to identify their CA125 level as the evidence of disease status. If it is low, they feel relieved and in control. They are safe to make plans and forget about their disease. If the level is elevated from prior levels, they know that the disease is back and must plan for more treatment. Unfortunately, even normal, insignificant fluctuations in CA125 level take on enormous meaning. As a result, emotional well-being may come to depend on lower CA125 values, even if these values remain in the normal range. Patients may find themselves on an 'emotional roller coaster', with ups and downs determined by the direction of serum blood levels.

The recent advent of treatments that prolong periods of disease-free survival for ovarian cancer patients has led to increased interest in assessing the psychosexual sequelae of ovarian cancer. Women often experience a long enough disease-free interval to gradually begin to refocus their energies from mortality concerns to rebuilding a sense of normal activity. Re-establishing sexual intimacy is an important part of this rehabilitation period. While studies of sexual dysfunction in the ovarian cancer population, specifically, have yet to be initiated, the incidence of sexual dysfunction after treatment for gynecological cancer has been established in studies assessing women with multiple gynecological tumor sites. Rates of sexual dysfunction in women with gynecological cancers have been found to be as high as 50%.[36] The most common sexual dysfunction experienced by gynecological cancer patients is low sexual desire. Vaginal dryness and dyspareunia are also frequently reported in women who have undergone treatment for gynecological cancer.[36] Attention toward rebuilding a satisfying sex life is important, because, when ignored, sexual problems do not improve and can have a damaging effect on the quality of a woman's relationship with her partner and her self-esteem.

In addition to the multiple painful issues that emerge during the post-treatment period, Ersek et al[31] documented some positive aspects of post-treatment survival that warrant attention. They found that women with ovarian cancer who were predominantly post treatment and free of disease reported appreciating life more, learning to live in the moment, experiencing improved relationships, enhanced appreciation of significant others, improved emotional health, and adoption of healthier lifestyles. The same patients reported continued uncertainty, fear of the future, perceived loss of control, anger, depression, and anxiety. Even though many women move forward with their lives after ovarian cancer, physical symptoms, psychological distress, uncertainty about the future, and interpersonal challenges continue to be very much a part of their lives.

What types of psychosocial intervention are appropriate?

Psychological interventions can facilitate adjustment and provide relief of psychological distress. Brief supportive psychotherapy provided in a group or individual setting can decrease psychological distress and prevent future treatment-related psychosocial morbidity. Two psychological intervention studies show effective relief of symptoms of psychological distress with brief treatment modalities. In a three-arm experimental design, Cain et al[12] evaluated a psychosocial support intervention for women with gynecological cancer. Ovarian cancer patients comprised 25% of the sample. Study participants received eight weeks of either group or individual structured 'thematic' counseling sessions, during which women shared information, expressed feelings, and resolved problems in areas of particular concern, such as body image, sexuality, diet, and exercise. Compared with a control group, women in the individual and group

therapy arms of the study acknowledged significant decreases in levels of anxiety and depression at two weeks and six months after the cessation of treatment. Another study with a similar population of patients assessed the efficacy of a four-session individual psychotherapy intervention in improving adjustment to diagnosis.[13] Patients received counseling immediately after initial cytoreductive surgery. Sessions focused on patient education and verbalization of feelings. Issues of femininity, self-esteem, and interpersonal relationships were emphasized in two of the sessions. Women who received the intervention reported a more positive self-image and better sexual functioning three months after treatment compared with a control group.

At what point is referral to a mental health care professional appropriate?

Receiving a referral to a mental health practitioner early in the treatment course reassures women that their psychological needs are important and will be addressed as an integral part of their medical care. Often, just one or two sessions of supportive, problem-focused psychotherapy can be of considerable help. During these sessions, it is useful to help patients anticipate problems, plan, problem-solve, identify distraction techniques and self-soothing activities, and enhance their appreciation of life 'in the moment'.

Creating barriers to social isolation is extremely important at this time, particularly for women. Many women resist shifting into the dependent role imposed by illness, as most struggle to maintain roles as caregivers in order to preserve important connections to children and others who depend on them. Many women report that they are frustrated by the need to take care of others while they are sick, but have trouble asking significant others for help. In order to meet the psychological and physical challenges brought on by ovarian cancer, however, women need to be able to taper some of their caregiving responsibilities, identify the reliable caregivers in their social support network, and rely on them for help when needed.

The importance of practical help cannot be overestimated.[37] One woman reported that having a friend bring meals to the house during the days after chemotherapy, for example, was just as important as having friends with whom she was able to share her emotional distress. It is also helpful for the patient to identify more than one individual who can help. Delegating responsibilities to several reliable significant others decreases the possibility that one friend will be overburdened by the patient's needs for emotional and practical support. Unfortunately, many friendships do not survive the initial phases of ovarian cancer because of the significant anxiety that the cancer evokes in others. As a result, many patients find some friends distancing themselves at the time when they are most needed. Support groups with an emphasis on peer support are helpful when this occurs.

New treatments for ovarian cancer have redefined the disease trajectory. It is now a chronic disease with recurrent episodes. Many women experience disease-free periods that last from months to years, during which they attempt to resume a normal life. Psychosocial rehabilitation is often needed during this period to control distress and help patients adapt to the multiple stress factors experienced as a result of the treatment and the disease itself. Individual psychotherapy, group therapy, or couples therapy aimed at resolving these issues is often helpful once the acute psychological distress has been adequately managed.[12,13] Psychotropic medications, particularly benzodiazepines and antidepressant medications, are often useful in limiting acute symptoms of depression and anxiety that emerge as a result of the stress of treatment.[38] Psychological support should be tailored to the patient's needs and degree of physical disability. Many women on chemotherapy, for example, benefit from brief face-to-face contact on the days they receive their treatment, followed by regular telephone sessions in between visits to the hospital. The majority of patients are too weak to attend weekly sessions of individual or group psychotherapy during this time.

LEARNING POINTS

❊ Women with ovarian cancer are most vulnerable to psychological distress after a disease recurrence.

❊ The management of acute psychological distress and physical pain are the primary goals in helping women adjust to their disease.

❊ Reassurance from her oncologist that a recurrence is not a 'death sentence' generates hope and motivation to continue therapy.

❊ Women experiencing a disease recurrence feel more hopeful when they receive information about all the treatments available – for example, what options are available if the current treatment is not effective.

❊ Anxiolytics, antidepressants, and hormone replacement therapy can be extremely helpful in treating anxiety, depression, fatigue, and sexual dysfunction, if not medically contraindicated.

❊ Referrals to mental health professionals are important, particularly for those suffering with moderate to severe symptoms of distress.

❊ Counseling is most effective when provided in a modality that suits the patient's particular life situation. Therapy can be provided in individual, couple, or group modalities, and can be ongoing or episodic, depending upon the needs of the patient.

REFERENCES

1. Ford D, Easton DF, Bishop DT et al, and the Breast Cancer Linkage Consortium, Risks of cancer in BRCA1 mutation carriers. *Lancet* 1994; **343**: 692–5.

2. Burke W, Daly M, Garber J et al, and the Cancer Genetics Studies Consortium, Recommendations for follow-up care of individuals with an inherited predisposition to cancer II. BRCA1 and BRCA2. *JAMA* 1997; **277**: 997–1003.

3. Bourne TH, Campbell S, Reynolds KM et al, Screening for early familial ovarian cancer with transvaginal ultrasonography and colour blood flow imaging. *BMJ* 1993; **306**: 1025–9.

4. Kramer BS, Gohagan J, Prorok PC, Smart C, A National Cancer Institute-sponsored screening trial for prostatic, lung, colorectal, and ovarian cancers. *Cancer* 1993; **71**: 589–93.

5. Robinson GE, Rosen BP, Bradley LN et al, Psychological impact of screening for familial ovarian cancer: reactions to initial assessment. *Gynecol Oncol* 1997; **65**: 197–205.

6. Blazer DG, Kessler RC, McGonagle KA, Swartz MS, The prevalence and distribution of major depression in a natural community sample: the national comorbidity survey. *Am J Psychiatry* 1994; **151**: 979–86.

7. Wardel J, Women at risk of ovarian cancer. *J Natl Cancer Inst Monogr* 1995; **17**: 81–5.

8. Aylard PR, Gooding JH, McKenna PJ, Snaith RP, A validation study of three anxiety and depression self-assessment scales. *J Psychosom Res* 1987; **31**: 261–8.

9. Zigmond AS, Snaith RP, The Hospital Anxiety and Depression Scale. *Acta Psychiatr Scand* 1983; **67**: 361–70.

10. Weisman AD, Worden JW, The existential plight in cancer: significance of the first 100 days. *Int J Psychiatry Med* 1976; **7**: 1–15.

11. Weisman AD, A model for psychosocial phasing in cancer. *Gen Hosp Psychiatry* 1979; **3**: 187–95.

12. Cain EN, Kohorn EI, Quinlan DM et al, Psychosocial benefits of a cancer support group. *Cancer* 1986; **57**: 183–9.

13. Capone MA, Good RS, Westie KS, Jacobson AF, Psychosocial rehabilitation of gynecologic oncology patients. *Arch Phys Med Rehabil* 1980; **61**: 128–32.

14. Guidozzi F, Living with ovarian cancer. *Gynecol Oncol* 1993; **50**: 202–7.

15. Kornblith AB, Thaler HT, Wong G et al, Quality of life of women with ovarian cancer. *Gynecol Oncol* 1995; **59**: 231–42.

16. Portenoy RK, Kornblith AB, Wong G et al, Pain in ovarian cancer patients: prevalence, characteristics, and associated symptoms. *Cancer* 1994; **74**: 907–15.

17. Lancee WJ, Vachon MLS, Ghadirian P et al, The impact of pain and impaired role performance on distress in persons with cancer. *Can J Psychiatry* 1994; **39**: 617–22.

18. Agency for Health Care Policy and Research, *Management of Cancer Pain*. Washington, DC: US Department of Health and Human Services, 1994.

19. Pearce J, Hawton K, Blake F, Psychological and sexual symptoms associated with the menopause and the effects of hormone replacement therapy. *Br J Psychiatr* 1995; **167**: 163–73.

20. Zweifel JE, O'Brein WH, A meta-analysis of the effect of hormone replacement therapy upon depressed mood. *Psychoneuroendocrinology* 1997; **22**: 189–212.

21. Schneider LS, Small GW, Hamilton SH et al, Estrogen replacement and response to fluoxetine in a multicenter geriatric depression trial. *Am J Geriatric Psychiatry* 1997; **5**: 97–106.

22. Barensten R, van de Weijer PH, Schram JH, Continuous low dose estradiol released from a vaginal ring versus vaginal cream for urogenital atrophy. *Eur J Obstet Gynecol Repro Biol* 1997; **71**: 73–80.

23. Henriksson L, Stjernquist M, Boquist L et al, A one-year multicenter study of efficacy and safety of a continuous, low-dose, estradiol-releasing vaginal ring (Estring) in post-

menopausal women with symptoms and signs of urogenital aging. *Am J Obstet Gynecol* 1996; **174**: 85–92.

24. Loprinzi CL, Pisansky TM, Fonseca R et al, Pilot evaluation of venlafaxine hydrochloride for the therapy of hot flashes in cancer survivors. *J Clin Oncol* 1998; **16**: 2377–81.

25. Wolkowitz OM, Prospective controlled studies of the behavioral and biological effects of exogenous corticosteroids. *Psychoneuroendocrinology* 1994; **19**: 233–55.

26. Fleishman SB, Lesko LM, Breitbart W, Treatment of organic mental disorders in cancer patients. In: *Psychiatric Aspects of Symptom Management in Cancer Patients* (Breitbart W, Holland JC, eds). Washington, DC: American Psychiatric Press, 1993: 23–47.

27. Weisman AD, Worden JW, The emotional impact of recurrent cancer. *J Psychosoc Oncol* 1986; **3**: 5–16.

28. Holland JC, Clinical course of cancer. In: *The Handbook of Psychooncology: Psychological Care of the Patient with Cancer* (Holland JC, Rowland JH, eds). New York, Oxford University Press, 1989: 75–100.

29. Andersen BL, Anderson B, deProsse C, Controlled prospective longitudinal study of women with cancer: II. Psychological outcomes. *J Consult Clin Psychol* 1989; **57**: 692–7.

30. Roberts CS, Rosetti K, Cone D, Cavanagh D, Psychosocial impact of gynecologic cancer: a descriptive study. *J Psychosoc Oncol* 1992; **10**: 99–109.

31. Ersek M, Ferrell BR, Dow KH, Melancon CH, Quality of life in women with ovarian cancer. *West J Nurs Res* 1997; **19**: 334–50.

32. Auchincloss SS, After treatment: psychosocial issues in gynecologic cancer survivorship. *Cancer* 1995; **76**(Suppl): 2117–24.

33. Anderson B, Lutgendorf S, Quality of life in gynecologic cancer survivors. *CA Cancer Clin* 1997; **47**: 218–25.

34. Andersen BL, Quality of life for women with gynecologic cancer. *Curr Opin Obstet Gynecol* 1995; **7**: 69–76.

35. Andersen BL, Anderson B, deProsse C, Controlled prospective longitudinal study of women with cancer: I. Sexual functioning outcomes. *J Consult Clin Psychol* 1989; **57**: 683–91.

36. Auchincloss S, Hamilton A, Management of sexual dysfunction. In: *Clinical Oncology* (Abeloff M, Armitage J, Lichter A, Niederhuber J, eds). New York: Churchill Livingstone, 2000: 2818–44.

37. Waxler-Morrison N, Hislop TG, Mears B, Kan L, Effects of social relationships on survival for women with breast cancer: a prospective study. *Soc Sci Med* 1991; **33**: 177–83.

38. Massie MJ, Shakin MD, Management of depression and anxiety in cancer patients. In: *Psychiatric Aspects of Symptom Management in Cancer Patients* (Breitbart W, Holland JC, eds). Washington, DC: American Psychiatric Press, 1993: 1–21.

19
Palliative care

Ilora Finlay

INTRODUCTION

The late presentation of many ovarian cancers means that palliative care must begin from the time of diagnosis in patients (Figure 19.1). For the majority, the disease will progress towards death, with remissions of varying length gained by relatively toxic chemotherapy. With the blow to body image through surgery, hair loss from chemotherapy and the often-constant fears of impending death, the woman and her family may well question whether all treatments were to no avail. It is almost impossible to say precisely when patients become 'terminally ill'. It is clear when the woman is dying, but concentration on the final days or weeks of her life may ignore major issues that needed to be addressed earlier. As treatment is often of necessity only palliative,

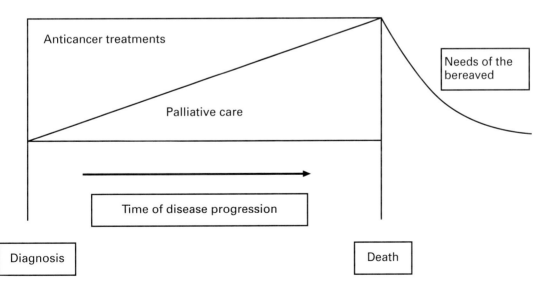

Figure 19.1
Patients' needs with time.

good symptom control and psychosocial support to the patient and family are paramount. As death approaches, specific ethical issues about cessation of anticancer treatment and the active management of emergencies can arise.

It is not uncommon for ovarian cancer to affect younger women, with all the social implications of a young mother dying. Changes that occur within a married couple facing the imminent death of one partner can be so devastating that they are unable to cope with the challenges of everyday living.[1-3]

Following magazine features on cancers, many women are increasingly aware of the genetic risk of breast cancer, and are sometimes also aware of its link with ovarian cancer. The association of ovarian cancer and breast cancer in some families makes establishment of a comprehensive family tree essential as a genetic and a social information tool.[4]

Some particular problems associated with ovarian cancer arise from the strong tendency for transcoelomic spread of tumour, which predisposes these women to bowel obstruction and ascites relatively early in the disease. Fistulation can also occur through necrosis of a metastatic deposit.

CASE HISTORY

Pat was 47 years old. For some months, she had noticed an increasing girth, and attributed it to her age. When eventually an ovarian tumour was diagnosed, she had a substantially sized carcinoma. She was devastated at the relatively matter-of-fact way that she was told the diagnosis, and drove home from the outpatient's clinic in a daze. With difficulty, she told her husband that she would need a hysterectomy and oophorectomy, but did not even recall the information she had been given about the extent of surgery.

Communication

Informing the patient of the initial diagnosis involves breaking bad news and sets the foundation for all future communication about the illness and its management. Recommended tactics for doing this include ensuring that news is broken in a quiet, comfortable, private location with enough uninterrupted time available with the patient.[5] There are no robust comparative trials, but recommended non-verbal strategies include face-to-face eye contact without physical barriers, such as a desk, between the doctor and patient. Although the patient may wish someone present who provides support, this is not always possible to set up without in the process creating a great deal of alarm. It can be helpful to explore the woman's own ideas of what is happening, perhaps even giving a 'warning' of the bad news, before imparting new information.

In a study of hospice patients, the need to maintain realistic hope was cited as very important in helping patients cope with their situation.[6] Patients can react and express emotion in very different ways, with a bland non-expressive exterior representing frozen shock rather than calm coping.

At the end of a consultation, it is helpful to briefly summarize the discussion, allow for questions and agree the proposed management plan with the patient herself. Although it may seem obvious, a warm, caring, empathic attitude by the physician is essential in demonstrating respect for the patient – so many patient complaints relate to an uncaring affect by the doctor. Language used should be straightforward, avoiding euphemisms and technical or medical jargon. Some patients will not take in the news given to them, and will need to revisit it several times as a part of the process of coming to terms with the situation.

Pat had extensive surgery, from which she appeared to make a recovery, but many changes occurred that were not easily perceived by those around.

She became quite depressed; her husband was tense and busied himself with the practicalities of running the household. Her 15-year-old son's schoolwork deteriorated rapidly, and he spent increasing amounts of time lounging around at home, avoiding going out with his friends and abandoning his football activities. Her 8-year-old daughter, Kim, woke several times a night, and often came through to her parents' room.

Pat's husband, Mike, feared to show affection for fear of his own emotional response, and they ceased any sexual relationships from the time of her surgery, using Kim's frequent night-time visits as their excuse to each other.

The family

In the context of a busy clinical service, it can be easy to overlook the needs of family, particularly the children, the woman's own parents if they are still alive, her siblings and even her grandchildren. There is no easy time to discuss what or how to 'tell the children', who are often forgotten by default. The children in a family, even the very young,[7] are usually very observant and rapidly become aware of what is happening. They rarely vocalize their feelings, may feel excluded from the family and may blame themselves for their mother's illness – e.g. 'if only I hadn't been naughty'. Meanwhile, parents, wanting to spare the child distress, avoid telling the child what is wrong. Parents need help to plan telling the children, as well as what to tell the child's school or college. It is easier to do these things in stages, stating the diagnosis and that treatment aims at 'getting better'; later informing that things are not going well, and speaking of death when it is imminent.

The child who is excluded from some knowledge of the illness will feel mistrustful, and may feel blamed and punished for the illness. Younger children are very likely to overhear conversations in the house or have remarks from classmates in the playground who have overheard adult conversations. Older children and adolescents may question what is being done and have views and fears related to decisions being taken; they need to be allowed to voice their opinions and be included in discussions. Adolescents are often aware of biomedical ethics, living wills and euthanasia; they also have particular difficulties about changes in the body image of the person they love, since they are so aware themselves about their own body image.[8]

Both children and adults may have difficulty in showing affection; such situations cause the patient great hurt and embarrassment, but are rarely spoken of unless given specific opportunities. People can have a range of emotions, including guilt and repulsion about the cancer, which can leave the woman feeling shunned by friends.

Marital relationships

Although relatively little has been written about sexual dysfunction following pelvic surgery, about 75% of women who have undergone radical pelvic surgery experience sexual problems,[9,10] with young single women a particularly vulnerable group. Although a stable marital relationship prior to the diagnosis of cancer helps the woman to cope, many women are strongly affected by their loss of fertility, disfigurement, depression and anxiety about their desirability as a sexual partner.[9]

In addition to problems associated with loss of fertility, sexual dysfunction and altered body image, other relationship problems occur as couples face death.[1] Couples cope by balancing their lives between the practicalities of daily living and the fears of what lies ahead, coping by making the illness a background rather than a foreground issue.

Changes in dynamics occur between couples who face death. Among them, about half have anxiety and/or depression, usually as a result of failure to cope with specific difficulties.[3] Relatives have very specific needs related to the process of loss and their anticipatory grief in contemplating the final parting through the woman's death. There is evidence of severe family anxiety existing in the relatives of terminally ill patients.[11] This anxiety may be expressed as anger, particularly towards health-care professionals, with relatives expressing a mistrust of clinical decisions.[12]

Spirituality

The term 'spiritual' embraces the essence of what it means to be human; thus holistic care requires open and honest attention to the spirituality of each patient. By remaining alert to the patient's turmoil, sensing her desire to open up, and creating an atmosphere of honest communication, the woman is helped to express her needs and to come to terms with progressing disease.[13] Debate over spiritual needs suggests that everyone has a spiritual dimension, entailing a search for meaning.[14]

After a period of stability following chemotherapy, Pat developed abdominal pain and increasing girth due to ascites.

After starting on morphine, she was constipated and had intermittent episodes of colic and nausea. Her appetite waned, and she felt increasingly weak. Her limbs became thinner, and she developed some leg oedema.

Symptom control

Accurate diagnosis of the cause of symptoms is the key to establishing symptom control. Poor symptom control is usually due to a failure in the process of diagnosis or the use of medications that are not based on applied pharmacology.

Pain

Pain is a complex phenomenon, caused by a noxious stimulus. The overall perception of pain is influenced by distress from other physical symptoms, and emotional, social or spiritual anguish (Figure 19.2).[15] Possibly the most potent modifier is fear, with irrational fears unvoiced unless directly sought by the attending professional.[13,16]

Patients may carry their guilt feeling about past life events, or their unresolved angers and griefs, as unexpressed burdens, which lower their pain threshold. Without sensitive communication skills to explore the patient's concerns and fears, the frightened or guilt-ridden patient may be unable to have her distress relieved.[16] Depression is known to occur in about 20% of cancer patients, is often undiagnosed, and undermines the woman's ability to cope.

A useful mnemonic for diagnosing the type of pain is PQRST (see Table 19.1), with a verbal (none/mild/moderate/severe/excruciating) or mnemonic (0–10) scale or pain impact score (see Table 19.2) to assess severity and evaluate ongoing treatment response.[17–19] Pain responses

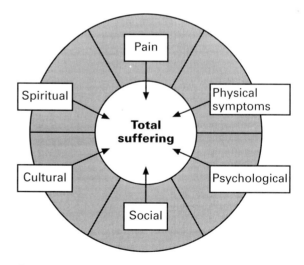

Figure 19.2
The components of suffering (after Woodruff[15]).

Table 19.1   Assessing pain: pain descriptors to help diagnose the cause of the pain (with examples)

P   **precipitating/relieving factors** (pain on movement from vertebral instability)

Q   **quality** (burning pain in area of sensory loss in neuropathic pain)

R   **radiation** (radicular thoracic pain as a pointer to spinal cord compression)

S   **severity** (scored from 0 to 10)

T   **time factors** (headache of raised intracranial pressure in the morning)

from an intact nervous system, when the pain is of recent onset, differ greatly from responses seen following protracted pain or when there is a degree of neuronal damage, as in neuropathic pain.

The use of analgesics according to the World Health Organization (WHO) guidelines,[20] with or without adjuvant drugs or co-analgesics, has been shown to adequately control pain in about 95% of the patients with cancer pain. Analgesic titration should begin with group 1 analgesics

(Figure 19.3), given regularly, and then adding a group 2 weak opioid analgesic, again taken regularly. If analgesia is incomplete, a strong opioid should not be withheld.[21] It is worth giving non-opioids in conjunction with opioids; their different modes of action mean they have an additive effect; of the non-opioids, paracetamol can be given with a non-steroidal anti-inflammatory drug (NSAID) to minimize the dose and hence lower the risk of adverse effects.

Morphine

Oral morphine is usually the drug of choice for those patients who can swallow. It should be started at a dose of about 5–10 mg 4-hourly regularly and reassessed every 24 hours. Dose increments of 30% should be used until pain is controlled. The duration of action of morphine means that 4-hourly dosing is required to maintain pain control; longer dose intervals will sentence the patient to repeated breakthrough pain. There is no maximum dose of morphine, although most pains are controlled by doses of about 30–100 mg of oral morphine 4-hourly (equivalent to 60–200 mg of diamorphine per 24 hours in a continuous infusion). When higher doses are required, but good analgesia is not

Table 19.2   The palliative care assessment tool[19]

Question to patient	Answer	Score
Q1: Do you have pain?	No	0
	Yes → Q2	
Q2: Does it affect your daily life?	No	1
	Yes → Q3	
Q3: Does it dominate your daily life?	No	2
	Yes	3

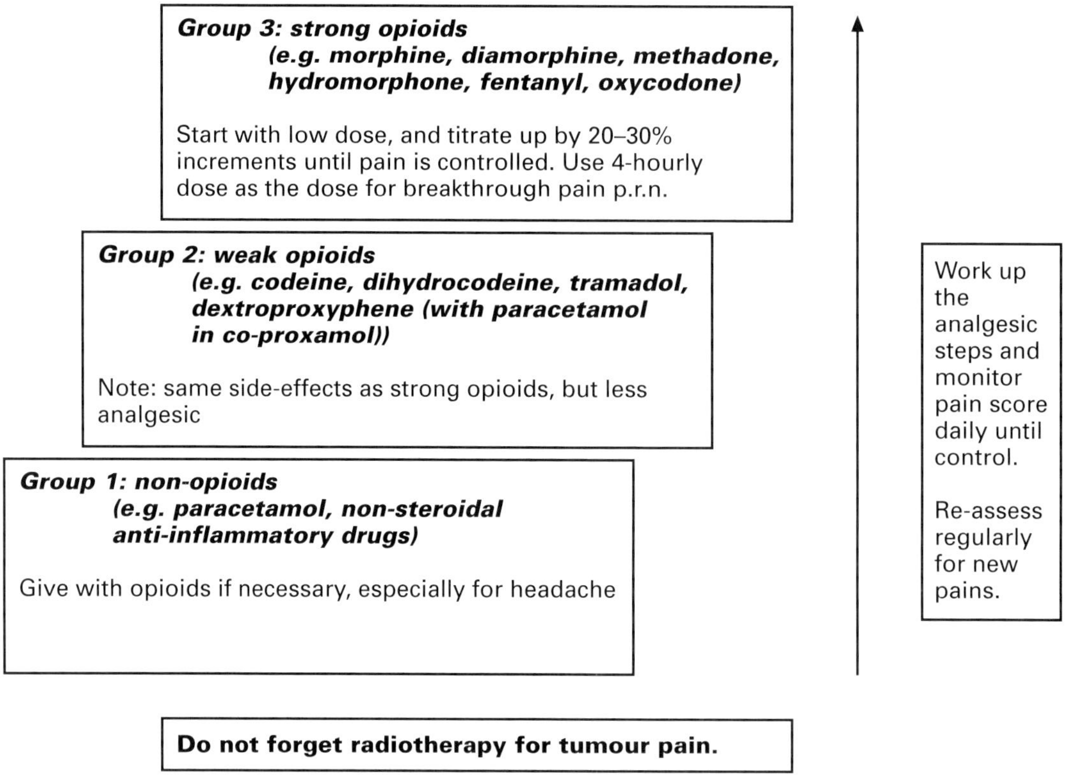

Group 3: strong opioids
        (e.g. morphine, diamorphine, methadone,
        hydromorphone, fentanyl, oxycodone)

Start with low dose, and titrate up by 20–30%
increments until pain is controlled. Use 4-hourly
dose as the dose for breakthrough pain p.r.n.

Group 2: weak opioids
        (e.g. codeine, dihydrocodeine, tramadol,
        dextroproxyphene (with paracetamol
        in co-proxamol))

Note: same side-effects as strong opioids, but less
analgesic

Group 1: non-opioids
        (e.g. paracetamol, non-steroidal
        anti-inflammatory drugs)

Give with opioids if necessary, especially for headache

Work up
the
analgesic
steps and
monitor
pain score
daily until
control.

Re-assess
regularly
for new
pains.

Do not forget radiotherapy for tumour pain.

Figure 19.3
Titrating analgesics.

achieved, it is likely that the pain is partly opioid-resistant and then requires other strategies. If the patient experiences repeated breakthrough pain, analgesic requirements are likely to escalate, as the pain experience is continually reinforced.

Once pain control has been achieved, the patient can change to a modified-release morphine preparation formulated to last either 12 hours or 24 hours. Importantly, the patient may still require additional 4-hourly normal-release doses for episodes of breakthrough pain.

There is no evidence that opioids given for cancer pain cause tolerance or addiction, or that they shorten life.[22] However, constipation is a serious side-effect in almost all patients on opioids, so a laxative must be prescribed concurrently.[23]

In bowel obstruction, the decreased peristalsis that occurs with morphine can be useful in the management of colic.

Fentanyl

The side-effects of sedation and constipation are significantly less with fentanyl than with morphine, making it particularly useful for long-term use in this group of patients, who are at such high risk of bowel obstruction. It is active at μ-1 opioid receptors, and has a short half-life and no active metabolite, making it relatively safe in renal failure. As it is less sedative than morphine, the first sign of toxicity may be slowing of the respiratory rate.[24]

Patients should have their analgesic requirement determined by titration on morphine and then can be switched to the equivalent transdermal fentanyl patch. The fentanyl is absorbed via a rate-limiting membrane and, being very lipophilic, forms a depot in subcutaneous tissues before being absorbed into the systemic circulation. After the first application of a patch, absorption takes about 12 hours until a steady-state blood level is reached. Therefore the last dose of regular 4-hourly morphine should be given as the patch is initially applied to avoid breakthrough pain occurring. Each patch lasts 72 hours. When a patch is removed, residual fentanyl from the subcutaneous depot is released into the systemic circulation for about 16 hours.

Inflammation and pain

Bone pain and pain in inflamed tissue may respond well to NSAIDs, since prostaglandins are probably involved in the mediation of the pain from the involved bone. In those also on steroids, a gastroprotective agent such as misoprostol or omeprazole should be given prophylactically to avoid gastrointestinal problems. The more potent NSAIDs should be used for pain, such as piroxicam, naproxen 500 mg b.d. or diclofenac 150 mg/day in divided doses.

Ketorolac, a potent NSAID with strong analgesic activity, can be given with opioids.[25] Its use for longer than five days carries a significantly increased risk of gastrointestinal bleeding.

Other opioids

Shorter-acting opioids such as pethidine are of no use in long-term pain control. Also, pethidine is metabolized to norpethidine, a central nervous system irritant, which accumulates and can cause convulsions.

Oxycodone, pharmacologically similar to morphine,[26] is useful for those fearful of morphine per se.

Hydromorphone is a synthetic opioid with morphine-like receptor affinity[27] but less dependence on renal excretion.

Drugs such as ketamine (a non-opioid) and methadone have high N-methyl-D-aspartate (NMDA) receptor affinity and may be useful in difficult neuropathic pain.[28–30] They should only be used under specialist palliative care supervision.

Neuropathic pain

Key diagnostic criteria for neuropathic pain include allodynia,[31] disordered temperature sensation, and a sensation of numb or burning pain. Allodynia is the perception of pain in response to a non-painful stimulus, such as stroking the skin.[32] This is similar to but different from hyperpathia, which is an abnormally prolonged and severe response to a stimulus that would normally be painful, such as a pinprick. It is relatively uncommon in patients with ovarian cancer, since the tumour does not invade the presacral plexus as aggressively as, for example, cervical tumours do. However, it should be suspected if pain control is difficult.

A recently described phenomenon with severe neuropathic pains is the effect of NMDA wind-up, which results in increasing morphine resistance with time.[33] Despite the incomplete effectiveness of many opioids in neuropathic pain, opioid titration remains the mainstay of pain control, even in neuropathic pain.[31] Co-analgesics such as low-dose amitriptyline, or other tricyclic antidepressants,[34] and anticonvulsants,[35] such as sodium valproate or carbamazepine, are useful in neuropathic pain. Their site of action is probably on inhibitory interneurones in the spinal cord, acting to 'close the gate' to impulse transmission, rather than affecting NMDA receptors directly.

Nerve blocks

Neurolytic superior hypogastric plexus block is reported as providing good analgesia in a large cohort of patients with pelvic pain from gynaecological malignancy.[36] Other types of block include a saddle block for perineal pain, and epidural or spinal infusions of opioids with a local anaesthetic at low dose.

Pat had pain control on controlled-release morphine 200 mg 12-hourly, amitriptyline 25 mg nocte, and diclofenac 50 mg 8-hourly. She took lactulose 10 ml daily and two co-danthrusate capsules daily, but remained severely constipated and had an episode of rectal bleeding which frightened her.

Constipation

Opioid-induced constipation is a very common complication of analgesic therapy. It requires stimulant laxatives and a faecal softener from the outset. Combined preparations can be too thick for some patients to swallow and co-danthramer can cause an anal rash; simple senna liquid 10 ml (as a stimulant) given with magnesium hydroxide mixture 10 ml (as a softener) once or twice a day is well tolerated by many patients. Some patients find lactulose a palatable alternative to the magnesium salt, but the breakdown of this non-absorbed sugar by gut flora produces flatus in many patients. Alternatives are sodium picosulphate solution as 5 mg in 5 ml given b.d. or t.i.d., which acts as a small bowel flusher, or various capsule preparations of co-danthrusate. Some patients also need a faecal softener; dry powder preparations of lactitol or lactulose-dry mix well in warm drinks or on food and cereals. It is important to check that patients have an adequate fluid intake to ensure that the faeces are not hardened in the colon.

Conventional therapy with stimulant and softening laxatives combined is often unpleasant to take, and may even induce colic, particularly in the patient at risk of subacute obstruction. Theoretically, the use of an opioid antagonist locally in the gut, such as oral naxolone, would seem to provide a potentially valuable therapy for opioid-related constipation;[37] initial data suggest that individual oral naloxone doses may be useful, but further trials are required.

Pat found that the smell of cooking in the house made her nauseated, and the family became increasingly concerned at her decreasing appetite. After about six weeks, she started to vomit occasionally after meals, but this gradually became more frequent and she would vomit large foul-smelling stagnant khaki-coloured vomits several times a day.

Nausea and vomiting

Nausea and vomiting are very common in women with advanced ovarian cancer. It is essential to identify the underlying cause in order to guide therapy;[38] in ovarian cancer bowel obstruction must always be considered, since it may coexist with other causes, such as hypercalcaemia or drug-induced vomiting. Emesis is a complicated process, often resulting from multiple afferent signals to the central vomiting centres. Afferent impulses from the chemoreceptor trigger zone receptors (drugs and toxins) are primarily dopaminergic. In the vomiting centre beneath the floor of the fourth ventricle, pathways involving antihistamines, acetylcholine and serotonin (5-hydroxytryptamine, 5-HT) receptors are important. Vagal afferents from splanchnic nerves and the gastrointestinal tract, including the liver, involve $5-HT_3$ receptors.[39] Vestibular sensitivity is increased in some patients, particularly after chemotherapy, predisposing them to travel sickness. This needs preventive management with a central antihistamine or anticholinergic antiemetic before the journey. Impulses from the cerebral cortex are also very important, since sounds, visual images and memories can all be emetogenic; several women with advanced malignancy appear to have hyperosmia and find the smell of food emetogenic.

Table 19.3 shows the sites of action, side-effects, dosages and uses of some antiemetics.

Table 19.3   Antiemetics

Drug	Site of action[a]	Side-effects	Dosage	Use
Metoclopramide	Gut 5-HT$_3$ receptors, VC dopamine receptors	Extrapyramidal in young occasionally	Up to 1 mg/ kg body weight	Prokinetic; second-line for drug-induced vomiting
Cyclizine	VC H$_1$ histamine receptors	Dry mouth, painful injection, antagonizes prokinetics	Up to 200 mg per 24 hours, s.c. infusion	With haloperidol in intestinal obstruction
Haloperidol	VC dopamine receptors	Parkinsonism in the elderly	2.5–10 mg as single dose or 24-hour s.c. infusion	Intestinal obstruction; drug-induced vomiting
Prochlorperazine	VC dopamine receptors	Sedative, dry mouth	5 mg 8-hourly	Vestibular sensitivity
Levopromazine (methotrimeprazine)	VC 5-HT$_2$, 5-HT$_4$ and dopamine receptors	Sedative, dry mouth	6.25–25 mg as single dose or 24-hour infusion	General
Domperidone	Gut dopamine receptors	No central action	10–30 mg 8-hourly	Hepatic and gut causes
Ondansetron, granisetron, etc.	Gut and VC 5-HT$_3$ receptors	Constipation	Variable	Chemotherapy; third-line for therapeutic trial in intractable vomiting

[a] VC, vomiting centres.

Bowel obstruction

As over 75% of ovarian cancers present as advanced stage III or IV,[40] bowel obstruction is a common complication due to transcoelomic spread.[40] It occurs in up to 42% of all patients,[41] but is not necessarily a terminal event.

Patients with bowel obstruction seem to fall into two main groups. Those who had had no anticancer treatment in the previous six months and are ascites-free have a better surgical prognosis than those with ascites and who have had recent treatment.[40] However, 62 patients followed prospectively by Fernandes et al[42] showed no survival-time difference between medically or surgically treated patients with bowel obstruction; the presence of ascites, hypoalbuminaemia and raised blood urea were bad prognostic indicators.[42] These findings suggest that conservative medical management is first-line in the poor-prognosis subgroup (see Chapter 13).

Patients with subacute obstruction often have diarrhoea as well as vomiting.[41] Upper bowel obstruction may result in large-volume bile-stained vomit; lower bowel obstruction can present with vomiting later. The foul, stagnant smell of the vomit can be diagnostic.

Octreotide is a somatostatin analogue that reduces the volume of intestinal secretions.[43] Its therapeutic role in intestinal obstruction has recently emerged. Octreotide has been reported as providing a complete response with cessation of vomiting in about 50–75% of patients, using a median dose of 0.3 mg/day.[44,45] However, octreotide is an expensive drug, and therefore, unless there is a good therapeutic response, it should not be continued without careful review. The ability of octreotide to decrease gastrointestinal tract secretions means that it also has a place in the treatment of diarrhoea caused by an enterocolic fistula.[43]

Cyclizine, a centrally acting H_1 histamine receptor antagonist, is useful in combination with centrally acting dopamine antagonists such as haloperidol in bowel obstruction. The drugs need to be given by continuous subcutaneous infusion in a patient who is vomiting; most women will require cyclizine 150–200 mg plus haloperidol 5 mg per 24 hours via syringe driver. For patients who find this combination too sedating, high-dose metoclopramide is an alternative, given as 1 mg/kg body weight per 24 hours as a subcutaneous infusion; its central dopamine antagonist effect provides effective antiemesis. The half-life of each drug warrants consideration. Oral haloperidol only needs to be administered once every 24 hours, whilst oral cyclizine should be given every 6–8 hours. Oral metoclopramide will need to be given every 6 hours. In acute vomiting, the intravenous route as a bolus of 10–20 mg is the most effective. Extrapyramidal reactions, reported more commonly in younger patients,[46] are very rare, and the lack of sedation with metoclopramide makes it a very useful antiemetic. Other antiemetics may need to be given at doses that are slightly sedative initially, but when the symptoms are controlled, women often require relatively low maintenance doses.

Most antiemetics, such as cyclizine, sting when injected, but subcutaneous injection is as effective as intramuscular and much less painful. Subcutaneous infusion over 24 hours is not painful, but it may be irritant, causing redness or sterile abscess. These irritant side-effects are often seen with levopromeprazine.

Levopromeprazine or methotrimeprazine, a phenothiazine with some evidence of analgesic properties,[47,48] is also a potent specific 5-HT_2 receptor antagonist.[51] At low dose (2.5–12.5 mg per 24 hours via continuous subcutaneous infusion), it has been shown to have good antiemetic properties; in a study of 23 terminally ill patients with refractory vomiting, 70% had good control at this dose without adverse effects.[49]

In some patients with intractable vomiting, a

therapeutic trial of a serotonin antagonist such as ondansetron or granisetron is warranted. However, if a response has not occurred within 48 hours, it is unlikely to do so. The drug is best administered initially as a bolus intravenous dose to ensure it has been absorbed and thereby to test efficacy.

Some patients, particularly those with hepatic deposits and multiple intraperitoneal deposits in carcinoma of the ovary, appear to show a response to steroids. The exact mechanism is unknown. Again, a therapeutic trial of dexamethasone at doses of 8–12 mg/day is warranted in the patient whose vomiting is not controlled with routine antiemetics as outlined above.[50] The evidence to support the use of steroids in bowel obstruction is inconclusive, but some reports suggest benefit in the resolution of the obstruction itself.[51]

When intestinal obstruction is not amenable to surgical correction, patients require symptom control until their death. In those whose nausea and vomiting has not been controlled by any medical means, the use of percutaneous endoscopic gastrostomy to decompress the upper gastrointestinal tract has been described as relieving the nausea, vomiting and abdominal pain caused by distended upper bowel,[52] but should only be considered when all other medical management has failed. A nasogastric tube is very uncomfortable and interferes with pharyngeal function, thereby increasing the patient's risk of an aspiration pneumonia;[53] there is no clear indication for a nasogastric tube, and most women prefer to tolerate the occasional vomit than have a tube down. Even if endoscopic percutaneous drainage is performed, the woman should be encouraged to continue with a soft diet and oral fluids, as there is some absorption from the upper gastrointestinal tract. There is no place for nil-by-mouth regimens, which can seem punitive and predispose to severe dehydration.

Hypercalcaemia

Hypercalcaemia, a common complication of malignancy, can present quite insidiously. The tumour releases a parathyroid-hormone (PTH)-related protein, leading to the hypercalcaemia.[54,55] Although minor levels of hypercalcaemia may be asymptomatic, when levels are significantly raised (e.g. >3.0 mmol/l), patients usually present with nausea, vomiting and constipation, which may mimic intestinal obstruction. They are often also drowsy, which can be wrongly attributed to the dehydration associated with nausea and vomiting. Dehydration is compounded by a direct effect of the PTH-related peptide on the kidney, where excess water and electrolytes are lost and calcium reabsorption in the proximal renal tubule is promoted. The calcium concentration must be corrected for any concomitant hypoalbuminaemia. Initial rehydration results in a temporary improvement, but rehydration should be followed by treatment with bisphosphonate to reverse the process – for example clodronate or pamidronate given intravenously, since drug absorption from the gut is unreliable.[56] Initial treatment with frusemide at the time of rehydration will reduce the serum calcium by only 15%,[56] and is not an alternative to treatment with bisphosphonate.

Steroids have no place in the modern management of cancer-related hypercalcaemia.

Without treatment, patients will become more drowsy and dehydrated. Confusion, sometimes with hallucinations, is common. Hypercalcaemic patients appear relatively analgesic-resistant; treatment of the underlying hypercalcaemia restores analgesic responsiveness. Some patients with marginally raised serum calcium levels seem to have a non-specific improvement in well-being when treated with hydration and an intravenous bisphosphonate infusion.

Nutrition

For a family, eating together can be the main social activity of the day, especially in some cultures. Preparing food is a way of showing love, fellowship and caring; the patient's inability to eat and enjoy the meal can cause tension, with the preparer feeling rejected and the patient feeling guilty and a burden. Preparing different foods can become very expensive for a family on a low budget.

Dilemmas over nutrition are one of the commonest problems in the nursing care of dying patients.[57] When the patient is dying, this must be clearly acknowledged, as otherwise the family can focus inappropriately on feeding in the belief that it is food that is keeping the patient alive.[58]

Different dietary supplements are available; their thick texture and synthetic taste is unpalatable to many patients, and there is no objective evidence of advantage over a normal diet. The consensus from the literature suggests that enteral and parenteral nutrition for cancer cachexia have very little place in advanced disease.[59] It is costly, has potential complications, and involves complex ethical issues in the decision to use it.

Chronic nausea often underlies anorexia, and requires treatment. Steroids are not recommended, since they potentiate weakness through muscle wasting. Megestrol acetate has been advocated as an appetite stimulant in cancer cachexia, but the cost-efficacy is unproven,[59] and metoclopramide, which has a gastrokinetic effect, is used in several palliative care units.

Prevention of malnutrition in advanced malignancy requires a simple, comforting approach to improve well-being. Good nursing practices, imaginative provision of food, and nutritious soups and drinks can do much to improve food intake.[60]

The ethical principles of non-maleficence and beneficence are crucial in decisions over nutrition and hydration interventions. Potential benefits may include preserving skin over pressure areas through maintained protein intake, not feeling hunger, alleviating the fear of starving to death and lessening weakness from protein catabolism.

Gastrostomy has sometimes been advocated for feeding. Many consider that feeding/gastrostomy tubes for nutrition are medical treatments and are warranted only when they make possible a quality of life in which the patient can reasonably be thought to have continued interest.[67]

Patients with advanced cancer generally do not experience hunger despite decreased food intake, and often experience early satiety. The legal and ethical ramifications around decisions to withhold or withdraw treatment from terminally ill patients have made nutrition a target of the debate. McCann et al[62] followed 32 patients who were terminally ill, and found that these patients had comfort despite minimal intake of food or fluids, consistent with the experience of others. A patient-centred team approach was required to help families understand that aggressive feeding would not alter the outcome.

Pat's ascites developed rapidly, and became tense and uncomfortable. She was unable to turn in bed at night. She had developed ankle oedema, which had initially been controlled with support hose, but the stockings became difficult to put on and were itchy.

She was pleased to have the ascites drained as an outpatient through a small peritoneal dialysis cannula. A total of 3200 ml was drained off, providing instant relief.

Ascites

Ascites is a particularly common complication of ovarian malignancy, often developing early in the disease. Treatment of the primary neoplasm provides improvement in most patients as part of initial therapy; in others, the ascites is severe and resistant, particularly when it recurs after treatment of the primary malignancy. Malignant ascites has been considered resistant to diuretics, but response has been reported to a combination of frusemide 20–80 mg and spironolactone 100–200 mg daily over several months.[67] In patients with resorbing ascites, the maximum fluid reabsorption rate is 930 ml per 24 hours,[64] so weight loss of over 1 kg per day in the patient would indicate intravascular fluid depletion and its concomitant risks. Diuretics should therefore be started at low dose and gradually increased.[63]

Paracentesis provides temporary relief, but the fluid rapidly reaccumulates. Many textbooks imply that haemodynamic changes are associated with large-volume drainage, but drainage of up to 9 litres has been reported as not causing serious hypotension, and the use of albumin infusion simultaneously with the drainage has been reported as protecting against this.[65] In a study of intraperitoneal pressures during drainage, the symptoms of tense ascites were completely relieved by drainage to pressures of approximately 13 cmH$_2$O, without symptoms or signs of hypovolaemia during or after total paracentesis.[66]

Peritoneo-venous shunting would seem a logical way to 'recycle' protein and decrease intraabdominal fluid volume; dissemination of metastases has not been reported as a problem.[67] However, complications of a shunt include blockage, disseminated intravascular coagulation, heart failure, venous thrombosis, sepsis, and peritoneal fibrosis with intestinal obstruction. Loculated effusions are unsuitable for shunt insertion. Other methods to decrease ascites have had little success; these include intraperitoneal *Corynebacterium parvum*, interferon, radiocolloid solutions of zinc and gold, and intraperitoneal chemotherapy.[63,68] Suppression of vascular permeability factor (VPF), which is thought to be involved in ascites formation in ovarian cancer, may provide a therapeutic tool.[70]

The mainstay remains drainage and diuretics. Good symptomatic control can sometimes be achieved with an implanted abdominal drain, but there is a risk of infection.[69]

Pat's leg oedema worsened dramatically over a few days, and the skin around her ankles began to ooze small beads of serous fluid. She also developed a hot red area on the skin of one leg, which appeared to be an early cellulitis.

Lymphoedema

Severe swelling of one or both legs is seen when tumour invades lymphatic vessels, causing lymphoedema; differential diagnosis includes deep vein thrombosis. The stagnant fluid is at risk of infection, and any skin break will provide an entry route for bacteria. Cellulitis should be treated with antibiotics immediately, since fibrosis after infection can worsen the lymphoedema in the long term. Hypoproteinaemia will also worsen the tissue swelling, since the intracapillary osmotic gradient is lost.

The increase in limb volume can be assessed by regular circumferential measurement using the Kuhnke method and the cylinder formula to calculate limb volume. The International Society for Lymphology has written assessment criteria, based on skin condition,[71] including the degree of fibrosis and the extent of pitting of the oedema. In general, more fibrosis and less pitting indicate a worse condition. Pain is sometimes secondary to the tissue distension pressure or the weight of the limb. Patients' body image is often severely disturbed, and anxiety and depression may be worsened.

Treatment must be aimed at providing gentle external support, care of the skin to avoid infection, and allowing the woman to express what the swollen limb means to her. External graded compression bandaging can be effective in reducing lymphoedema, although great care must be exercised; application of the bandaging is a specialized technique, and lymph drainage is aided by the massage technique of efflurage.

Malignant pericardial effusion

Pericardial effusion due to pericardial tumour deposits is a very rare but rapidly fatal complication of malignancy, unless treated. Cardiac tamponade usually presents with respiratory symptoms, often misdiagnosed as pulmonary disease.[72] Pulsus paradoxus, tachycardia, hypotension and increased jugular venous pressure are classic signs of cardiac tamponade, but may not all be present.[73] Diagnosis may be confirmed by echocardiography and treatment is by pericardiocentesis, initially by simple sub-xiphoid drainage. Creation of a pericardial window should be considered for longer-term control.[72]

On checking Pat's serum albumin, the laboratory reported that the urea and creatinine were both rising. She asked for the results and wanted to know what could be done to prolong her life, even by a few weeks.

Renal failure

Renal failure can provide a therapeutic dilemma: an obstructive nephropathy can be managed by insertion of a ureteric stent or a nephrostomy; for the majority of terminally ill patients with a renal insufficiency, haemodialysis is inappropriate.[74,75] The decision must be taken in the context of the overall disease process and the patient's social situation,[75,76] requiring open and honest discussion with her. Nephrostomy may buy some time to allow affairs to be put in order, but should not be used as a mechanism to resuscitate patients for them to 'die again' from more distressing complications.

Harrington et al[77] suggest that the patients most likely to benefit from urinary diversion are those for whom therapeutic options are available for treatment of the underlying malignancy. Percutaneous nephrostomy may be indicated when ureteric stenting has failed;[78] in a study of 42 patients, 40% survived for over six months when urinary diversion by percutaneous nephrostomy or JJ ureteric stents was used. However, infection, septicaemia and re-obstruction are common complications.

Pat became more ill, and her children indicated to her that they knew she was dying. They wanted to stay home with her all the time, and the older child begun searching on the Internet for a cure for her cancer. He found a therapy in the USA and began to ask if she would go there for treatment. He wanted to fundraise through the local newspaper and at school for her to go to the USA.

Children of a dying parent

Adults usually seriously underrate children's awareness of death and its implications. Children over 8 years of age generally have concepts similar to an adult; they are aware of the finality and irreversibility of death. They often have been excluded from the illness of their parents, since they are considered by others to be too young. This can result in much anger and resentment in bereavement, since the child has not been allowed to show love and caring for the relative in life and has been isolated in grief. This suppressed emotion in children and teenagers can result in behavioural disturbances, such as tempers or mood swings. Children at this stage require counselling to help resolve the grief – otherwise they remain at high risk of depression in later life.

Children under the age of five often have a great deal of fantasy and magical thinking in their interpretation of events. They can seem very pragmatic about the hard facts of death, but tend to think of death as somehow reversible. Between 5 and 8 years, children feel that someone might escape death, although they are aware of its finality.[79] They are often interested in the ceremonies surrounding death, whereas younger children tend to be more inquisitive about what actually happens to the body of the dead person. Children often blame themselves for the illness or accident that caused the death, and may repeatedly reiterate questions, which may not directly address their real concerns. Those under about 8 years can find the abstract concept of heaven very difficult to comprehend.[79]

The dying parent may find it helpful to create a memory box for the child to have in later years. Letters to be opened on key birthdays can also be a helpful way for the dying mother to feel she has some influence in the future and is not completely leaving the lives of her children.

Ethics

Some principles in medical ethics are invaluable in helping ensure that clinical decisions are appropriate for a patient and are not based on dogma, whim or paternalism. These principles are not absolutes; their relative weights have to be compared whenever a clinical decision is taken. The fundamental principle of 'respect for life' underlies the ethos of medical practice.[80] It does not allow the doctor the right to impose life-prolonging treatment on the competent patient who refuses consent to such treatment, and nor should the doctor 'strive unofficiously to keep alive' when treatment is futile and undermines a patient's dignity by causing a lingering death.

Autonomy

Patient autonomy can only exist if the patient can exercise autonomy and if that autonomous wish can be respected. Patient autonomy cannot be exercised in isolation, since each person has the right to autonomy. Thus the patient does not have an absolute right to demand from the doctor treatment that the doctor and healthcare team feel strongly is harmful to the patient.

The principle of informed consent comes from the principle of autonomy; it also depends on both beneficence and non-maleficence, since the information given to a patient must be in a form that can be understood and that the patient can cope with. The question of the patient's competence relates to each specific task undertaken; consent is a continuum throughout the period of care, during which time the patient's needs and comprehension may fluctuate. Every intervention requires consent; it is only for major procedures that written consent is sought, but this written consent is of no value if the procedure has not been adequately explained to the patient and the patient has not understood the explanation. Taking medication requires consent; by swallowing a tablet or allowing an injection, the patient is consenting to a therapeutic intervention.

Before seeking consent, it is important that the doctor has evaluated the reasonableness of the proposal to be put to the patient. Informed consent is not an excuse for the doctor to abdicate the responsibility of appropriately weighing up the treatment options to be discussed and the information to be given. Medico-legal considerations have driven the trend to overload the patient with information and then expect the bewildered person to make a rational choice.

For those with expressive or receptive communication disorders, the difficulties are enormous. Discussion is impaired or impossible, and the patient, sensing the doctor's workload, may be reluctant to demand more time than appears to be allotted. Many fears, hopes and beliefs, crucial to making informed choices, are unexpressed. The professional is in danger of second-guessing the patient's wishes or taking the relatives' expressed view as if it is the wish of the patient. However, studies have shown that relatives and healthcare professionals are poor proxies for patients,[81] and sadly sometimes are ill intentioned.

Confidentiality

Confidentiality also arises from the principle of autonomy; the patient has the right to knowledge of his or her condition and to decide who should be informed.

A very small number of patients will opt not to have their diagnosis and treatment options discussed with them and to hand the responsibilities onto a spouse; it is very important to ensure that this is truly the patient's express wish. For the majority, this is not the case, but the cultural practice within a family may be to discuss the diagnosis with a relative such as the eldest son. This may respect autonomy if the routes of communication have been condoned by the patient, but can cause difficulties over confidentiality.

Non-maleficence and beneficence

To do no harm and to do good may seem obvious and straightforward. However, they require a careful assessment of the risks involved and the burdens to the patient of a proposed course of action to be carefully weighed against the potential benefits for that patient.

Justice

The principle of justice requires that the patient have the best possible treatment within the resources available and that the resources be equitably and fairly distributed according to need. Expensive futile treatment takes resources away from others and cannot be justified; when resources are scarce, this rationing can pose major dilemmas for the clinician. If the 'benefits' versus 'risks and burdens' equation is applied to each situation, it can be much easier to make fair decisions and justify the decisions to others in the multiprofessional team.

Pat's symptom control was quite good for two weeks, and she enjoyed visits from other members of the family. She even managed a short trip to a wedding anniversary party at her cousin's house. Although she complained of little, her mouth was dry and her lips and tongue were so dry that talking was difficult for her unless she took frequent sips of water.

Mouth problems

Xerostomia affects more than three-quarters of terminally ill patients,[82] and many drugs produce xerostomia.[83] Treatment with artificial saliva has no great benefit over frequent sips of water.[84] Most artificial saliva preparations contain carboxymethylcellulose, which has a short-lived effect. Preparations containing porcine mucin as a lubricant must be prescribed with care, since some patients have serious religious or dietary objections. Some xerostomic patients gain benefit from sialogues. Sugar-free chewing gum, pilocarpine tablets (5–10 mg t.i.d.)[73] and anetholetrithione all act by increasing salivary gland excretion; the effect comes on gradually and depends on the patient having an intact duct and gland. Benefit from lubricants and artificial salivas is increased by coating the whole of the oral mucosa; slow-release devices in appliances such as partial dentures can be helpful.[85]

Candida species have been isolated from the mouths of over 85% of terminally ill patients.[86] They contribute to loss of taste, angular stomatitis and dysphagia.[82,87] Topical nystatin preparations need a long mucosal contact time to be effective. This means rigorous regular dosing, and the benefit may not come on for several days. The newer systemic fungal agents (fluconazole and itraconazole) are safer than ketoconazole, which is associated with some liver enzyme disturbance when used in high dose for a prolonged period of time. Fluconazole can be given as a single dose of 150 mg and will have a therapeutic action for about six weeks.[88] Unfortunately, not all candidiasis is due to *Candida albicans*; other species such as *C. glabrata*, *C. tropicalis*, *C. parapsilosis* and *C. krusei* have differing spectra of sensitivity to antifungal agents,[89,90] and fluconazole-resistant *Candida* species are increasingly found. They should be suspected whenever a patient with clinical candidiasis does not respond to standard antifungal therapy.[91]

Pat began to look very pale, and her haemoglobin was 10.5 g/dl. She had a light ooze from an umbilical lesion. She had commented that she had difficulty when trying to write the letters for her children in the future, and so she had dictated them onto a tape. A friend of hers had offered to type them out. However, Pat was worried that she was unable to concentrate and at times she felt a little muddled.

Fungating wounds

Although fungation is not common, a secondary deposit in the umbilicus will often break down, leading to smell and a serosanguinous discharge. Management of a fungating wound becomes time-consuming, with a disproportionate amount of staff time spent on physical, rather than psychosocial, care. Colonization of the surface by anaerobic organisms results in the offensive smell of rotting flesh. Many patients are themselves aware of the smell, but are too embarrassed to mention it to their doctor or nurse; topical metronidazole (0.75% or 0.8%) can dramatically decrease smell and discharge from the tumour surface without the side-effects, particularly nausea and vomiting, of systemic metronidazole.[92] Radiotherapy to the lesion to decrease the exudate should also be considered.

Confusion

Dysgraphia may be the first sign of confusion; it is easily detected by asking patients to write their own name and address.[93] As confusion becomes more overt, the distress to the patient is compounded by distress caused to the family. The commonest causes are drugs, infection, hypercalcaemia and cardiorespiratory insufficiency causing some cerebral anoxia. Anxiety should not be blamed as a cause of confusion. It is often a secondary symptom of a developing underlying toxic delirium. In an agitated delirium, the patient may require treatment to settle whilst other underlying causes are sought and treated. Although many drugs should usually be stopped, haloperidol, a butyrophenone, is probably the drug of choice to decrease agitation.[93]

It is important to avoid escalating sedation inappropriately in a patient who needs to talk. Apparent terminal agitation can result from the inappropriate use of drugs and anxiety in the patient who has unfinished business and affairs to put in order; this requires rapid efficient support – not sedation.[94]

Anaemia

In anaemia from malignancy, blood transfusion is indicated for patients with symptoms attributable to the anaemia with a haemoglobin below 9 g/dl and preferably with a life expectancy of two weeks or more.[95] In those patients with a shorter life expectancy, careful consideration is needed to balance the fair distribution of scarce resources (distributive justice) against the rights of the individual.[96] However, Gleeson and Spencer[97] have suggested that symptomatic improvement in breathlessness and weakness in patients with anaemia is independent of the level of pretransfusion haemoglobin. In 246 terminally ill cancer patients, subjective well-being was reported the day after transfusion in 51.4%,[98] unrelated to the severity of dyspnoea or fatigue.

Pat became very ill and was drinking little. Her son asked why she did not have an intravenous fluid infusion, and wanted to have his mother in hospital, but Pat had clearly expressed a wish to remain at home with her family around her.

Hydration

When patients are in the very last hours of life, cessation of all measures, other than those required directly for comfort, is not a contentious issue.[99] However, earlier in the course of a terminal illness, the place of alimentation in care has been widely debated,[99] and many patients receive artificial hydration as death approaches. There is little definitive research on rehydration in the terminally ill.[99]

A study of 32 patients with malignant disease at St Christopher's Hospice, London found that artificial intravenous hydration did not significantly relieve a dry mouth (present in 87%) or a feeling of thirst (present in 83%). When the patients died, their respiratory tract secretions and 'death rattle' were not associated with their level of hydration.[100] However, some patient's families will wish intravenous hydration,[101] and each patient's management must be guided by their expressed wish and the expectations and attitudes within their family.[102–104]

Oliver[105] found that in 22 patients dying within 24 hours of admission to a hospice inpatient unit, approximately half had essentially normal blood biochemical parameters and the other half had only moderate changes in serum urea and calcium levels. A sample of 82 patients at St Christopher's Hospice[100] with a median survival of two days had no biochemical markers of dehydration. Together, these findings demonstrate a greater degree of biochemical normality than might be predicted, suggesting that a specific form of salt and water deficiency, so-called terminal dehydration, may be occurring.[106] Some hold that there is no difference ethically between withholding and withdrawing treatment. Once a treatment confers no benefit or the benefits are outweighed by the burdens, it is difficult to justify continuing or initiating a treatment. But judgement of benefits is complex, and requires experience, compassion and an appreciation of the patient's viewpoint.

The patient's view is often difficult to ascertain, since the dying patient is frequently drowsy.

The existence of an advance directive may be helpful, or a close family member or friend may act as a proxy guide to the patient's preference. Clinical experience suggests that the grieving process may be smoother if the family are involved in decisions at the end-stage, but the physician must guard against 'sacrificing the interests of our patient to the emotional distress of the relatives'.[99,107]

Non-resuscitation orders and advance directives

An advance directive will allow a patient, when competent, to express their wishes for their management once they are no longer able to give informed consent. It forms part of an ongoing dialogue. Although the legal status of a written advance directive varies between different countries, good open communication is the cornerstone of care. The dialogue over each intervention ensures that consent and good written clinical records will protect the professional. The advance directive should ensure that the management is in the best interests of the patient, and the physician must be wary of pressure from family or others. Early in the course of disease, it is worth trying to raise options over treatment and management; the patient's wishes should be clearly recorded in the notes, and witnessed if possible. The wish to not be resuscitated needs clarifying; does the patient mean all supportive interventions, such as an intravenous infusion, are forbidden, or does the patient want to exclude cardiopulmonary resuscitation in the event of cardiac arrest? What about giving antibiotics in the event of infection, and for what type of infection?

There is evidence to suggest that in the terminally ill patient, cardiopulmonary resuscitation is futile, since it almost invariably fails to re-establish cardiac function, or succeeds only to result in further cardiac arrest with no intervening hospital discharge.[108–110] This is different from a patient who is undergoing active anti-cancer treatment, when resuscitation may be successful.

Pat was confined to bed at home. She spent much of the day drowsy and barely responsive, but from time to time had short periods of being alert. Her drugs had been converted to administration via a syringe driver. She had diamorphine 200 mg and cyclizine and haloperidol over 24 hours.

As death approaches

When a patient is in the last days of life, the focus of care alters. The family needs clear explanation and warning that the decline appears inevitable. It may be only at that time that the reality of the situation hits them. People of different faiths have different needs.[111] It is very important to check with the family whether there are any particular customs or rituals that they wish to have observed around the time of death. Even within a religious denomination, there can be wide variation in cultural requirements and expectations between different families. Although arrangements should have been made for care of any surviving children, for ensuring that a will is properly drawn up and for settling any other affairs, it is not too late to sort out any unfinished business. As the patient becomes more ill, the threat to her dignity becomes greater,[112] requiring sensitive nursing care.

The focus of drug therapy also alters. Much of the medication can be stopped: for example, anti-coagulants that had previously been maintained for a deep vein thrombosis may now be futile. Blood tests may be unnecessary. However, turning a patient continues to be important, since pressure sores develop very rapidly in patients who are extremely ill.[113,114] Hydration of the oral mucosa can be maintained using small shards of broken ice gently placed in the patient's mouth or by moistening the mouth using a small swab. Glycerine should be avoided on the oral mucosa, since it tends to dehydrate the superficial epithelium.

As the woman is dying she may become restless. This is most easily managed with a small dose of benzodiazepine such as midazolam 5 mg statim, followed by 10–30 mg as a subcutaneous infusion over 24 hours. If she develops a bubbly chest and a 'death rattle', hyoscine may be given subcutaneously; the effect can be maintained by repeated dosing, or adding the drug to the contents of a 24-hour syringe pump. Alternatively, glycopyronium 0.2 mg subcutaneously appears to be as effective as (or more so) than hyoscine and the duration of effect is longer. The dose should be repeated after 4–6 hours, or 0.4 mg can be put in the subcutaneous infusion with midazolam if necessary.

Frusemide should be given if there is an element of cardiac failure. Vigorous suction of a patient may be distressing, and does not remove endotracheal secretions. Careful positioning of the patient allows postural drainage from the main bronchi and trachea, but a significant worsening of the death rattle may cause distress to relatives and is not warranted. The relatives must live in their grief with the memory of her dying hours; the memory of a calm peaceful death appears to contribute to relatives' ability to cope in bereavement.

Pat died peacefully at home with her family present. About two hours before she died, the district nurse thought she was developing a bubbly chest, and so gave her a single subcutaneous injection of hyoscine. After Pat's death, her son shouted out that the injection had killed his mother.

Double effect and questions about euthanasia

There may be times when a treatment is instigated with the intention of relieving a symptom, but in the process an unforeseen complication arises. An example of this is where a drug such as morphine is given to relieve pain, but it suppresses cough and pneumonia develops, which may prove fatal. In this case, the intent is to relieve the distressing symptom and not to kill the patient; the benefit precedes the adverse effect. The adverse secondary and potentially fatal effect is a secondary or 'double effect', and is not passive euthanasia.[80]

When medication is withdrawn because it is having no clear benefit, this also is not passive euthanasia.[115] The cessation of futile treatments is justified; they are burdens to the patient without benefit. Futile treatments are also contrary to 'justice', since they do not represent a just allocation of resources. Using the framework of beneficence and non-maleficence, it is easier to take decisions to cease futile treatments, such as chemotherapy in the patient with advancing disease.

Bereaved children

There are some books available to help children understand death and bereavement. There is no substitute for a caring adult sitting down with the child and carefully addressing the topic, answering the child's questions, and allowing the child to be as much or as little involved with the dying parent and in the funeral as he or she wishes.[79] Choosing flowers for the coffin and drawing a picture to go inside the coffin with the body or to be put on the grave can be important ways of helping the child express grief and feelings. Children who wish to attend the funeral should be allowed to do so; those who do not wish to should not be pushed.

Adolescents have particular difficulty when they lose a parent. The disruption to their development is so severe that they may well continue to search throughout their adult life for a replacement for the person they have lost, often idealizing the dead person in their memory. Rapport with a bereaved adolescent can be established through the type of music that is prominent in their life.[116]

Bereavement support

Care of the terminally ill patient does not end with the patient's death. A significant morbidity and mortality in the bereaved is associated with failure to grieve normally.

Often the bereaved have many unanswered questions relating to the illness and to its outcome. Some of these questions only arise after the death, when there are news reports of 'wonder drugs' or the chance inappropriate remark of a friend may act as a trigger. The many losses associated with bereavement and the social hardship that is associated with loss of income and of the family structure only impact after the death. An invitation to interview with the consultant who provided care, or a letter on the anniversary of the death, can be very supportive.

There are some important pointers to indicate that a person is at risk of complicated, or abnormal, grief in bereavement.[117] These include the loss of a child, however old the parent losing their child may be. Those who have experienced multiple bereavements recently and those who had a very interdependent or ambivalent relationship with the person who is dying tend to adapt less well to their loss. Death that was disfiguring, distressing, untimely or unexpected is more likely to result in complicated grief. Identification of those at risk and provision of bereavement support is an integral part of the care of the patient herself.

LEARNING POINTS

✻ Listen to the patient and to her family – never assume that your agenda and hers are the same.

❋ Define the patient's problem list before planning the next stage of management, remembering that all problems have a psychosocial domain and that fears are often unvoiced unless the patient feels really safe to talk about them.

❋ If there is no improvement in a patient's distress within 48 hours, ask for advice from a specialist in palliative care.

❋ Pain has many causes; if titrating up an opioid is not having a benefit, consider whether there is a neuropathic element to the pain.

❋ Nausea and vomiting from bowel obstruction can be well controlled with antiemetics via a subcutaneous infusion; 'drip and suck' is not necessary.

❋ The children in a family have needs that must be addressed early in the course of a patient's illness, particularly when they face the death of their mother.

REFERENCES

1. Lewis FM, Deal LW, Balancing our lives: a study of the married couple's experience with breast cancer recurrence. *Oncol Nurs Forum* 1995; **22**: 943–53.

2. Stedeford A, Couples facing death. I – Psychosocial aspects. *BMJ* 1981; **283**: 1033–6.

3. Stedeford A, Couples facing death. II – Unsatisfactory communication. *BMJ* 1981; **283**: 1098–101.

4. Dept SW, Family trees. In: Document from St Christopher's Hospice, London, 1991.

5. Ptacek JT, Eberhardt TL, Breaking bad news. A review of the literature. *JAMA* 1996; **276**: 496–502.

6. Finlay I, Ballard P, Jones N et al, A person to have around. *J Healthcare Chaplaincy* 2000; **3**: 41–52.

7. Nelson E, Sloper P, Charlton A, While D, Children who have a parent with cancer: a pilot study. *J Cancer Educ* 1994; **9**: 30–6.

8. Gordon A, The tattered cloak of immortality. In: *Adolescents and Death* (Corr C, McNeil JN, eds). New York: Springer-Verlag, 1986: 25.

9. Corney RH, Crowther ME, Everett H et al, Psychosexual dysfunction in women with gynaecological cancer following radical pelvic surgery. *Br J Obstet Gynaecol* 1993; **100**: 73–8.

10. Crowther ME, Corney RH, Shepherd JH, Psychosexual implications of gynaecological cancer. *BMJ* 1994; **308**: 869–70.

11. Higginson I, Priest P, McCarthy M, Are bereaved family members a valid proxy for a patient's assessment of dying? *Soc Sci Med* 1994; **38**: 553–7.

12. Weiss R, Separation and other problems that threaten relationships. *BMJ* 1998; **316**: 1011–13.

13. Hilliard N, Spirituality in hospice care. *Palliat Care Today* 1998; **6**(4): 52–3.

14. Walter T, The ideology and organization of spiritual care: three approaches. *Palliat Med* 1997; **11**: 21–30.

15. Woodruff R, *Palliative Medicine*. Melbourne: Aspergula Press, 1997.

16. Maguire P, Faulkner F, Regnard C, Eliciting the current problems of the patient with cancer – a flow diagram. *Palliat Med* 1993; **7**: 151–6.

17. Cleeland CR, Ryan KM, Pain assessment: global use of the brief pain inventory. *Ann Acad Med* 1994; **23**: 129–38.

18. Walker VD, Webb P, Pain assessment charts in the management of chronic cancer pain. *Palliat Med* 1987; **1**: 111–16.

19. Ellershaw JE, Peat SJ, Boys LC, Assessing the effectiveness of a hospital palliative care team. *Palliat Med* 1995; **9**(2): 145–52.

20. World Health Organization, *Cancer Pain Relief and Palliative Care*. Geneva: WHO Technical Report 804, 1990.

21. EAPC (Expert Working Group of the European Association for Palliative Care), Morphine in cancer pain: modes of administration. *BMJ* 1996; **312**: 823–6.

22. Twycross R, *Introducing Palliative Care*. Oxford: Radcliffe Medical Press, 1995: 83–5.

23. Portenoy R, Management of common opioid side effects during long-term therapy of cancer pain. *Ann Acad Med* 1994; **23**: 160–70.

24. TTS–Fentanyl Multicentre Study Group (Ahmedzai SA, Fallon E, Finlay M et al), Transdermal fentanyl in cancer pain. *J Drug Dev* 1994; **6**: 93–7.

25. Gillis JC, Brogden RN, Ketorolac. A reappraisal of its pharmacodynamic and pharmacokinetic properties and therapeutic use in pain management. *Drugs* 1997; **53**: 139–88.

26. Bruera E, Belzile M, Pituskin E et al, Randomized, double-blind, cross-over trial comparing safety and efficiency of oral controlled-release oxycodone with controlled-release morphine in patients with cancer pain. *J Clin Oncol* 1998; **16**(10): 3222–9.

27. Ellershaw J, Hydromorphone: a new alternative to morphine. *Prescriber* 1998; **Feb**: 21–6.

28. Mercadante S, Lod F, Sapio M et al, Long-term ketamine subcutaneous continuous infusion in neuropathic cancer pain. *J Pain Symptom Manage* 1995; **10**: 564–8.

29. Manfredi PL, Morrison RS, Meier DE, The rule of double effect. *N Engl J Med* 1998; **338**: 1390.

30. Gannon C, The use of methadone in the care of the dying. *Eur J Palliat Care* 1997; **4**: 152–8.

31. Twycross RG, Neuropathic pain. *Palliat Care Today* 1992; Autumn: 55–7.

32. Sykes J, Johnson R, Hanks GW, ABC of palliative care. Difficult pain problems. *BMJ* 1997; **315**: 867–9.

33. Mao J, Price DD, Mayer DJ, Mechanisms of hyperalgesia and morphine tolerance: a current view of their possible interactions. *Pain* 1995; **62**: 259–74.

34. McQuay HJ, Moore RA, Antidepressants and chronic pain. *BMJ* 1997; **314**: 763–4.

35. McQuay H, Carroll D, Jadad AR et al, Anticonvulsant drugs for management of pain: a systematic review. *BMJ* 1995; **311**: 1047–52.

36. Plancarte R, de Leon-Casasola OA, El-Helaly M, Allende S, Lema MJ, Neurolytic superior hypogastric plexus block for chronic pelvic pain associated with cancer. *Reg Anaesth* 1997; **22**: 562–8.

37. Sykes N, An investigation of the ability of oral nalozone to correct opioid related constipation in patients with advanced cancer. *Palliat Med* 1996; **10**: 135–44.

38. Rousseau P, Antiemetic therapy in adults with terminal disease: a brief review. *Am J Hospice Palliat Care* 1995; **12**: 13–18.

39. Hesketh PJ, Gandara DR, Serotonin antagonists: a new class of antiemetic agents. *J Natl Cancer Inst* 1991; **83**: 613–20.

40. Zoetmulder FA, Helmerhorst TJ, van Coevorden F et al, Management of bowel obstruction in patients with advanced ovarian cancer. *Eur J Cancer* 1994; **30A**: 1625–8.

41. Ripamonti C, Management of bowel obstruction in advanced cancer. *Curr Opin Oncol* 1994; **6**: 351–7.

42. Fernandes JR, Seymour RJ, Suissa S, Bowel obstruction in patients with ovarian cancer: a search for prognostic factors. *Am J Obstet Gynecol* 1988; **158**: 244–9.

43. Mercadante S, Treatment of diarrhoea due to enterocolic fistula with octreotide in a terminal cancer patient. *J Pain Sympt Manag* 1992; **6**: 257–9.

44. Riley J, Fallon MT, Octreotide in terminal malignant obstruction of the gastrointestinal tract. *Eur J Palliat Care* 1993; **1**: 23–5.

45. Khoo D, Hall E, Motson R et al, Palliation of malignant intestinal obstruction using octreotide. *Eur J Cancer* 1994; **30A**(1): 28–30.

46. Kris MG, Tyson LB, Gralla RJ et al, Extrapyramidal reactions with high-dose metoclopramide. *N Engl J Med* 1983; **309**: 433–4.

47. McGee JL, Alexander MR, Phenothiazine analgesia – fact or fantasy? *Am J Hosp Pharm* 1979; **36**: 633–40.

48. St John AB, Born CK, Characterization of analgesic and activity effects of methotrimeprazine and morphine. *Res Commun Chem Pathol Pharmacol* 1979; **26**: 25–34.

49. Twycross R, Barkby GD, Hallwood PM, The use of low dose levomeprazine

[methotrimeprazine] in the management of nausea and vomiting. *Prog Palliat Care* 1997; **5**: 49–53.

50. Twycross R, Back I, Nausea and vomiting in advanced cancer. *Eur J Palliat Care* 1998; **5**: 39–45.

51. Feuer DJ, Broadley KE, Systematic review and meta-analysis of corticosteroids for the resolution of malignant bowel obstruction in advanced gynaecological and gastrointestinal cancers. Systematic Review Steering Committee. *Am Oncol* 1999; **10**: 1035–47.

52. Campagnutta E, Gallo A, Zarrelli A et al, Palliative treatment of upper intestinal obstruction by gynaecological malignancy: the usefulness of percutaneous endoscopic gastronomy. *Gynecol Oncol* 1996; **62**(1): 103–5.

53. Campagnutta E, Cannizzaro R, Gallo A et al, Palliative treatment of upper intestinal obstruction by gynaecological malignancy: the usefulness of percutaneous endoscopic gastrostomy. *Gynecol Oncol* 1996; **62**(1): 103–5.

54. Watters J, Gerrand G, Dodwell D, The management of malignant hypercalcaemia. *Drugs* 1996; **52**: 837–48.

55. Ralston SH, Pathogenesis and management of cancer associated hypercalcaemia. *Cancer Surv* 1994; **21**: 179–96.

56. Kovacs CS, MacDonald SM, Chik CL, Bruera E, Hypercalcemia of malignancy in the palliative care patient: a treatment strategy. *J Pain Symptom Manage* 1995; **10**: 224–32.

57. Copp G, Dunn V, Frequent and difficult problems perceived by nurses caring for the dying in the community, hospice and acute care settings. *Palliat Med* 1993; **7**: 19–25.

58. Boyd KB, Beeken L, Tube feeding in palliative care: benefits and problems. *Palliat Med* 1994; **8**: 156–8.

59. Fainsinger R, The modern management of cancer related cachexia in palliative care. *Prog Palliat Care* 1997; **5**: 191–5.

60. Powell-Tuck J, Nutrition support in advanced cancer. *J R Soc Med* 1997; **90**: 591–2.

61. Gillon R, Withholding and withdrawing life-prolonging treatment – moral implications of a thought experiment. *J Med Ethics* 1994; **20**: 203–4, 222.

62. McCann RM, Hall WJ, Groth-Juncker A, Comfort care for terminally ill patients. The appropriate use of nutrition and hydration. *JAMA* 1994; **272**: 1263–6.

63. Sharma S, Walsh D, Management of symptomatic malignant ascites with diuretics: two case reports and a review of the literature. *J Pain Symptom Manage* 1995; **10**: 237–42.

64. Lifshitz S, Ascites, pathophysiology and control measures. *Int Radiat Oncol Biol Phys* 1982; **8**: 1423–6.

65. Ginés P, Arroyo V, Quintero E, Comparison of paracentesis and diuretics in the treatment of cirrhotics with tense ascites: results of a randomised study. *Gastroenterology* 1987; **93**: 234–41.

66. Gotlieb WH, Feldman B, Feldman-Moran O et al, Intraperitoneal pressures and clinical parameters of total paracentesis for palliation of symptomatic ascites in ovarian cancer. *Gynecol Oncol* 1998; **71**: 381–5.

67. Souter RG, Wells C, Tarin D, Kettlewell MG, Surgical and pathologic complications associated with peritoneovenous shunts in management of malignant ascites. *Cancer* 1985; **55**: 1973–8.

68. Stuarat GC, Nation JG, Snider DD, Thunberg P, Intraperitoneal interferon in the management of malignant ascites. *Cancer* 1993; **71**: 2027–30.

69. Yukita A, Asano M, Okamoto T, Mizutani S, Suzuki H, Suppression of ascites formation and re-accumulation associated with human ovarian cancer by an anti-VPF monoclonal antibody in vivo. *Anticancer Res* 2000; **20**: 155–60.

70. Kerr-Wilson R, Terminal care of gynaecological malignancy. *Br J Hosp Med* 1994; **51**: 113–18.

71. Casley-Smith J, Alterations of untreated lymphedema and its grades over time. *Lymphology* 1995; **28**: 174–85.

72. Shepherd AF, Malignant pericardial effusion. *Curr Opin Oncol* 1997; **9**: 170–4.

73. Vassilopoulos PP, Nikolaidis K, Filopoulos E et al, Subxiphoidal pericardial 'window' in the management of the malignant pericardial effusion. *Eur J Surg Oncol* 1995; **21**: 545–7.

74. Rouseau P, Pilocarpine in radiation-induced xerostomia. *Am J Hospice Palliat Care* 1995; **12**: 38–39.

75. Smith P, Bruera E, Management of malignant ureteral obstruction in the palliative care setting. *J Pain Symptom Manage* 1995; **10**: 481–6.

76. Finlay I, Difficult decisions in palliative care. *Br J Hosp Med* 1996; **56**: 264–7.

77. Harrington KJ, Pandha HSP, Kelly SA et al, Palliation of obstructive nephropathy due to malignancy. *J Urol* 1995; **76**: 101–7.

78. Emmert C, Rassler J, Köhler U, Survival and quality of life after percutaneous nephrostomy for malignant ureteric obstruction in patients with terminal cervical cancer. *Arch Gynecol Obstet* 1997; **259**: 147–51.

79. Raphael B, The bereaved child. In: *The Anatomy of Bereavement*. London: Routledge, 1985: 74–138.

80. Walton J, Report of the Select Committee on Medical Ethics. London: House of Lords, HL Paper 21-1, 1994.

81. Higginson IW, McCarthy M, Palliative care views of patients and their families. *BMJ* 1990; **301**: 277–81.

82. Jobbins J, Bagg J, Parsons K et al, Oral carriage of yeasts, coliforms and staphylococci in patients with advanced malignant disease. *J Oral Pathol Med* 1992; **21**: 305–8.

83. Cooke CA, Ahmedzai S, Mayberry J, Xerostomia – a review. *Palliat Med* 1996; **10**: 284–92.

84. Wiesenfeld D, Stewart AM, Mason DK, A critical assessment of oral lubricants in patients with xerostomia. *Br Dent J* 1983; **155**: 155–7.

85. Tenovuo J, Söderling E, Chemical aids in the prevention of dental diseases in the elderly. *Int Dent J* 1992; **42**: 355–64.

86. Aldred MJ, Addy M, Bagg J, Finlay I, Oral health in the terminally ill: a cross-sectional pilot survey. *Spec Care Dent* 1991; **11**: 59–62.

87. Finlay IG, Oral *Candida* and symptoms in the terminally ill. *BMJ* 1986; **292**: 592–3.

88. Regnard C, Allport S, Stephenson L, ABC of palliative care. Mouth care, skin care, and lymphoedema. *BMJ* 1997; **315**: 1002–5.

89. Samaranayake LP, Jacob HP, The classification of oral candidosis. In: *Oral Candidosis* (Samaranayake LP, MacFarlane TW, eds). London: Wright, 1990: 124–31.

90. Arendorf TW, Walker DM, Oral candidal populations in health and disease. *Br Dent J* 1979; **147**: 267–72.

91. Finlay I, Oral fungal infections. *Eur J Palliat Care* 1995; **2**(Suppl 1): 4–7.

92. Finlay IG, Bowszyc J, Famalu C, Gsiezdzinski MD, The effect of topical 0.75% metronidazole gel on malodorous cutaneous ulcers. *J Pain Symptom Manage* 1996; **11**: 158–61.

93. Macleod AD, Whitehead LE, Dysgraphia and terminal delirium. *Palliat Med* 1997; **11**: 127–32.

94. Adam J, ABC of palliative care – The last 48 hours. *BMJ* 1997; **315**: 1600–3.

95. Finlay IG, Jenkins MJ, 6 year audit of blood transfusion for hospice patients: simple criteria increase benefit. In: *Proceedings of 5th European Association for Palliative Care Congress, 1997*. London: EAPC, 1997: 294.

96. Gillon R, The principle of double effect and medical ethics. *BMJ* 1986; **292**: 193–4.

97. Gleeson CS, Spencer D, Blood transfusion and its benefits in palliative care. *Palliat Med* 1995; **9**: 307–13.

98. Monti M, Castellani L, Berlusconi A, Cunietti E, Use of red blood cell transfusions in terminally ill cancer patients admitted to a palliative care unit. *J Pain Symptom Manage* 1996; **12**: 18–22.

99. Dunphy K, Finlay I, Rathbone G et al, Rehydration in palliative and terminal care: If not – why not? *Palliat Med* 1995; **9**: 221–8.

100. Ellershaw JE, Sutcliffe JM, Saunders CM, Dehydration and the dying patient. *J Pain Symptom Manage* 1995; **10**: 192–7.

101. Craig G, Is sedation without hydration or nourishment in terminal care lawful? *Med Leg J* 1994; **62**: 198–201 [erratum 1995; **63**: 31].

102. Craig G, Thirst and hydration in palliative care. *J Med Ethics* 1996; **22**: 361.

103. Craig GM, On withholding artificial hydration and nutrition from terminally ill sedated patients. The debate continues. *J Med Ethics* 1996; **22**: 147–53.

104. Joint Working Party of National Council for Hospice and Specialist Palliative Care Services and Ethics Committee of the Association for Palliative Medicine of Great Britain and Ireland. Artificial hydration for people who are terminally ill. *Eur J Palliat Care* 1997; **4**: 124.

105. Oliver D, Terminal dehydration. *Lancet* 1994; **ii**: 531.

106. Billings J, Comfort measures for the terminally ill: Is dehydration painful? *J Am Geriatr Soc* 1985; **33**: 308–10.

107. Wilkes E, Withholding nutrition and hydration in the terminally ill: Has palliative medicine gone too far? A commentary. *J Med Ethics* 1994; **20**: 144–5.

108. Dautzenberg PL, Broekman TC, Hooyer C et al, Review: Patient-related predictors of cardiopulmonary resuscitation of hospitalised patients. *Age Ageing* 1993; **22**: 464–75.

109. Bedell SE, Delbanco TL, Cook EF, Epstein FH, Survival after cardio-pulmonary resuscitation in the hospital. *N Engl J Med* 1983; **309**: 569–75.

110. Ebell MH, Pre-arrest predictors of survival following in-hospital cardio-pulmonary resuscitation: comparison of two predictive instruments. *Resuscitation* 1994; **28**: 21–5.

111. Neuberger J, *Caring for Dying People of Different Faiths*, 2nd edn. London: Mosby, 1994.

112. De Raeve L, Dignity and integrity at the end of life. *Int J Palliat Nurs* 1996; **2**: 71–6.

113. Bale S, Purcell P, Finlay I, Harding KG, Pressure sores in advanced disease: a flow diagram. *J Wound Care* 1995; **3**: 263–5.

114. Bale S, Finlay I, Harding KG, Pressure sore prevention in a hospice. *J Wound Care* 1995; **4**: 465–8.

115. Finlay IG, *Submission from the Ethics Group of the Association for Palliative Medicine to The Select Committee of the House of Lords on Medical Ethics*. Southampton: Association for Palliative Medicine of Great Britain and Ireland, 1993.

116. Attig T, Death themes in adolescent music. In: *Adolescents and Death* (Corr CA, McNeil JN, eds). New York: Springer-Verlag, 1986: 32–53.

117. Parkes CM, Bereavement in adult life. *BMJ* 1988; **316**: 856–9.

SECTION 6: Management of the Internet Surfer

20

Management of the Internet surfer

Beth A Morrison, Kenneth D Swenerton

INTRODUCTION

Nearly half of adult Internet users in the USA have recently accessed health and medical Websites.[1] There has been an explosion of information produced in electronic format. Much of the Web is entertainment or commercial, but there is also a great deal that is informational and educational. A cynic would add that greater quantity leads to lesser quality. The good news is that there is a lot of information out there; the bad news is that there is a lot of information out there!

The exponential growth of the World Wide Web has greatly accelerated the evolution of the relationship between physician and patient. Historically, the physician's role was to direct care and make decisions on their patient's behalf.[2] Since mid-century, the public's attitude has been changing from one of passive compliance with medical authority towards one of active partnership. Until recently, medical information has remained largely inaccessible to the public. Suddenly, the Web allows egalitarian access to vast resources of medical information. People are empowered with genuine participation in medical care.

CASE HISTORY

A 45-year-old woman has stage III ovarian cancer with bulky residual disease after primary surgery. She received chemotherapy with six courses of paclitaxel (Taxol)–cisplatin, and achieved a radiologically complete remission, but the CA125 (initially 5000 U/ml) was still raised at 200 U/ml. Her husband, a successful businessman, has researched treatment options on the Internet, and requested treatment with high-dose chemotherapy.

What would you do?

How do we respond to this or any other treatment proposal? Information is of little use without context – in this case, a fairly detailed knowledge of the natural history of advanced ovarian cancer. The disease recurs in the majority of patients, and even if further responses are obtained, it ultimately becomes refractory to all available treatment. This reality establishes the appropriate goal for therapy in advanced disease: to prolong life while maximizing the quality of life remaining.

As early in the process of care as possible, it is the physician's responsibility to communicate this reality to the patient and those close to her. This need not dash hopes, since outcomes can be gratifying, but can avoid sustaining any unrealistic expectations.

At the beginning of the therapeutic relationship, the physician should promise candour, encourage questions and offer access to reliable medical information. The Internet is not the sole source of information and support. Useful videos, books and audiotapes are also available. Telephone 'Help Lines' are another valuable resource, as are local support groups (see the appendix to this chapter). The doctor and others in the health-care team must demonstrate a willingness to listen, despite time constraints.

In this case, high-dose chemotherapy has been suggested. This tactic has well-documented effectiveness in certain diseases, such as relapsed Hodgkin's disease. However, there are no convincing data to recommend this tactic in the setting of advanced ovarian cancer (and the results of its use in breast cancer are discouraging).[3–6] We would review other options, distinguishing between those of established benefit, the experimental, and the more speculative.

A full discussion took place with the patient and her husband. The uncertainties of the management of persisting disease were outlined. Options included observation or further courses of chemotherapy with carboplatin. High-dose chemotherapy was ruled out because there is no evidence of benefit from randomized trials. After discussion, treatment with three further courses of carboplatin was given. The CA125 level fell to normal, but four months later there was evidence of relapse with symptoms of intestinal obstruction. Treatment with paclitaxel, and then topotecan, proved ineffective. The patient's husband then called with Internet information on a new treatment that targets the p53 gene.

What would you do now?

Whereas we had been dealing with the primary management of advanced disease, we now face the even more difficult circumstance of relapse. At this especially stressful time for the patient and her family, the involvement of a multidisciplinary team can be reassuring, demonstrating that many are committed to her care. The physician should recognize that the needs of the patient may differ from those close to her. In this case, the husband's search for information may not reflect his wife's concerns (or his, for that matter!).

We need a framework to evaluate the overall usefulness of treatment – one that promotes consideration not only of 'efficacy' but of 'acceptability' as well. Efficacy can be reflected by parameters such as survival and response rate; acceptability by safety (which means tolerable and predictable toxicity), treatment convenience and affordability. The relative importance of these factors varies according to the circumstances of the patient (see Table 20.1).

In this case, the patient has recurrent, symptomatic disease. Palliation is essential; cure is not yet possible. Desirable treatment would offer a realistic opportunity to achieve a symptom-relieving response and be free of substantial toxicity, inconvenience or expense.

Treatment that targets *p53* has been suggested. Expression of aberrant *p53* is a marker of poor prognosis, associated with more virulent disease and resistance to cytotoxic drugs.[7] The introduction of wild-type *p53* into tumour cells may induce sensitivity to cytotoxic agents and enhance apoptosis.[8] This novel strategy is conceptually attractive, and an appropriate subject for study. However, its clinical usefulness has yet to be demonstrated. In general, it is entirely reasonable to discuss the possibility, availability and limitations of such phase I and II trials.

In such desperate situations, it is important to reassess the potential value of 'standard' therapies. In this case, since the disease had continued to respond to carboplatin and paclitaxel through-

Table 20.1   Patient circumstances and the evaluation of treatment[22]

Patient circumstance	Measure of treatment value				
	Efficacy		Acceptability		
	Survival	Response	Safety	Convenience	Affordability
Early disease	+++		++	+	+
Advanced disease	++	++	++	++	++
Recurrent disease	+	++	+++	+++	+++

+++   of greatest importance;
++   of importance;
+   of less importance.

out the course of primary treatment, re-introduction of carboplatin (with or without paclitaxel) could still be beneficial.

Motivation of the Internet surfer

Many motives may underlie the search for Web-based medical information.

Conviction that the Web has all the answers

There is a widespread misconception that the Web contains the accumulation of all information and knowledge, and that it is always up to date. This is patently false: data is bountiful, knowledge is scarce. However, many people remain convinced that the answers are 'out there' on the Web.

Helpfulness

Patients and families want to be helpful in a constructive way. They have the time and motivation to search the Web. Often they do find good information, and it obviously should be exploited!

Suspicion

Some people feel suspicious about medical care. Even if they like and trust the physician, they may not be convinced that their oncologist is knowledgeable about the latest treatments. They may feel that better treatments are available elsewhere but are unavailable to them locally because of treatment rationing.

Control

Some Web searchers want *all* of the information, unfiltered. They may not want a 'scientific' judgement of the information. They recognize that 'highly recommended' Websites, produced by organizations with establishment credentials, may justifiably lean towards the conservative, shying away from the more controversial or the less well substantiated. They want to know about all the latest treatments, including the unconventional and experimental.[9]

What is the Web?

The World Wide Web is one part of the Internet, which is a worldwide network of networks of

---

Box 20.1

Bulletin boards are 'places' on the Internet where people can post notes, essays or letters on a stated topic, much like a real bulletin board. Once you post a message, others can come and look at the posting. *Warning:* Postings stay on the bulletin board until the owner removes them.

Listservs are like group E-mail that requires subscription. If you send a message to your listserv, it is distributed to every subscriber on the list. Each listserv has a theme and a moderator, who may exert much or little control over content.

Online chat rooms are places where groups of people can virtually congregate and 'chat' in real time. It is not E-mail – when you type your words and hit the Enter button, the message is read simultaneously by all the people in the 'room'. Smaller groups can break off and go into a side room for a private chat if they choose. Imagine a cocktail party with small groups constantly forming and re-forming.

---

computers that can all recognize the same computer language.[10] Some other parts of the Internet are newsgroups, E-mail and listservs (see Box 20.1). Anyone can publish or post information on the Internet for a very low cost, and, once published, that information is instantly available to anyone in the world who is connected to the Internet.

Governments as well as businesses have cut costs by publishing on the Web rather than in more traditional formats, and organizations large and small have followed suit. This has led to a proliferation of information on the Web by organizations, governments, businesses and individuals.

Health on the Web

Health-related information on the Web has grown tremendously in the last few years. Some estimate that 38% of all Websites provide health or medical information, and as many as 24% of all Web inquiries are health-related.[11]

The US National Library of Medicine has now made Medline freely available on the Web (http://www.ncbi,nlm.nih.gov/PubMed/) and has recently begun a consumer health initiative called MedlinePlus (http://www.nlm.nih.gov/medlineplus/) (see Box 20.2). This reflects a major shift in US government policy. Medline and the other medical databases produced by the US government have always been produced solely for health-care professionals. This new project shows that they recognize the growing concern over the availability of reliable, current consumer health information. As stated earlier, nearly half of adult US Internet users have recently accessed health-related Websites. 'The surveyors extrapolate from their data that this figure represents some 15.6 million people – a formidable potential audience that includes patients, their families, and "well consumers".'[1]

One of the most interesting features of the Web has been the proliferation of online support groups (see the appendix to this chapter). Using bulletin boards, listservs and online chat rooms, patients and family members are now able to connect with people everywhere who have the same or similar conditions. They can:

1. Discover and compare diagnoses, treatments and doctors;

Box 20.2   Consumer Health from the US National Library of Medicine

MEDLINEplus
(http://www.nlm.nih.gov/medlineplus/)

is designed to assist you in locating appropriate, authoritative health information sources. To accomplish this, NLM creates and maintains web pages that point to selected web sites. Our emphasis is on information available from NLM and NIH. We include links to searches of MEDLINE, our database that indexes medical literature, and to the many full-text publications produced by the NIH institutes. We organize the information to help you locate the specific information you need. The information includes sections on health topics, dictionaries and glossaries for finding definitions of medical terms, links to major associations and clearinghouses, publications and news items, directories of health professionals and health facilities and libraries that provide health information services for the public.

MEDLINEplus is not a list of every web page on health, but is a selected list of quality sources. The selection guidelines we use in evaluating web pages are listed below.

- **Quality, authority and accuracy of content**
  The source of the content is established, respected and dependable.
  A list of advisory board members or consultants is published on the site.
  The information provided is appropriate to the audience level, well-organized and easy to use.
  Information is from primary sources (i.e., textual material, abstracts, web pages).
  Lists of links are evaluated/reviewed/quality-filtered.
- **The purpose of the web page is educational and is not selling a product or service.** Most content is available at no charge.
- **Availability and maintenance of the web page**
  The web site is consistently available.
  Links from the site are maintained.
  The source for the contents of the web page(s) and the entity responsible for maintaining the web site (webmaster, organization, creator of the content) is clear.
  Information is current or an update date is included.
- **Special features**
  The site provides unique information to the topic with a minimum of redundancy and overlap between resources.
  The site contains special features such as graphics/diagrams, glossary, or other unique information.
  The content of the site is accessible to persons with disabilities.

---

2. Identify resources;
3. Share emotional support;
4. Disseminate information about new treatment options.

They can dispel myths, but they can also spread misinformation and perpetuate myths.[12-15] Some listserv owners report that occasionally someone will sign-up, ostensibly as a patient, and then try to sell alternative therapies to the listserv members. When the sales pitch becomes obvious, they are usually 'unsubscribed' by the listserv owner. However, these messages may have been forwarded to so many places that they may never be erased completely from the Web.

For a fee, there are services on the Web that offer to send the best and latest information on your disease. Some of these services seem legitimate and some do not. There are huge legal, ethical and practical implications for anyone providing advice through the use of E-mail.[1] It is not yet possible for any Internet advisor to receive enough information about the patient through E-mail alone. The electronic patient record may change this, making E-mail consultations more reliable, but confidentiality of records may remain problematic.

Caveat emptor

The Internet is anarchic. Logical progression has nothing to do with information-seeking on the Web. Web pages can be accessed through the 'back door', and disclaimers and warnings on home pages of Websites may be missed. The Web searcher therefore may not be able to place information in context, risking misinterpretation.[16]

Medical information found on the Internet can be misleading, naive, unscientific, proselytising, erroneous, fraudulent and often maddeningly plausible even to healthcare professionals. Perhaps there should be a warning label that the 'Internet can be hazardous to your health'.[17]

The Internet is unpoliced. Since there are no rules or systematic peer-review processes, the reliability of information is suspect. It is sometimes impossible to assess the quality of a Website or its information, because authentication is lacking.[17,18]

The unsophisticated reader of technical material can gloss over important facts, limiting under-standing of complex issues. There is also the danger of false inferences from even reliably accredited information; facts taken out of context can be misinterpreted.[16] Also, Web searchers may not recognize important deficiencies but treat all Website information equally.[19]

Unconventional therapies and quackery abound on the Web. The scientific community might expect that therapies touted on the Web would seem suspect to a public grown jaded with mass advertising, but this is not always the case. A Web page confronts the viewer with only one product or line of products at a time. The impact can be much greater than if seen amidst other promotional material. Further, the technical language and posture of the advertisers can be seductive to the scientifically naive (visit http://www.americanbiologics.com/Hospital/ABIMCnotice.htm). Unfortunately, those skilled at flitting through the Web may have very little understanding of the scientific method. Even the Web searcher with a scientific background can be led astray by the sophistication of some sites.

Computer-literate physicians will more easily appreciate the dichotomy between the erratic nature of the Web and the formal structure of science. A simple explanation of the scientific method that can be recommended to Web searchers is at http://pc65.frontier.osrhe.edu/hs/science/pmethod.htm.

Evaluating information on the Web

How can patients and healthcare professionals judge information found on the Internet?[20] Evaluating information, and sources of information, is a valuable skill. There are some instruments on the Web which try to rate medical information by giving awards, by declaring a site 'best', or by using a quality rating system. 'However, if the instruments used to produce the ratings are flawed (e.g., if they are produced to sell specific products or if they do not have any discriminatory power), they may mislead or misinform health care providers or consumers.'[9]

Different models have been proposed for evaluating medical information on the Web (see Box 20.3). One model is for external organizations to accredit Websites. Health on the Net (http://www.hon.ch/) is one such organization. Another model is for disinterested organizations to develop tools for searchers to evaluate Web-sites or the information on websites. The Health Summit Working Group (http://hitiweb.mitretek.org/) is one such organization. A second is DISCERN (http://www.discern.org.uk/). But these require work, and are unlikely to be used by any but the most diligent searcher. Many common-sense evaluative tools have also been developed (Box 20.4). Most are designed to teach critical thinking and provide cautionary checklists.

Box 20.3   Assessing information on the web: the three organizations below have each taken a slightly different approach to evaluating health information found on the Web

Health On the Net (http://www.hon.ch/) HON's mission is to help individuals, medical professionals and healthcare providers to realize the potential benefits of the World Wide Web. It is a leading certifier of the reliability and authority of health-related information on the Internet. Organizations agreeing with and honouring the principles of their code of conduct may display the HON symbol on their Website.
(http://www.hon.ch/HONcode)

The HON Website offers individuals suffering from a specific illness or disability access to relevant information and links to support communities. HON's server also provides a detailed listing of papers from relevant medical conferences and other recognized sources.

Health Information Technology Institute (http://hitiweb.mitretek.org/) is a non-profit company that provides a public benefit through the application of science and technology. It convened a Health Summit Working Group to develop a set of criteria for use in assessing the quality of health information on the Internet. The Working Group has developed a tool to evaluate websites, not the information the Website provides. This tool leads the evaluator through a series of questions about the Website in order to judge it.

DISCERN (http://www.discern.org.uk/) has developed a brief questionnaire that provides users with a valid and reliable way of assessing the quality of written information on treatment choices for a health problem. Information providers can use DISCERN to evaluate the quality of their written product. Consumers, family, friends and carers can use it to assess the quality of written information and to increase involvement in decisions about treatment by raising issues to discuss with health professionals. It can also be used as a training tool for health professionals to improve communication and shared decision-making skills.

Box 20.4   Diving goes deeper than surfing: evaluating medical information on the Web (BA Morrison, 1999)

Trustworthy
- Cite their sources of information
- Biographical information for author/creator is given
- Organizational information is given if no individual author/creator is listed
- Reputation/experience/job title of author/creator is clearly stated and checkable
- Information is taken from books/journals that are credible
- Refereed journal/information
- Corroboration of other sources – more than two more sources agree on this information

Not trustworthy
- Anonymous author/creator
- Lack of quality control is evident
- Numbers or statistics presented without source being cited
- Lack of corroboration from other sources
- No bibliography or documentation

Accurate
- Audience and purpose for information is clear
- Information has date of updating or posting attached
- Comprehensive – includes all important aspects to consider – may even include opposing viewpoints if relevant

Not accurate
- No date on the information
- An old date on information known to change rapidly
- Very one-sided view that does not acknowledge opposing views or respond to them
- Bad grammar and/or misspellings

Sensible
- Consistent
- Fair
- Objective
- Moderate
- Bias of author is clearly stated

Not sensible
- Extreme language
- Overstating claims
- Vague or sweeping generalizations
- Conflict of interest
- Seem to be biased against conventional medicine

Public health issues

Our ageing population means a higher incidence and prevalence of cancer. We are at the beginning of a swelling wave of patients who are more questioning about diseases, tests and therapies. These factors have major consequences for oncologists' schedules. In the past, the occasional information-hungry patient could be accommodated within a doctor's routine. Quite simply, it is not cost-effective for physicians to assume sole responsibility as 'quality filters' of patient information. Other models must be found to respond to this change in expectations.

CONCLUSIONS

Good communication is fundamental to a successful relationship between physician and patient. 'Reviews of the legions of studies which have associated patient–physician communication and subsequent patient adherence identified these 4 dimensions associated with increased

---

Box 20.5   A model for a cancer information service

The British Columbia (BC) Cancer Agency in Vancouver, Canada has a Library/Cancer Information Centre (CIC), which has served our physicians, staff, medical researchers and the people of British Columbia for over 20 years. Anyone asking for information is referred to the Library/CIC.

The Library/CIC arranges for oncologists to write lay-level information regarding the different types of cancer, risk factors, diagnostic tests and treatment options. This regularly updated material is available to everyone, in person, by phone, by mail, by E-mail and on our Website (http://www.bccancer.bc.ca/).

For more in-depth information, there is a non-technical collection of books and videos. While basic information in lay terms is enough for most people, many patients and family members pursue more technical information with the help of medical librarians. Medline, CancerLit, PDQ and the Internet are some of the tools the Library might use to help someone find information.

The partnership between the Library/CIC and BCCA healthcare professionals is a close one. Physicians and staff often refer patients to the librarians, and, in turn, the librarians often ask physicians, pharmacists or dietitians to help answer questions.

After questions about cancer and its treatment, the most popular services provided are the relaxation tapes and coping books. There is extensive information about unconventional remedies. The manual *Unconventional Cancer Therapies* that the Library/CIC has produced is also in electronic format on the Website. The Audiovisual Room houses the Humour Room collection of humorous videos, books and audiotapes.

Physician–patient communication is improved when the patient has a basic understanding of terminology and treatment options. Patients ask more intelligent questions of their oncologist, and have a better understanding of the answers.

Patient trust is enhanced by the knowledge that the Library and its information resources are the same as those used by the staff. The Library/CIC is a highly appreciated service, which helps patients and the public, and serves the BC Cancer Agency in a cost-efficient way.

adherence to treatment protocols: clear information and patient education, mutual expectations, an active role for the patient, and positive affect of the practitioner.'[21] Patients and family members may well provide good information. The physician should be willing to explore alternatives with the patient before they act independently on any information they may have found.

Quality filtering is an increasingly important concept in consumer health information. It must become an integral part of health care to provide, to help locate and to evaluate information.

We can meet increasing demands from patients and families for information with less costly resources than physicians (see Box 20.5). Medical librarians are skilled in evaluating information sources. Other professionals can be excellent quality filters and patient educators, particularly nurses, dietitians, pharmacists and counsellors.[23] It should always be kept in mind that Websites and other multimedia resources are of limited use for teaching. For a thorough understanding of medical information, personal discussion is essential.

Shared with sensitivity, knowledge provides protection from unrealistic expectations and unwarranted fears. A trustful relationship is the best foundation for hope in the face of uncertainty.

LEARNING POINTS

✱ The threshold has been crossed. The public accesses vast amounts of health information on the Web.

✱ Good information is a boon. Bad information is wasteful and potentially dangerous. Even the sophisticated surfer may not be able to differentiate.

✱ Health care must provide, help locate and help evaluate information for patients. Diving goes deeper than surfing!

REFERENCES

1. McLellan F, 'Like hunger, like thirst': patients, journals, and the internet. *Lancet* 1998; **ii**: 39–43.

2. Deber RB, Physicians in health care management: 7. The patient–physician partnership: changing roles and the desire for information. *CMAJ* 1994; **151**: 171–6.

3. Bezwoda WR, Randomised, controlled trial of high dose chemotherapy (HD-CNVp) versus standard dose (CAF) chemotherapy for high risk, surgically treated, primary breast cancer. *Proc Am Soc Clin Oncol* 1999; **18**: 2.

4. Results from a randomized adjuvant breast cancer study with high dose chemotherapy with CTC-b supported by autologous bone marrow stem cells versus dose escalated and tailored FEC therapy. The Scandinavian Breast Cancer Study Group 9401. *Proc Am Soc Clin Oncol* 1999; **18**: 2.

5. Peters WP, Rosner G, Vredenburgh J et al, A prospective, randomized comparison of two doses of combination alkylating agents (AA) as consolidation after CAF in high-risk primary breast cancer involving ten or more axillary lymph nodes (LN): preliminary results of CALGB 9082/SWOG 9114/NCIC MA-13. *Proc Am Soc Clin Oncol* 1999; **18**: 1.

6. Stadtmauer EA, O'Neill A, Goldstein LJ et al, Phase III randomized trial of high-dose chemotherapy and stem cell support (SCT) shows no difference in overall survival or severe toxicity compared to maintenance chemotherapy with cyclophosphamide, methotrexate and 5-fluorouracil (CMF) for women with metastatic breast cancer who are responding to conventional induction chemotherapy: the 'Philadelphia' Intergroup Study (PBT-1). *Proc Am Soc Clin Oncol* 1999; **18**: 1.

7. Buttitta F, Marchetti A, Gadducci A et al, p53 alterations are predictive of chemoresistance and aggressiveness in ovarian carcinomas: a molecular and immunohistochemical study.

Br J Cancer 1997; **75**: 230–5.

8. Song K, Li Z, Seth P et al, Sensitization of cis-platinum by a recombinant adenovirus vector expressing wild-type p53 gene in human ovarian carcinomas. *Oncol Res* 1997; **9**: 603–9.

9. Jadad AR, Gagliardi A, Rating health information on the Internet: navigating to knowledge or to Babel? *JAMA* 1998; **279**: 611–14.

10. Simmler MC, Dessen P, The internet for the medical and scientific community. *Mol Hum Reprod* 1998; **4**: 725–30.

11. Lewis D, The Internet as a resource for health-care information. *Diabetes Educ* 1998; **24**: 627–30, 632.

12. McLeod SD, The quality of medical information on the Internet. A new public health concern. *Arch Ophthalmol* 1998; **116**: 1663–5.

13. Smith J, Members only: electronic support groups closed to the average surfer. *J Natl Cancer Inst* 1998; **90**: 1696.

14. Smith J, 'Internet patients' turn to support groups to guide medical decisions. *J Natl Cancer Inst* 1998; **90**: 1695–7.

15. Eng TR, Maxfield A, Patrick K et al, Access to health information and support: a public highway or a private road? *JAMA* 1998; **280**: 1371–5.

16. Eysenbach G, Diepgen TL, Towards quality management of medical information on the internet: evaluation, labelling, and filtering of information. *BMJ* 1998; **317**: 1496–500.

17. Larkin M, Internet can be hazardous to your health. *Newsday* 1996; Tuesday, March 26.

18. Muir Gray JA, Hallmarks for quality of information. *BMJ* 1998; **317**: 1500–1.

19. Ling CA, Guiding patients through the maze of drug information on the Internet. *Am J Health Syst Pharm* 1999; **56**: 212–14.

20. Gorman C, A web of deceit; the latest e-mail campaign attacks an artificial sweetener. Here's how to find the truth. *Time* 1999; **153**(5).

21. Stewart M, Brown JB, Boon H et al, Evidence on patient–doctor communication. *Cancer Prev Control* 1999; **3**: 25–30.

22. Swenerton KD, The emerging role for paclitaxel in the treatment of epithelial ovarian cancer. *Indian J Med Paed Oncol* 1994; **15**: 20–7.

23. Davidoff F, Florance V, The informationist: a new health profession? *Ann Intern Med* 2000; **132**: 996–8.

APPENDIX

Cancer information for patients: some good Websites and telephone numbers

The following information is not intended to be comprehensive. These are what we consider to be some of the best sources. We regret any omissions. (This was last updated in July 2000.)

Canada

Canadian Cancer Society, Cancer Information Service: 1-888-939-3333

BC Cancer Agency: http://www.bccancer.bc.ca/

P.O.W.E.R. Surfers: http://www.city.windsor.on.ca/wpl/power/beginsearch.html

Manitoba Cancer Treatment and Research Foundation:
http://www.mctrf.mb.ca/PatientResources.htm

UK and Europe

Ovacome: http://www.ovacome.org.uk

Cancer Research Campaign:
http://www.crc.org.uk

CancerLink: http://www.cancerlink.org

CancerBACUP Help Line: 0808 800 1234

CancerBACUP Home Page:
http://www.cancerbacup.org.uk/

CancerWeb (Gray Laboratory):
http://www. graylab.ac.uk/cancerweb.html

Imperial Cancer Research Fund:
http://www. icnet.uk/

European Organization for Research and Treatment of Cancer: http://www.eortc.be

European Society for Gynaecological Oncology:
http://www.esgo.com

USA

National Cancer Institute, <u>Cancer Information Service</u>: 1-800-4-CANCER (1-800-422-6237) TTY 1-800-332-8615: <u>http://www.nci.nih.gov</u>
CancerNet (NCI) <u>http://cancernet.nci.nih.gov/</u>
E-mail: cis@icic.nci.nih.gov
Oncolink (University of Pennsylvania): <u>http:// cancer.med.upenn.edu/</u>
Memorial Sloan-Kettering Cancer Center: <u>http://www.mskcc.org/ti.htm</u>

Directories – Where is it?

Consumer health libraries – Consult your local public library to direct you to the nearest one.
Cancer centres <u>http://www.cancerdirectory.com/hospital.htm</u>
A Website that lists online support groups <u>http://www.acor.org/</u>

Appendices

The illustrations in Appendix 1 and Appendix 2 are reproduced with permission from MSKCC Medical Illustration and Graphics.

Appendix 1

FIGO (International Federation of Gynaecological Oncology) staging of ovarian cancer

I Growth limited to the ovaries.

IA   Growth limited to one ovary; no ascites. No tumour on the external surface, capsule intact.

IB   Growth limited to both ovaries; no ascites. No tumour on the external surface, capsule intact.

IC   Tumour either stage IA or IB, but with tumour on the surface of one or both ovaries, or with capsule ruptured, or with ascites present containing malignant cells, or with positive peritoneal washings.

II Growth involving one or both ovaries with pelvic extension.

IIA   Growth involving one or both ovaries with pelvic extension.

IIB   Extension and/or metastases to the uterus and/or tubes.

IIC   Tumour either stage IIA or IIB, but with tumour on the surface of one or both ovaries, or with capsule(s) ruptured, or with ascites present containing malignant cells, or with positive peritoneal washings.

III Tumour involving one or both ovaries, with peritoneal implants outside the pelvis and/or positive retroperitoneal or inguinal nodes. Superficial liver metastases equal stage III. Tumour is limited to the true pelvis, but with histologically verified malignant extension to small bowel or omentum.

IIIA   Tumour grossly limited to the true pelvis, with negative nodes but with histologically confirmed microscopic seeding of abdominal peritoneal surfaces.

IIIB   Tumour of one or both ovaries, with histologically confirmed implants of abdominal peritoneal surfaces, none exceeding 2 cm in diameter. Nodes negative.

IIIC   Abdominal implants greater than 2 cm in diameter and/or positive retroperitoneal or inguinal nodes.

IV Growth involving one or both ovaries, with distant metastasis. If pleural effusion is present, there must be positive cytologic test results to allot a case to stage IV. Parenchymal liver metastasis equals stage IV.

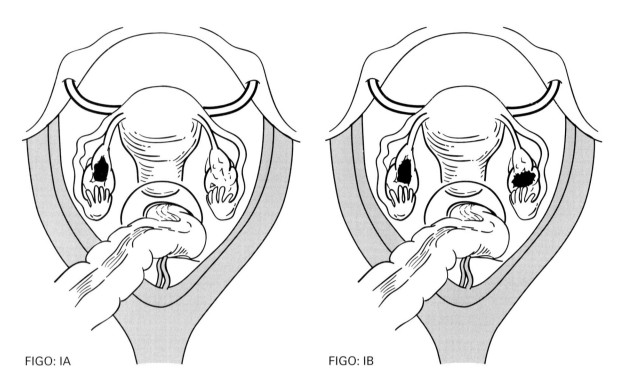

FIGO: IA

FIGO: IB

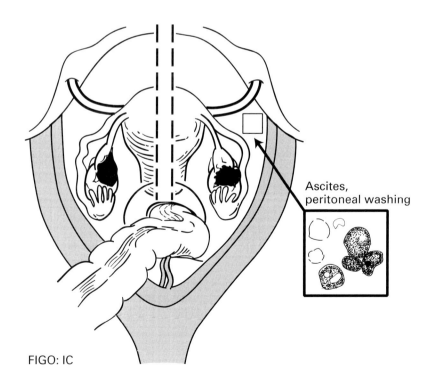

FIGO: IC

Ascites,
peritoneal washing

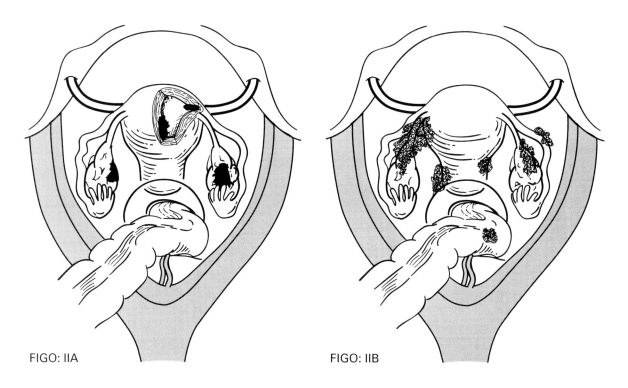

FIGO: IIA

FIGO: IIB

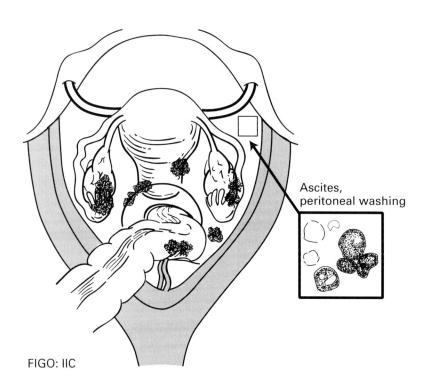

FIGO: IIC

Ascites,
peritoneal washing

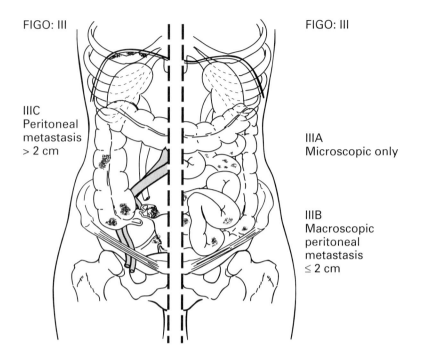

FIGO: III

FIGO: III

IIIC
Peritoneal
metastasis
> 2 cm

IIIA
Microscopic only

IIIB
Macroscopic
peritoneal
metastasis
≤ 2 cm

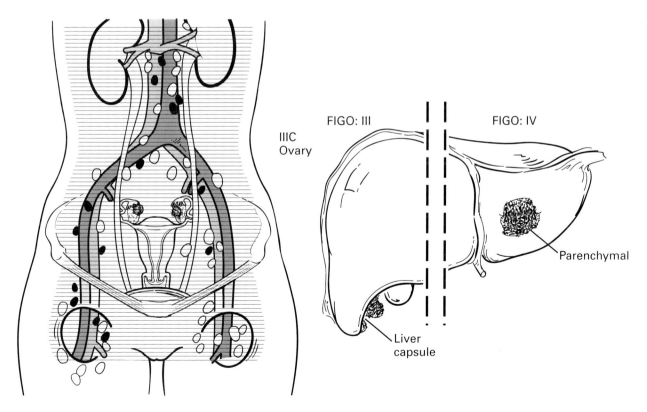

IIIC
Ovary

FIGO: III

FIGO: IV

Parenchymal

Liver
capsule

Appendix 2

FIGO (International Federation of Gynaecological Oncology) staging of fallopian tube cancer[a]

---

0   Carcinoma in situ (limited to tubal mucosa).

I   Growth limited to fallopian tubes.

    IA   Growth limited to one tube, with extension into submucosa and/or muscularis but not penetrating serosal surface; no ascites.

    IB   Growth limited to both tubes, with extension into submucosa and/or muscularis but not penetrating serosal surface; no ascites.

    IC   Tumor either stage IA or IB, but with extension through or onto tubal serosa, or with ascites containing malignant cells, or with positive peritoneal washings.

II   Growth involving one or both fallopian tubes, with pelvic extension.

    IIA   Extension and/or metastasis to uterus and/or ovaries.

    IIB   Extension to other pelvic tissues.

    IIC   Tumor either stage IIA or IIB and with ascites containing malignant cells or with positive peritoneal washings.

III   Tumor involving one or both fallopian tubes, with peritoneal implants outside pelvis and/or positive retroperitoneal or inguinal nodes.

Superficial liver metastasis equals stage III. Tumor appears limited to true pelvis, but with histologically proved malignant extension to small bowel or omentum.

    IIIA   Tumor grossly limited to true pelvis, with negative nodes but with histologically confirmed microscopic seeding of abdominal peritoneal surfaces.

    IIIB   Tumor involving one or both tubes, with histologically confirmed implants of abdominal peritoneal surfaces, none exceeding 2 cm in diameter. Lymph nodes are negative.

    IIIC   Abdominal implants greater than 2 cm in diameter and/or positive retroperitoneal or inguinal nodes.

IV   Growth involving one or both fallopian tubes, with distant metastases. If pleural effusion is present, cytological fluid must be positive for malignant cells to be stage IV. Parenchymal liver metastasis equals stage IV.

Note: Staging for fallopian tube cancer is by the surgical pathological system. Operative findings designating stage are determined before tumour debulking.

---

[a] Taken with permission from Pettersson F, Staging rules for gestational trophoblastic tumors and fallopian tube cancer. *Acta Obstet Gynecol Scand* 1992; **71**: 224–5.

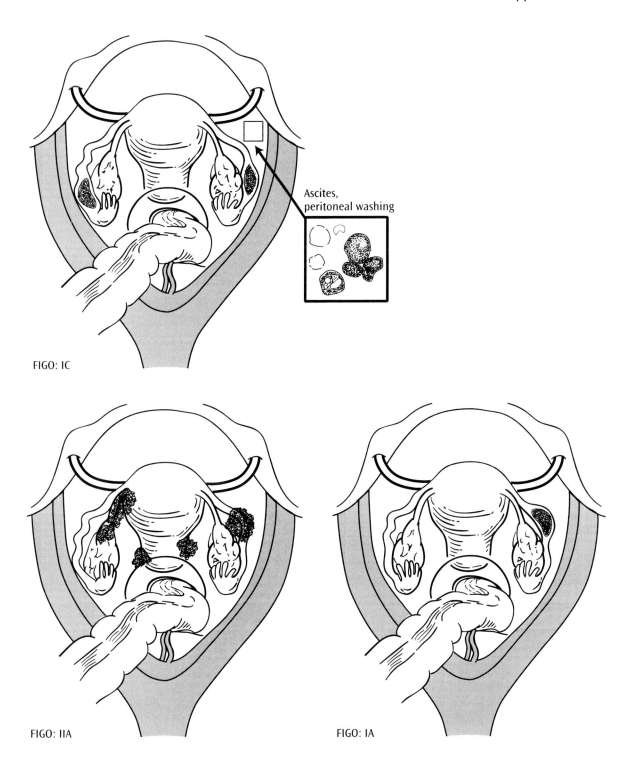

Ascites,
peritoneal washing

FIGO: IC

FIGO: IIA

FIGO: IA

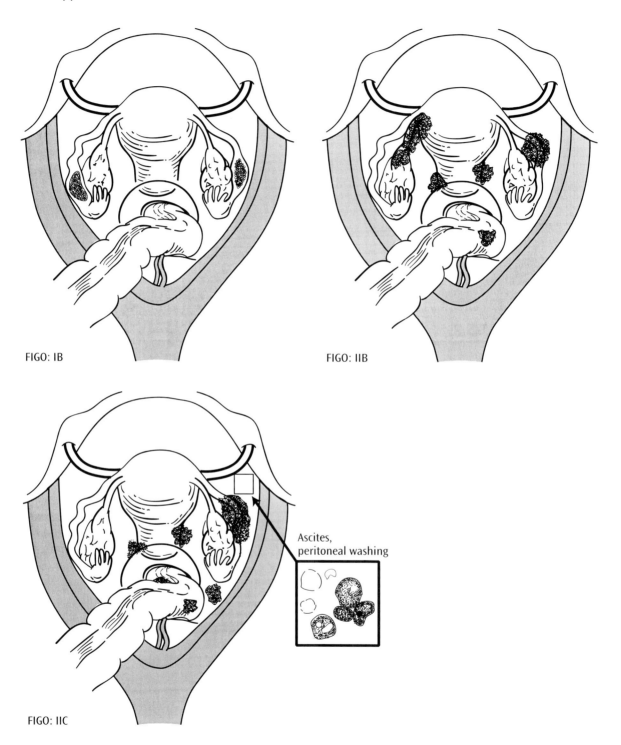

FIGO: IB

FIGO: IIB

FIGO: IIC

Ascites,
peritoneal washing

FIGO: III and IV – see figures for Ovary, Stages III and IV.

Appendix 3

Eastern Cooperative Oncology Group (ECOG) Performance Status Scale

ECOG scale	Performance status
0	Fully active, able to carry out all pre-disease performance without restriction.
1	Restricted in physically strenuous activity, but ambulatory and able to carry out work of a light or sedentary nature, e.g. light housework, office work.
2	Ambulatory and capable of all selfcare, but unable to carry out any work activities. Up and about more than 50% of waking hours.
3	Capable of only limited selfcare, confined to bed or chair more than 50% of waking hours.
4	Completely disabled. Cannot carry out any selfcare. Totally confined to bed or chair.

Note: The grades of the WHO Performance Status Scale are equivalent to those of the ECOG scale.

Index